ReadingsPLUS with 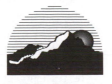 WebLinks

Issues in
Women's Health and Wellness
97/98

*Current and controversial readings
with links to relevant Web sites*

Readings and World Wide Web Sites
Edited and Selected by

C. Amanda Rittenhouse, Ph.D.

Morton Publishing Company
925 W. Kenyon Avenue, Unit 12
Englewood, CO 80110
800/348-3777

About the Editor   C. Amanda Rittenhouse is a community college instructor with a background in health education and research in women's health. She currently teaches at City College of San Francisco and Diablo Valley College in Pleasant Hill, California. She received a B.A. in Anthropology from the University of California-Berkeley and a Master's degree in Public Health from Berkeley. After completing her M.A., she attended the University of California-San Francisco and received a Ph.D. in medical sociology with an emphasis in women's health. She returned to Berkeley the following year to complete post-doctoral training in alcohol and drug studies with an emphasis on gender issues. Her research interests include premenstrual syndrome, human sexuality, and drug and alcohol issues. Her teaching philosophy is oriented toward empowering students and encouraging critical thinking. She hopes that her students not only gain knowledge but also learn the skills necessary to question what they read and to formulate their own opinions on health matters.

Credits:
Cover Design: Sandy Burr
WebLinks Logo: Laura Patchkofsky

ReadingsPLUS with WebLinks: Issues in Women's Health and Wellness, 97/98
Copyright © 1997, Morton Publishing Company
925 W. Kenyon Avenue, Unit 12
Englewood, Colorado 80110
800/348-3777

ISBN: 0-89582-348-9

5   4   3   2   1

We make a sincere effort to ensure the accuracy of the material described herein; however, Morton Publishing Company makes no warranty, express or implied, with respect to the freedom from error of this document. Neither Morton Publishing Company nor its distributors shall be liable to the purchaser or any other person or entity with respect to any liability, loss, or damage caused or alleged to have been caused directly or indirectly by this book.

All terms mentioned in this book that are known to be trademarks or service marks have been appropriately capitalized. Morton Publishing Company cannot attest to the accuracy of this information. Use of a term in this book should not be regarded as affecting the validity of any trademark or service mark.

Printed in the United States of America.

WebAdvisory Board

Members of the WebAdvisory Board provide feedback on readings and World Wide Web sites, and generally advise the editor and the publishing staff. WebAdvisory Board Members are drawn from colleges and universities throughout the United States and Canada. They are academics with a variety of specialties and teaching experiences.

Because Morton Publishing Company also values the perspective students bring to course materials, student advisors are instrumental in shaping *ReadingsPLUS with WebLinks*.

Linda Amankwaa
Florida State University

Barbara Bragonier
California State University-Long Beach

Susan Cataldo
Student Advisor
CUNY-Hunter College

Joanne Chopak
Georgia Southern University

Olivia Cousins
CUNY-Borough of Manhattan
    Community College

Susan Crawford
Simon Fraser University

Maureen Edwards
Montgomery College-Rockville

Sharon Garcia
Diablo Valley College

Cathy Gaul
University of Victoria

Barbara Horn
SUNY-Nassau Community College

Dorothy Rentschler
University of New Hampshire

Robin Roth
City College of San Francisco

Robin Saltonstall
University of Colorado

Preface

Women represent the majority of patients in the health care system, and if you were to look at *all* health professions, women would also be the majority of providers. However, women are still in the minority when it comes to being doctors and researchers. This fact has affected not only the delivery of health care to women but also women's participation in research studies. Historically, women have not been included in drug trials and research studies dealing with general health issues. Most research on and discussions about women and health have tended to focus on reproductive functions. Yet recent research shows that women react differently than men to many drugs, such as painkillers, and that certain medical treatments that work for men may not work as well for women. Women's health is now being studied in its own right, in part due to the creation of a women's health branch at the National Institute on Health (NIH).

As a result of this effort, we are learning more about women's health. And more information on topics in women's health is appearing in both popular and academic publications. However, getting this information out to a student audience in an easy-to-follow format has not been done. There are wonderful books for students, such as *Our Bodies, Ourselves,* by the Boston Women's Health Collective; however, these books cannot always provide current and updated information about all topics. Thus, there is a need for a volume such as *ReadingsPLUS with WebLinks.* This collection takes various current and controversial readings in women's health from the popular press and from academic sources and brings them together in one affordable publication. Because it is updated annually, *ReadingsPLUS with WebLinks* can provide students with information that would not otherwise be available to them. Also, it provides links with the World Wide Web, which increasingly will play a role in accessing information on all topics.

The readings and Web sites selected for this volume were chosen for their quality and their timeliness. Some of the readings as well as some of the Web sites were chosen to provide a general overview of a topic, while others focus on a specific issue or area in women's health. Also, some of the readings are highlighted as controversial. These readings present issues over which there has been some debate, and are ones that can be used in the classroom as source material for debates or discussions. This volume can be used on its own as a means of facilitating discussion or in conjunction with other texts in health and women's health. Also, it is hoped that students will think critically about these issues and formulate their own opinions on each of these topics. The diversity of readings provides a variety of points of view, and should illustrate the complexity of the field of women's health.

— C. Amanda Rittenhouse

A Note from the Publisher

Welcome to *ReadingsPLUS!*

Alert and adventurous readers are important to us in keeping this volume up-to-date and accurate. So if you would like to recommend a timely reading on an important topic in women's health, or if you happen upon a great World Wide Web site with compelling resources, or even if you discover an error (it happens), we'd appreciate hearing from you. Our phone number is 1-800-348-3777. Or just drop us a line at:

Morton Publishing Company
✉ 925 W. Kenyon Avenue, Unit 12
Englewood, Colorado 80110

Fax: 303-762-9923

e E-mail: morton@morton-pub.com

💻 Web address: http://www.morton-pub.com

What You Will Find in This Book

This book contains **45 current and controversial readings** on topics in women's health and wellness. The readings are drawn from a mix of professional journals and popular, high-quality magazines and newsletters. The readings that are controversial carry the label *A Reading for Critical Thinking*. In addition to the readings, you will find:

"Health Information On-Line"

This introductory reading at the front of the book (see pp. xx–xxiv) will provide you with a general overview of the World Wide Web (what it is and how to use the Web as a resource). This reading also contains excellent suggestions for how to evaluate online sources of information on any topic.

WebLinks: A Directory of Annotated World Wide Web Sites

(See Appendix A at the back of the book on pp. 185–191.) Here you will find World Wide Web sites that contain information and resources relevant to the issues discussed in the readings. The Web addresses have been fully verified, and all the sites are briefly described. The Web sites are organized alphabetically by site name, and each site has been numbered for easy reference and referral. The Quick Reference Guide to Topics/Readings/World Wide Web Sites (which is described in detail below) will let you quickly match a reading with the Web sites that are relevant to it. However, please note that the Guide, while extensive, is not exhaustive in linking readings with Web sites, and you may want to explore sites on your own and make your own connections between readings and Web sites. The brief description of each Web site can also assist you in deciding which sites to consult.

Quick Reference Guide to Topics/Readings/World Wide Web Sites

The Quick Reference Guide correlates topics on women's health and wellness with the readings and World Wide Web sites found in the book. (See pp. xv–xix.) It can be used for easy reference to locate readings and Web sites. In addition, the Quick Reference Guide makes it possible to integrate readings and Web sites with any course syllabus or textbook. The Guide can also be used to make class assignments. Although it is not comprehensive in its scope (i.e., there may be topics addressed in the readings and Web sites that are not listed in the Quick Reference Guide), it can still serve as a convenient starting point.

Web Journal

(See Appendix B at the back of the book on pp. 193–198.) Use these pages to make note of sites you have visited. You could record your reactions to a site, or briefly note what information you found there. Is the site worth a repeat visit in your opinion? Could you use it for personal reference? Could you use it for a research assignment? Who runs the site? Where is it located? You may want to develop the habit of evaluating both the content at a site and how well the site operates. Ask yourself, is the site easy to navigate? Are the graphics odd or are they appropriate? Are there any special features that you particularly like? How does the information at a site compare with what you have learned in a reading? If you write up your visit to a site, you will have a record of where you have been on the Web. Use these pages as you would any journal or lab manual. It is a place for you to make personal observations about your Web experiences, and to raise issues you would like to discuss in class about a site. (Should you run out of Web Journal pages, you may Xerox the Web Journal for your own personal use.)

Other Features

You will also find an annotated table of contents at the front of the book, which highlights key sentences from the readings, and *ReadingsPLUS with WebLinks* is fully indexed.

Suggestions for Accessing a Web Site

WebLinks: A Directory of Annotated World Wide Web Sites contains sites that relate to the topics covered in the readings. You will see that each Web site has been assigned a descriptive heading and a number. For each site, the exact address, or Universal Resource Locator, is provided. (Here is an example of a site's descriptive heading with its assigned number: *Web of Addictions, No. 93.* Its address or URL is http://www.well.com/user/woa.). To access a Web site, you will need to be at a computer that is hooked to the Internet and has a graphical browser—that is the software that allows you to access the World Wide Web. (The most popular browsers are Netscape and Mosaic). Once you have opened Netscape or Mosaic, delete the address that appears in the Location bar. Then, *carefully* type the address or URL of the Web site into the Location bar (or Go To bar) on the screen and press the Enter key.

The screen may look something like the one below after you have typed in the address.

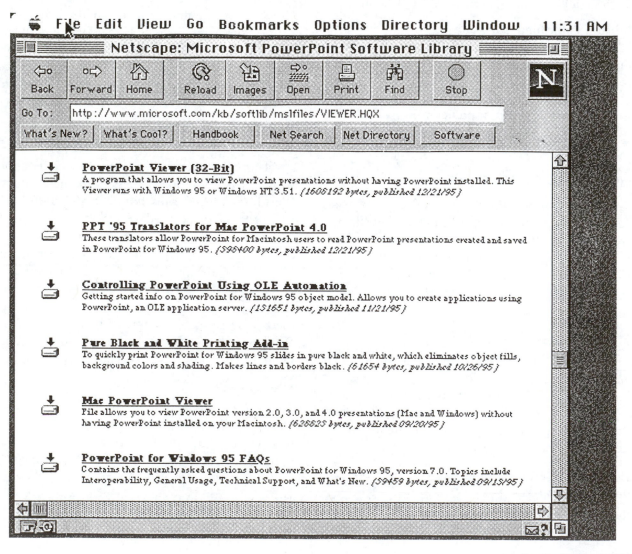

There are many ways to visit cyberspace, and the WebLinks Directory is designed to be a guide to academically appropriate Web sites on issues related to women's health. Use it for research for class assignments, or to follow your own interests.

A Word About Critical Thinking

ReadingsPLUS with WebLinks: Issues in Women's Health and Wellness introduces you to a wide variety of current and controversial readings on topics in women's health, and there are over 100 World Wide Web sites for you to consult as well. All the readings have been selected with care to provide you with a wide range of perspectives on important topics in women's health. The readings that are labeled "A Reading for Critical Thinking," however, are ones that are especially designed to encourage your critical thinking skills. To arrive at a thorough understanding of a topic, you will need to think critically about what you are reading (both in print and on screen). Critical thinking skills are increasingly important, particularly as the amount of information available to the average person keeps expanding. To be a critical thinker, you will need to learn how to ask questions, and to consider not only what is said (or written) but what is not said (or implied). You may want to consider taking a course in critical thinking. And we recommend the following print and online resources:

In Print

M. Neil Browne and Stuart M. Keeley, *Asking the Right Questions: A Guide to Critical Thinking*, 2nd ed. (Prentice-Hall, 1986).

Vicent Ryan Ruggiero, *Becoming a Critical Thinker*, 2nd ed. (Houghton Mifflin, 1996).

Glen Thomas and Gaye Smooth, "Critical Thinking: A Vital Work Skill," *Trust for Educational Leadership* (February/March 1994), pp. 34-38.

Online

Critical Thinking: A Vital Work Skill

http://www.enc.org/online/ENC2315/2315.html

Provided by the Eisenhower National Clearinghouse for Mathematics and Science Education, this site highlights a U.S. Department of Labor report that says that today's jobs demand higher-order thinking skills. Page is co-written by the director of the Curriculum Framework and Textbook Development Unit of the State Department of Education and a consultant for the unit. An excellent site for research with documented facts. Links to a searchable catalog of curriculum resources.

The Critical Thinking Community

http://www.sonoma.edu/CThink/

This site is maintained by Sonoma State University's Center for Critical Thinking. Site provides educators, students, and the public with a wealth of information about the theory and practice of critical thinking, concepts and definitions, techniques for learning and teaching, and classroom exercises that implement the principles. Other features include weekly updates, an Educator's Resource Guide for integrating critical thinking into the curriculum, a collection of critical thinking articles, and a list of conferences. Links to online discussion groups. The site is directed by Richard Paul, Ph.D., and comments are invited thru E-mail addresses provided. Also offers links to a sampling of critical thinking offices nationwide.

Mission Control

http://www.sjsu.edu:80/depts/itl/

This site is produced by the Institute for Teaching and Learning at San Jose State University. Its goal is to create a "virtual lab" capable of familiarizing users with the basic concepts of critical thinking in a self-paced, interactive environment. Comments and reactions are encouraged, and an E-mail address is provided. Site includes links to each step in the process plus exercises for the student to do. A good online way to become a critical thinker.

Your Thoughts Are Important to Us

Our mission in developing *ReadingsPLUS with Web-Links* is simple: to make the resources of the popular press and the World Wide Web accessible and usable within a course specific context. By carefully selecting current, academically appropriate readings from high-quality popular press sources, and by filtering and organizing World Wide Web sites, we can help you keep up-to-date and current, and we can assist you in incorporating new technology into your courses. We sincerely welcome your feedback, and please contact us with your suggestions and recommendations.

Contents

 indicates a controversial reading

PART I *Women and the Health Care System, 1*

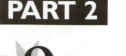
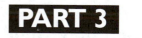
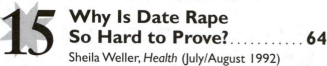
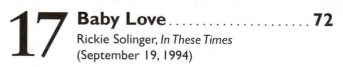

PART 4 · *Reproductive Choices, 90*

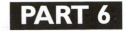
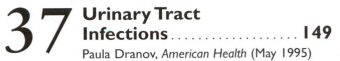

42 Women and Heart Disease 171
UC Berkeley Wellness Letter (February 1992)

"The myth that heart disease is something that happens only to men—especially busy executives—seems to be at last on its way to oblivion. There's a growing awareness that the prevention of cardiovascular disease is—or ought to be—a pressing personal concern not only for men but for women, too."

43 Hormone Replacement Therapy: Frequently Asked Questions 174
UC Berkeley Wellness Letter (October 1995)

"Most doctors think you should begin HRT at menopause and continue for the rest of your life in order to get the greatest protection against heart disease and osteoporosis. You certainly get your greatest gains if you start at menopause, though there's some evidence that HRT can also be beneficial if started later."

44 Bone Medicine 177
Burkhard Bilger, *Health* (May/June 1996)

"Some 25 million Americans have dangerously thin bones; osteoporosis causes 1.5 million fractures, runs up $10 billion in health care costs, and ends the independence of tens of thousands of elderly people every year. Yet women like Sylva have long been offered only two troublesome options. Calcitonin had to be injected in the thigh daily, so it had few takers. Estrogen helps prevent heart disease as well as osteoporosis, but it can also cause menstruation to resume (when taken with progestin), and it may encourage cancer."

45 Positive Passage 181
Lonnie Barbach, Ph.D.,
San Francisco Focus (September 1993)

"Some women tell me that while they didn't enjoy the symptoms they experienced during The Pause, it caused them to change their diet, increase their exercise, and reduce their stress. As a result, they felt better than they had in many years, and looked forward to a longer, healthier life."

Quick Reference Guide
to Topics/Readings/WWW Sites

Topic Area	Treated in: Reading	Treated in: Web Site
Abortion	22. Blood and Tears	Women and Health Resources, No. 95 Yahoo: Reproductive Health Links, No. 109
	23. Diminished Choice	Interactivism, No. 51 National Abortion Rights Action League, No. 63 National Women's Health Organization, No. 70 Women Leaders Online Website, No. 99
Aging/Menopause	42. Women and Heart Disease	American Heart Association, No. 2
	43. Hormone Replacement Therapy	Harvard Women's Health Watch, No. 43 Women at Wellness Web, No. 98
	44. Bone Medicine	Doctor's Guide to Osteoporosis, No. 23 MenoTimes, No. 59 Osteoporosis and Related Bone Disease, No. 77
	45. Positive Passage	Menopause Matters, No. 58 Power Surge, No. 83
Birth Control	21. Still Fumbling in the Dark	Birth Control Trust, No. 13 Family Health International, No. 27 Feminist.com, No. 31 Women's Health Resources OnLine, No. 103 Depo-Provera, No. 21 Planned Parenthood, No. 82
	24. Norplant Suits Allege Severe Side Effects	American Civil Liberties Union, No. 1
	25. The Pill	Ann Rose's Ultimate Birth Control Links, No. 6 Birth Control Pills, No. 12
Body Image/ Weight Control	9. Diet Pills	Nutrition HomePage, No. 73
	12. Body Mania	American Society for Clinical Nutrition, No. 4 Internet Mental Health Resources, No. 52 Nutrition Sites on the Internet, No. 74 Yahoo: Weight Links, No. 111
	13. Who's the Healthiest of Them All?	Cyberdiet, No. 20 Fitness Issues, No. 35 Fitness World, No. 37 Food Safety and Nutrition Information, No. 38 Hardin Meta Directory, No. 41 Harvard University's Health Publications, No. 42 National Agricultural Library, U.S. Dept. of Agr., No. 64
Cancer	6. Primary Care of Lesbian Patients	National Gay and Lesbian Task Force, No. 67 Sexuality Information and Education Council, No. 89 WWWomen, No. 108

ReadingsPLUS with WebLinks

Health Information

On-Line

By Marilynn Larkin

Consumers are using the Internet to get information about health. How reliable is this information? That's not an easy question to answer.

It's no secret that the Internet — especially its graphics portion, the World Wide Web — is enjoying unprecedented popularity in business and professional communities, and in homes across America. A recent survey by the Times Mirror Center for the People & the Press revealed that the number of Americans subscribing to on-line services jumped from 5 million at the end of 1994 to nearly 12 million in mid-1995, while an additional 2 million people have direct connections to the Internet.

Among people with home offices, approximately one-third have access to the Internet, and, of these, about 10 percent have a home page on the Web, according to a survey conducted by the Gallup Organization and reported in the Dec. 19, 1995, issue of *PC Magazine.*

Another survey, by CDB Research & Consulting, indicates that consumers are showing a growing inter-

> The FDA home page provides an excellent jumping off point for those who want to learn more about the agency and the drugs, food supplements, and medical devices it regulates.

est in obtaining information about health and beauty aids on-line as a means of supplementing traditional medical counsel. The company speculates that the discretion and convenience of the on-line environment may hold special appeal to people with disabilities and chronic illnesses.

However, easy access to virtually limitless health and medical information has pitfalls, experts caution. "My advice to consumers about information on the Internet is the same as it is for other media: You can't believe everything you see, whether it's in a newspaper, on TV, or on a computer screen," says Bill Rados, director of FDA's Communications Staff. Since anyone — reputable scientist or quack — who has a computer, a modem (the device that permits a computer to dial and connect to the Internet or an on-line service), and the necessary software can publish a Web page, post information to a newsgroup, or proffer advice in an on-line chat room, "you must protect yourself by carefully checking out the source of any information you obtain."

WORLD WIDE WEB

By far, the most consumer-friendly part of the Internet is the World Wide Web. It is also the newest part of the Internet, having become accessible only in the past couple of years, with the wider availability of browsers such as Mosaic and Netscape Navigator. While the rest of the Internet displays text only, the Web, as it has come to be called, has the ability to display colorful graphics and multimedia (sounds, video, virtual reality) to complement text-based information. For example, sites that offer medical information on neurological diseases, such as stroke, may also contain images of the brain showing which areas are affected by disease or may have downloadable (files that can be copied from one computer to another) "movies" of actual magnetic resonance imaging (MRI) exams pinpointing blockages in blood vessels.

From *FDA Consumer* (June 1996), pp. 21-25.

Many legitimate providers of reliable health and medical information, including FDA and other government agencies, are taking advantage of the Web's popularity by offering brochures and in-depth information on specific topics at their Web sites. Material may be geared to consumers as well as industry and medical professionals (see "Sources of Internet Health Information").

But con artists have also infiltrated the Web. "A physician was browsing the Web when he came across a site that contained a fraudulent drug offering. He called us to report it," says Roma Jeanne Egli, a compliance officer in FDA's division of drug marketing. "The person who maintains the site claimed he had a cure for a very serious disease, and advised those with the disease to stop taking their prescription medication. Instead, they were told to buy the product he was selling, at a cost of several hundred dollars."

More details can't be released because FDA has a case pending against the Web site owner who, according to Egli, has a history of marketing bogus cures. She advises consumers to be skeptical when someone advocates a purported "cure" to be purchased and taken in lieu of prescribed medicine.

If you come across a suspected fraudulent offering on the Internet, alert FDA by E-mail: *otcfraud@cder.fda.gov*.

If con artists and scientists have equal publishing rights on the Internet, what's to keep a health-conscious consumer from getting sidetracked by an official looking page offering unsound advice?

"This is a real concern," says Valencia Camp, of FDA's Office of Information Resources Management. "Although the Internet can be a reliable source of information, it is important to be aware that what is found there is only as good as the quality and integrity of the original information. What you find cannot be taken as gospel. It should be checked out and supported by other sources." (See "Is This Site Reliable?")

FDA ON-LINE

The FDA home page provides an excellent jumping off point for those who want to learn more about the agency and the drugs, food supplements, and medical devices it regulates. "Twenty-five cents of every dollar spent by consumers goes for something that FDA regulates," Rados notes. These products "could be used more safely and more effectively if people know more about them." Because it is expensive to print and mail materials, FDA offers many of its publications on the Internet.

FDA material can be downloaded to a home or office computer and then printed out. Those who don't have a personal computer can try accessing the Internet from their local library or from a community organization. If you have a computer but do not have Internet access, you can receive text from FDA's site (no graphics) by dialing by modem the agency's bulletin board service (BBS): (1-800) 222-0185; type "bbs" and select the information you want from the menu.

If you come across a suspected fraudulent health or medical offering on the Internet, alert FDA by E-mail: otcfraud@cder.fda.gov

---

"Our goal is to have virtually all consumer education material available on the Internet," says Rados. "Every new piece we publish is immediately placed on our Web site. We now have more than a hundred different publications to choose from." FDA also has a "comments" button on many of its Web pages so that visitors can offer suggestions and feedback. However, questions about specific drugs, devices, or food supplements should be addressed to the agency in writing at FDA (HFE-88), Rockville, MD 20857, or by calling your local public affairs specialist listed under "FDA" in your local phonebook, Rados adds. Before beginning any particular therapy, however, consult with your doctor or pharmacist.

In addition to providing consumer education materials, the FDA site also offers technical information to help industry professionals file regulatory materials.

EXCHANGING INFORMATION

In Internet "newsgroups," such as Usenet groups, people post questions and read messages much as they would on regular bulletin boards. Through "mailing lists," messages are exchanged by E-mail, and all messages are sent to all group subscribers. In "chat" areas on some services and on the Internet's IRC (Internet Relay Chat) users can communicate with each other live.

Assessing the value and validity of health and medical information in news and chat groups demands at least the same — and maybe more — discrimination as for Web sites, because the information is more ephemeral and you often can't identify the source. Although these groups can provide reliable information about specific diseases and disorders, they can also perpetuate misinformation.

"Around Christmas time last year, I saw a whole bunch of messages implying that mistletoe has anti-cancer properties," recalls Serena Stockwell, editor of the medical trade publication *Oncology Times* and longtime user of various cancer-related forums and resources on one of the commercial on-line services. "I wondered where this was coming from, since it seemed a little odd."

Stockwell did some digging and discovered that in an announcement of a new drug to treat lung cancer, "one of the researchers had a slip of the tongue and said the drug was derived from mistletoe instead of periwinkle. As a result, the word soon spread to the newsgroups, where people inadvertently perpetuated the mistake."

In another instance, Stockwell saw that the herbal tea Essiac was being touted in a newsgroup as a cancer remedy. "Doctors were being questioned about it, so I assigned a reporter to cover the story," she says.

As it turned out, there is no evidence to support this claim.

As with all health and medical information in cyberspace, advice in newsgroups "should not be taken by itself," Stockwell says. "As a writer and editor, I find newsgroups useful for keeping in touch with topics of conversation among patients, doctors and researchers. But to determine whether the information is trustworthy, I'd want to document it in the usual ways."

Other information services are commercial on-line services, fee-charging companies that provide vast amounts of proprietary information. They often include health and medical databases, electronic versions of popular newspapers and magazines, and

---

Is This Site Reliable?

FDA staff and others familiar with Internet medical offerings suggest asking the following questions to help determine the reliability of a Web site:

- Who maintains the site? Government or university-run sites are among the best sources for scientifically sound health and medical information. Private practitioners or lay organizations may have marketing, social or political agendas that can influence the type of material they offer on-site and which sites they link to.

- Is there an editorial board or another listing of the names and credentials of those responsible for preparing and reviewing the site's contents? Can these people be contacted by phone or through E-mail if visitors to the site have questions or want additional information?

- Does the site link to other sources of medical information? No reputable organization will position itself as the sole source of information on a particular health topic.

   On the other hand, links alone are not a guarantee of reliability, notes Lorrie Harrison of FDA's Center for Biologics Evaluation and Research. Since anyone with a Web page can create links to any other site on the Internet — and the owner of the site that is "linked to" has no say over who links to it — then a person offering suspect medical advice could conceivably try to make his or her advice appear legitimate by, say, creating a link to FDA's Web site. What's more, health information produced by FDA or other government agencies is not copyrighted; therefore, someone can quote FDA information at a site and be perfectly within his or her rights. By citing a source such as FDA, experienced marketers using careful wording can make it appear as though FDA endorses their products, Harrison explains.

- When was the site last updated? Generally, the more current the site, the more likely it is to provide timely material. Ideally, health and medical sites should be updated weekly or monthly.

- Are informative graphics and multimedia files such as video or audio clips available? Such features can assist in clarifying medical conditions and procedures. For example, the University of Pennsylvania's cancer information site, called OncoLink, contains graphics of what a woman can expect during a pelvic exam.

   Bear in mind, however, that multimedia should be used to help explain medical information, not substitute for it. Some sites provide dazzling "bells and whistles" but little scientifically sound information.

- Does the site charge an access fee? Many reputable sites with health and medical information, including FDA and other government sites, offer access and materials for free. If a site does charge a fee, be sure that it offers value for the money. Use a searcher (see "Sources of Internet Health Information") to see whether you can get the same information without paying additional fees.

   If you find something of interest at a site — say, a new drug touted to relieve disease symptoms with fewer side effects — write down the name and address of the site, print out the information, and bring it to your doctor, advises Valencia Camp of FDA's Office of Information Resources Management. Your doctor can help determine whether the information is supported by legitimate research sources, such as journal articles or proceedings from a scientific meeting.

   In addition, your doctor can determine if the drug is appropriate for your situation. Even if the information comes from a source that is reputed to be reliable, you should check with your doctor to make sure that it is wise for you to begin a certain treatment. Specific situations (such as taking other drugs) may make the therapy an inadvisable choice. Your doctor can decide whether the drug is suitable for you and may be able to offer more appropriate alternatives.

— M. L.

Sources of Internet Health Information

There are literally thousands of health-related Internet resources maintained by government agencies, universities, and non-profit and commercial organizations. Following are the addresses of Usenet groups (newsgroups), mailing lists, and reputable sites that link to other sites with medical information. This list is by no means complete; it is offered as a jumping-off point.

Usenet Groups

(Access is through the Internet provider)

bionet. immunology
(immunology research and practice)

bionet.aging
(issues related to aging theory and research)

misc.health.diabetes
(discussion of diabetes management in daily life)

sci.med diseases.cancer
(cancer treatment and research)

sci.med. vision
(treatments for vision problems)

Mailing Lists

(to subscribe, send an E-mail message to the address given; in the message area type "subscribe," followed by the name of the list and then your name)

Alzheimer's Disease
List name: ALZHEIMER
Subscribe:
listserv@wubois.wustl.edu

Breast Cancer
List name: BREAST-CANCER
Subscribe:
listserv@MORGAN.UCS.MUN.CA

Stroke
List name: STROKE-L
Subscribe:
listserv@UKCC.UKY.EDU

Geriatrics
List name: GERINET
Subscribe:
listserv@UBVM.CC.BUFFALO.EDU
(Source: *A Guide To Healthcare and Medical Resources on the Internet* by Michael S. Brown)

World Wide Web Sites

American Cancer Society:
http://charlotte.npixi.net/acs/.facts.html

American Heart Association:
http://www.amhrt.org/ahawho.htm

American Medical Association:
http://www.ama-assn.org/

Centers for Disease Control and Prevention: *http://www.cdc.gov/*

Department of Health and Human Services: *http://www.os.dhhs.gov/*

Food and Drug Administration:
http://www./fda.gov/

National Cancer Institute:
http://www.nci.nih.gov/

National Institutes of Health:
http://www.nih.gov/

National Institute for Allergies and Infectious Diseases:
http://www.niaid.nih.gov/

National Library of Medicine:
http://www.nlm.nih.gov/

Oncology Data Base/University of Pennsylvania (ONCOLINK):
http://cancer.med.upenn.edu/about_oncolink.html

SEARCH PROGRAMS

Because the Internet contains no central indexing system, getting the information you want quickly can be a major challenge. That's where search engines come in. These powerful tools can help narrow the field if you have a specific topic to pursue, or the name of a specific organization but no address for its site. Input a few words that describe what you're looking for, and the searcher returns a list of sites related to your query.

Be aware, however, that although a searcher can point the way, it does not evaluate the information it points to. For example, a search on the words "breast cancer" is just as likely to point to a page advertising a reconstructive surgeon or a health food store's article on the purported benefits of phytochemicals as it is to the National Cancer Institute. The reason? Scott Stephenson, production engineer and spokesman for Webcrawler, one of the popular searchers, explains. "Webcrawler scans documents and counts the number of times a particular word or expression searched for appears on a Web page. That alone determines whether the page is listed in our results and where it appears on the list." This means that by mentioning, say, breast cancer many times in the Web page copy, a savvy marketer of bogus medicinals could draw a lot of people to his or her site. It is up to the visitor to evaluate the information the site contains. Here are a few of the many search engines:

Alta Vista:
http://www.altavista.digital.com/

Excite: *http://www.excite.com/*

Lycos: *http://www.lycos.com/*

Webcrawler:
http://www.webcrawler.com/

Yahoo:
http://www.yahoo.com/Health/Medicine/

— M. L.

their own chats and newsgroups, as well as Internet access.

The fact that information may be screened by a commercial service does not necessarily make it more reliable than other sources. And most services do not verify what is posted in their newsgroups, nor control what is "said" in chat rooms. Health and medical material obtained through services also should be corroborated by your physician or other medical sources.

REGULATORY CONCERNS

The fact that it is easy to publish health and medical information and reach vast audiences without having the information verified by other sources presents potential issues for FDA and other government agencies, according to Melissa Moncavage, a public health advisor in FDA's division of drug marketing, advertising, and communications. FDA has created a working group from each of its divisions to address the issues that fall within the agency's purview.

"We are working together to determine the scope and type of product information that is going directly to consumers. Product information on the Internet is unlike traditional forms of advertising and labeling. Current regulations on prescription drug advertising differ between print and broadcast media. The Internet presents additional challenges," Moncavage says.

While regulatory agencies try to devise ways of ensuring that accurate and well-balanced health and medical information is presented on the Internet, consumers "will have to use a lot more discretion in evaluating what they see," Moncavage says. "A Web page can be changed very quickly. It is easy to put up, and easy to take down. There is no guarantee that what you see one day will be there the next." So on the Internet, as elsewhere, "caveat emptor" — let the buyer beware — are watchwords for the foreseeable future.

Marilynn Larkin is a medical writer whose Web site links to the Web sources of health information listed in this article: http://members.gnn.com/mlco

PART I

Women and the Health Care System

There are many changes occurring in the delivery of health care in the United States and Canada as a result of cost containment pressures. These changes are having an impact upon the delivery of health care for women. For example, there has been a lot of media attention given to the controversy about the length of hospital stays for women and their newborn babies, and the number of days health maintenance organizations (HMOs) will pay for. For some women and babies, leaving the hospital 12 hours after birth is fine. For others, it is not. Another recent controversy concerns the emerging practice of performing mastectomies on women diagnosed with

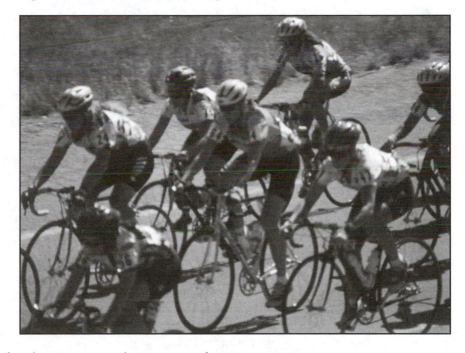

breast cancer on an outpatient basis. Again, this may be fine for some women, but certainly not for all. These issues got media attention and the attention of politicians. There is a concern that patient care is being sacrificed for cost containment. Health care delivery is changing, how it will change is not yet clear. And how those changes will directly impact women is less clear, although a cause for concern.

This section pulls together readings that introduce a broad range of issues and topics in women's health. The readings include ones that offer advice about seeking quality health care, as well as those that cover some of the controversial issues that have emerged in the debates over women and the health care system. The readings and World Wide Web sites chosen for this Part serve the purpose of giving you a solid background for understanding issues in women's health. Several readings and WWW sites also offer practical information women can use for protecting and maintaining good health. (Please see **Quick Reference Guide to Topics/Readings/WWW Sites** and **Appendix A: WebLinks: A Directory of Annotated World Wide Web Sites** to select WWW sites that coordinate with the readings in this part.)

A Reading for Critical Thinking

prescription for change

A new generation of patients and doctors is changing the politics of women's health.

by Marilee Strong

Joan Chambers epitomizes "aging gracefully." At sixty-two, the former school-district administrator from Menlo Park regularly bikes and even Roller blades with a club of gray-haired skaters known as the "Silver Streaks." She sailed through menopause fifteen years ago without any symptoms, has never been hospitalized except for an auto accident in college, and has the lowest cholesterol count her doctor said she had ever seen. Yet when Chambers asked for a bone-density scan to check if her diet and exercise regimen were successfully staving off osteoporosis, her doctor refused to give her the test unless she agreed in advance to go on estrogen.

Dell, a Humboldt County woman who asked that her full name not be used, got both too much and too little attention from the health-care system. She was just thirty-seven when doctors removed her uterus because she had an overgrowth of fibroid tumors. She accepts the decision as the prevailing wisdom of the time, even though doctors now believe that fibroids have only a .1 percent chance of turning cancerous. What she does not accept, twenty years later, is the continued intransigence of the medical establishment. For the past year she complained to her general practitioner of persistent burning in her vagina. When test after test came up negative, the physician turned to what was — in his mind — a more likely explanation.

"He'd pat me on the hand and ask me with this sardonic sense of humor, 'How are things at home? Are you still communicating with your husband?'" says Dell, now fifty-seven. "Yes, my marriage was kaput. There had been a few recent deaths in the family. But I knew something was chronically wrong with me. At my age, if I don't know my body, I'm not paying much attention."

After a year of "bludgeoning" her doctor for a referral to a specialist, Dell was diagnosed with a human papilloma virus, a sexually transmitted gift from her soon-to-be ex-husband. In some strains the virus can cause cervical cancer. Fortunately hers was not one of those strains, "but for a year I've been dinking around with my GP who didn't have the good sense to send me to a gynecologist," says Dell.

Experiences like those of Joan and Dell are all too common. Women are by far the biggest medical consumers in the United States, accounting for two-thirds of all visits to doctors and medicines prescribed. But their health concerns have been so ignored and underestimated by the medical establishment that a gender gap exists between men and women — with deadly results — where medical care and medical research are concerned. More women than men die from cardiovascular disease each year, for example, yet nearly all the research on prevention and treatment has been

From *San Francisco Focus* (September 1993), pp. 69-71, 115-120. Reprinted by permission of Marilee Strong, a newspaper and magazine writer and the recipient of numerous honors, including a National Headliner Award and The Society of Professional Journalists Enterprise Award.

done exclusively on men. Similar statistics exist in other areas of medicine.

The seeds of the gender gap, according to an increasingly vocal number of women patients, physicians, and health care advocates, are sown in society's view of women and nurtured in medical training, practice, and research.

Doctors are trained in the United States to look at women's health in terms of disease rather than natural body processes or life stages. The managing of childbirth and menopause are good examples: American medicine and the insurance system emphasize drugs and surgery (hormone-replacement therapy, hysterectomies, cesarean sections) instead of prevention and nonmedical healing (from nutrition and exercise to midwifery and home birth).

"We talk about the American health system being the best in the world," says Dr. Karen Johnson, assistant clinical professor of psychiatry at the University of California, San Francisco, and the nation's most outspoken critic of women's second-class health status. "My response is, "For whom?""

The recognition of women's second-class status in medicine reached critical mass in 1990 with the publication of a General Accounting Office (GAO) report documenting women's exclusion from research at the National Institutes of Health, the principal federal agency supporting biomedical research. Women's health issues accounted for less than 14 percent of the agency's budget, and only three of the NIH's two thousand researchers specialized in the one field dedicated to women's health needs: obstetrics and gynecology.

There are signs that the tide is beginning to turn, however, as women move into positions of power within the medical establishment and the government agencies that oversee health care and research. Women now constitute 38 percent of the medical students being trained in the United States and 18 percent of practicing physicians, according to the American Medical Association. During the past few years women have been appointed to many of the top scientific posts in the country: from Bush appointees Bernadine Healy and Surgeon General Antonia Novello to Clinton's Health and Human Services Director Donna Shalala and Surgeon General appointee Joycelyn Elders.

Other efforts are under way. The NIH has established the largest clinical trial ever conducted in this country, focusing on women's health issues, and has also taken steps to ensure the inclusion of women in government-sponsored research. The Food and Drug Administration has plans to reverse its prohibition against some women participating in drug trials. And several medical schools are developing women's health centers and even a separate specialty to focus on women's health.

Still, until these nascent efforts bring forth real progress, women will continue to receive less than equal attention from the medical world.

THE DISEASE-CENTERED VIEW

"When I was an intern at UCLA," recalls Dr. Ricki Pollycove, an obstetrician-gynecologist at California Pacific Medical Center, "there was a joke going around: 'What are the indications for a hysterectomy in Beverly Hills?' Answer: 'The presence of a uterus and monthly bleeding' — meaning anything."

GENDERCIDE?

The medical establishment's treatment of women as a group, in terms of care and research can be seen over the years as a long-term policy of malignant neglect. The statistics are alarming:

- More women than men die from cardiovascular disease each year, yet nearly all the research on both prevention and treatment has been done exclusively on men.

- Lung cancer is the deadliest cancer in both women and men, yet men are twice as likely as women to be screened for the disease.

- Gastrointestinal disease is three times more common in women than men, yet has been almost completely unstudied in women.

- Women with kidney disease are less likely to receive dialysis or transplants than their male counterparts.

- Many immune-system disorders strike women at a higher rate than men — autoimmune thyroid diseases, fifteen to one; lupus, nine to one; systemic sclerosis, four to one; and rheumatoid arthritis, three to one — yet doctors haven't studied these diseases enough to know why.

- Depression is twice as common in women. Yet again, doctors are at a loss to explain why.

- Overall, women suffer from acute conditions, chronic illness, and short-term and long-term disabilities at higher rates than do men. While they outlive men on average by seven years, their final years are often unhappy ones. They outnumber men in nursing homes three to one and are more prone to such chronic debilitating illnesses as osteoporosis, Alzheimer's disease, Parkinson's disease, blindness, and hearing loss. Of the seven million women over age seventy-five in 1990, almost 30 percent were partly or completely disabled.

The medical establishment has long taken a less-than-enlightened view of women in general and diseases exclusive to women. "Most medical students have never felt an ovary by the time they finish medical school," says Pollycove.

Consider some other facts:

- Two decades ago, one in twenty American women could expect to be diagnosed with breast cancer during her lifetime. Today the odds are one in nine. Yet a study that would have examined the role that diet plays in prevention was killed by the NIH because researchers said that women could not be trusted to accurately report their diet.

- Ovarian cancer continues to be the deadliest reproductive cancer in women, striking some 22,000 American women per year, yet no effective screening exists to detect it.

- Little research has been done on fibroids even though they strike a third of all premenopausal women and are the most common reason for hysterectomies.

"Why do we know so little about uterine fibroids when the treatment is removing a major organ from a woman's body?" asks Johnson. "Can you think of a single benign disease in men, let alone one in the genital region, for which organ removal is the treatment of choice?"

The hysterectomy, the medical "treatment of choice" for fibroid tumors, is the third most common surgical procedure performed in the United States. (In fact, six of the twenty most common surgical procedures are performed only on women.) Thirty-seven percent of American women will undergo a hysterectomy by age sixty-five, yet only 10 percent of the 650,000 operations performed each year are done because of cancer or some other life-threatening condition. Not only do women lose some or all of their reproductive organs, the procedure also can create health problems of its own. Removal of a woman's uterus can double her risk of suffering a heart attack, and nearly half of all women will suffer surgical complications from the operation such as infection, urinary tract complications, or hemorrhaging.

"When I was a resident, it was not hard to convince me that a hysterectomy for a few fibroids was essential," says Dr. Katherine O'Hanlan, associate director of the Gynecological Cancer Service at Stanford University Medical Center. "Nor was it hard to convince me that a hysterectomy was essential for a woman who had spotting three times in a row. This was 1980 through 1984, and I was a respectful physician. Yet I thought that way because that's how I was trained."

Medical schooling can be so narrowly focused that women's health problems are overlooked. "Barely hours into our training we were already being taught that there was nothing to be learned from examining breasts," wrote Dr. Adriane Fugh-Berman, a 1988 graduate of Georgetown University Medical School, in *The Nation* last year. Instead, she wrote, her anatomy professor instructed students to cut off their cadaver's breasts and throw them away.

Now a physician practicing in Washington, DC, Fugh-Berman continues, "How many of my classmates currently in practice, I wonder, regularly examine the breasts of their female patients?"

"If one in nine men were dying of a disease to a part of the male anatomy, I can't imagine that part getting lopped off and thrown in the trash can," adds Johnson. "It would be unthinkable."

What gets learned in medical school, of course, gets put into practice. In the examination room, women's complaints are too easily dismissed as psychological or hormonal. A computer programmer from San Ramon is still stunned by the diagnosis she received after her hands became so crippled from repetitive typing that she could no longer even comb her hair. The only way she could work her computer was to grip a pencil and poke one key at a time. The company doctor told her that her ailment was "probably hormonal."

Janet, another computer programmer, actually had a hormonal problem: profuse bleeding — the result of hormone-replacement therapy, initiated at her doctor's insistence, five years after she went through menopause. "It was taking over my life," says the fifty-three-year old. "It was like having the first day of your period every day for four months. I didn't want to go anywhere because I thought I'd get up and leave a pool of blood behind. But every time I called the doctor he said, 'You're fine. It's just your imagination.'"

The same bias that leads doctors to view natural female conditions as "diseases" may make those same doctors dismiss serious symptoms when they point to an illness not perceived as traditionally "female." Cardiovascular disease is perhaps the prime example of this.

Women suffering heart attacks have been sent home from emergency rooms because doctors did not even suspect cardiovascular disease, still viewing it largely as a male problem even though women have outnumbered men in deaths from cardiovascular disease for the past nine years.

Doctors used to think heart attacks were more fatal in women because, on average, women were struck by them ten or twenty years later than men. But a study of nine hundred hospitals released earlier this year found that women who suffer heart attacks are more likely to die, at any age, than are their male counterparts.

Researchers speculated that differences in medical care are responsible for the deadly disparity: Women are not taken seriously at hospitals, they don't present the same symptoms as men, and drugs approved through studies on men are less effective in women. A 1987 American Medical Association study found that female cardiac patients were twice as likely as male patients to have the abnormal results of a treadmill test attributed to psychiatric or other noncardiac causes.

Two other studies, including one that videotaped patient visits to doctors' offices, found (in cases matched for every variable but gender) that men were twice as likely as women to be referred to a specialist. Women, complaining of the same symptoms, were more likely to be referred to a psychotherapist.

"If a woman comes in and says, 'I'm too tired to do my work,' she'll be diagnosed as depressed," says Dr. Iris F. Litt, director of Stanford's Institute for Research on Women and Gender. "If a man tells his doctor he can't play eighteen holes of golf anymore, he'll be sent to a cardiologist."

NO WOMEN ALLOWED

"There are two reasons women don't get good medicine," says O'Hanlan, "societal sexism and medical elitism."

To O'Hanlan's list, a third reason should be added: Call it separatism. The systematic exclusion of women as subjects in medical research and drug trials has left even the most benevolent physicians operating largely in the dark when it comes to treating women patients. Diseases that are the major cause of death and disability in women, even some that predominately strike women, have been studied almost exclusively in men alone. What little research has included women has focused almost entirely on reproduction.

"It's long been thought that the only health problems women have are related to making babies," says Litt.

The assumption that what's good for the gander is good for the goose leads many doctors to dispense advice, treatment, and drugs that may not be effective for women — and may even be dangerous.

Perhaps nowhere has the exclusion of women from research had a more dire effect than in the area

The medical establishment has long taken a less-than-enlightened view of women in general and women's diseases. "Most medical students," says one female ob-gyn, "have never felt an ovary by the time they finish medical school."

of cardiovascular disease, the leading cause of death for women in the United States.

Differences between women and men abound in both screening and treatment. The treadmill, the major diagnostic test for heart disease, is less accurate in women. Women are less likely than men to receive cardiac catheterization, angioplasty, or bypass surgery. And when they do get surgery, women are more likely to die in the operating room. (Researchers speculate that one reason might be that most operating technologies were developed for men's larger arteries.) Even some heart drugs, such as beta blockers, can be less effective and more dangerous in women, bringing on such side effects as fatigue and depression without improving arterial flow in some cases.

Yet nearly all the major studies on prevention and treatment have looked only at men. Will an aspirin a day keep the heart attack away? Yes, doctors concluded from a study of 22,000 men and no women. Can too much coffee increase the risk of heart attacks? No, according to a study of 45,000 men and no women (although we know caffeine contributes to ovarian and breast cysts in women).

Studies on oat bran, cholesterol-lowering drugs, the benefits of cardiac surgery, Type-A behavior, and such risk factors as hypertension, smoking, high cholesterol, and obesity have been performed on men only. Even a government-sponsored study of estrogen, which doctors believe helps women stave off heart disease until after menopause, was conducted only on men. The study was aborted after the men began developing breasts and blood clots.

The exclusion of women from medical research was no oversight. It was deliberate, according to the NIH, because of cost, fear of liability should a woman become pregnant during a trial, and a belief that women's fluctuating hormones during the menstrual cycle would throw off test results. Under the same rationale, women capable of becoming pregnant have been excluded from trials of new drugs until the final stage of testing, by which time many drugs that might have proved effective for women have been rejected as ineffective.

The fear of risk and inaccurate results would be compelling if it weren't for the fact that once drugs are approved, they are put on the market and prescribed to women even if they haven't been proven safe or effective in women. DES, or synthetic estrogen, was given to between three million and six million women from 1941 to 1971 to prevent miscarriages. But the drug had never been tested for use by pregnant women. Today many of the daughters of women who took DES show an increased risk of both vaginal and breast cancer.

Men and women simply are not the same physiologically and do not always tolerate drugs or procedures in the same way. "Brain structures, body weights, and cerebral blood flow, which can influence blood metabolism, are different in women and men," says Dr. Susan Blumenthal, chief of behavioral medicine at the National Institute of Mental Health. Women given the antidepressant bupropion suffered seizures because the initial recommended dosage had been established by tests in men with greater body weights. Significant differences show up also in how men and women metabolize cardiovascular, central nervous system, and nonsteroidal, anti-inflammatory medications, and women have twice the number of fatal drug reactions that men do.

OFFICIAL STEPS

"Every drug prescribed to women needs to be tested in women. To not do so is to practice bad medicine," says Litt. "I think there needs to be a lot more research about the normal physiology of women throughout their life span."

In an effort to end the practice of "bad medicine," patients and advocacy groups are lobbying at the grassroots level, with the help of some powerful congressional allies. Slowly, the doors that locked women out of the health-care system are being broken down.

In 1985, the NIH adopted a policy requiring women and minorities to be included in research studies, but it did little to enforce the policy — even neglecting to change grant application criteria to reflect the mandate. After the GAO report came out in 1990 documenting the institute's continued poor record, Representative Pat Schroeder of Colorado and her Congressional Caucus for Women's Issues pressured the NIH to increase funding for women's health.

In 1991, ten days after her confirmation as the first woman to head the NIH, Bernadine Healy announced the Women's Health Initiative, the largest clinical trial ever to be undertaken in the United States. The fifteen-year, $625 million project will involve 160,000 women in a series of studies on the causes and prevention of cardiovascular disease,

Women have been systematically excluded from medical research. Even a government-sponsored study on estrogen, which doctors believe helps women stave off heart disease until menopause, was conducted only on men.

cancer, and osteoporosis, the major causes of death, disability, and frailty in women. Researchers will look specifically at the effects of a low-fat diet, calcium, and other vitamin supplements, and the risks and benefits of hormone-replacement therapy.

While no Women's Health Initiative trials are underway yet, several Bay Area hospitals are involved in other studies. Stanford is participating in the DEER trial (415/723-3337), looking at the effects of diet and exercise on heart disease, and the HERS trial (415/723-4589), investigating hormone-replacement therapy on the prevention of heart disease. Tamoxifen, a drug researchers are exploring as the first preventive therapy for women at high risk for breast cancer, is being tested at many hospitals around the Bay Area. (For information, call 800/283-9765.)

Healy was not George Bush's first choice for the job. (It was rumored that six men turned down the job before her.) But by the time the Cleveland, Ohio, cardiologist stepped down from her post last June she had done perhaps more than any other woman to raise women's health issues to a higher place on the national agenda.

Pressure from Pat Schroeder's Congressional Caucus for Women's Issues also led to the establishment of the NIH's Office of Research on Women's Health to ensure the inclusion of women in all government-sponsored research and implement a ten-year agenda of research priorities to address the biggest gaps in knowledge about women's health. Grants from the office are funding studies of lung, breast, cervical, and ovarian cancer as well as hypertension, diabetes, AIDS, and Alzheimer's.

This year President Clinton proposed spending $662 million of the NIH's fiscal 1994 $10.7 billion budget on women's health research. The budget proposal was criticized by some lawmakers for increasing funding for two diseases with growing lobbies — AIDS and breast cancer — while cutting back on funding for a traditional sacred cow among medical researchers: heart disease.

"We left researchers to their own devices for decades, and they left out major portions of the population," said Health and Human Services Director Donna Shalala, defending the budget.

The Food and Drug Administration plans to drop its prohibition of women capable of becoming pregnant participating in early phases of drug trials. It also plans to encourage drug manufacturers to include women in "reasonable numbers," providing the agency with data on any different responses noted between men and women.

"While the FDA still believes that protecting fetuses from potentially toxic agents is an important principle, the agency concluded that fetal protection can be achieved by measures short of excluding women from early trials," an FDA release explained. Those measures include pre-enrollment pregnancy testing, use of contraception, and education about the risks.

"There is a price you pay for including women in research," says Dr. Mary Lake Polan, chair of the department of gynecology and obstetrics at Stanford and cochair of the task force on opportunities for research on women's health for the NIH. "It isn't right to say we want to be included, but we don't want to pay for it and we don't want to take on any risk."

TOWARD WOMEN'S HEALTH

"Recently, a psychiatrist at the National Institute of Mental Health was talking to a male colleague about a patient of hers who was depressed because she'd been raped," says Dr. Karen Johnson. "The male doctor replied, 'Sure, it would be demoralizing to be raped, but it wouldn't cause depression.' Tell me we don't need a specialist in women's health."

Johnson applauds the Women's Health Initiative as a step in the right direction. But she thinks it will take a radical reorganization of the way medicine is taught and delivered in order to legitimize women's health concerns and fuel research on an ongoing basis.

From her first day of medical school in 1972, Johnson was amazed by the misconceptions doctors and their physicians-in-training held about women patients. On hospital rounds, she noted what little attention doctors paid women patients and what little effort was made to educate them about their condition or ways to improve their health. In the doctors' lounge she was shocked by the mechanistic way her male colleagues debated radical mastectomies versus lumpectomies "as if a breast was not attached to a human being."

She got a taste of the medicine she was being trained to dispense when she visited the hospital for her own gynecological exam. Without asking her permission, the doctor brought in another medical student to view the exam. "They talked *at* my pelvic area," recalls Johnson. "I felt so disembodied."

As women move into positions of power in the medical establishment and government agencies, the doors that locked them out of the health-care system are being broken down. Some feel the system will change if only out of doctors' self-interest.

The problem, says Johnson, goes to the structure of medical education. Students spend two of their four years in medical school in the classroom and two years seeing patients in clinical rotation. The only required rotation with any emphasis on women is obstetrics and gynecology — a six-week session. Unless they choose an ob-gyn residency, that's the only specialized training they will get in women's health.

To correct the situation, Johnson, who trained in family practice before switching to psychiatry, has proposed establishing a multidisciplinary medical specialty in women's health. A women's health specialist would be a primary care physician for women — as pediatricians are for children and gerontologists are for the elderly — and would have specialized training in everything from managing menopause and spotting signs of physical abuse to understanding how drugs and diseases act differently in women and men.

Johnson envisions a three- or four-year residency program that would give the new specialists experience in "every area of medicine with a focus on women." She also envisions graduates teaching a basic level of women's health care to all medical students.

Such a specialty would correct the arbitrary division of women's bodies among the specialists who treat them.

"Take domestic violence, for example," says Johnson. "Depending on how the injured woman enters the health-care system, she may be treated by an emergency room physician for fractures, an ob-gyn for vaginal lacerations and repeated infections, or a psychiatrist for panic attacks and depression. Each clinician sees only a fragment of the overall problem and may have neither the knowledge nor the resources to intervene effectively."

The proposal has received both support and opposition, the latter mostly from gynecologists, family practitioners, and internists who feel they already provide good, comprehensive care to women. One prominent critic, psychiatrist Michelle Harrison of the University of Pittsburgh School of Medicine, is a strong advocate for women's health care but fears a specialty would "ghettoize" that care.

"A field created for the nonsurgical routine care of women, whose practitioners would invariably be mostly female, would likely become a relatively low-paid, low-status field with little or no opportunities for advancement or access to power within universities or specialty societies," says Harrison.

"Women's health would become a marginalized area for a few dedicated physicians," Harrison continues. "Meanwhile, the rest of medicine would continue as it is, with both the male body and male psyche the standard of normality and health."

But Johnson counters that prediction. "It's already ghettoized in a very destructive way," she says. "Women's health has been pushed into the field of obstetrics and gynecology, which is a surgical specialty. But ob-gyns are trained to deal with women's reproductive health, period. It's no accident that when we have a medical problem it ends up being cut out because it's in the hands of surgeons. People tend to do what they were trained to do."

If the proposal gathers momentum, it would probably be at least a decade or more before the specialty is considered by the American Board of Medical Specialties.

A few medical schools are already offering electives or postgraduate fellowships in women's health. Cornell University Medical College professor Lila Wallis has developed a curriculum organized around the life stages of women, which will be offered to practicing physicians this fall at New York Hospital–Cornell Medical Center. For each age the curriculum covers standard medical problems as well as specific issues such as sexuality, violence, abuse, and mental health. The University of Washington, the Medical College of Pennsylvania, and the Medical College of Virginia are all developing multidisciplinary women's health centers for patient care and doctor training.

In the end, Johnson believes the system will change, if only out of doctors' self-interest. "Medicine is already under siege," she says. "Doctors feel very threatened because their incomes have been reduced by managed care. But their incomes will be reduced more if the majority of their women patients abandon them and go to a women's health specialist.

"Let's face it: If we had to choose from among three doctors — a physician trained in internal medicine based only on research with men, an ob-gyn who focuses only on our reproductive organs, or a physician who has been comprehensively trained in women's health — whom would we go to? I know whom I'd choose."

How to Find a Doctor Who Really Cares

by Rhoda Donkin Jones

Do you feel your doctor doesn't take you seriously — or have enough time for you? Studies suggest that many women are being shortchanged. But you can get good care, if you know what to look for.

Karen Martin* made an appointment with a new physician when she developed cramps and heavy vaginal bleeding. "He gave me an internal exam and said I had fibroid tumors," she says. "Then he turned to his nurse and told her to schedule me for a hysterectomy."

Upset and confused, Martin, age 41, asked for an explanation of the tumors. She didn't realize fibroids aren't malignant or life threatening. Instead of reassuring her, the doctor gave her a booklet about hysterectomies. Martin, whose parents had both died of cancer that year, pressed the doctor to tell her whether she was

Name changed for privacy.

at risk for ovarian cancer. "If you're worried about that, we can remove your ovaries too," was the doctor's reply. Martin left the office humiliated and scared.

Experiences like Martin's aren't that uncommon. In fact, many women say they're dissatisfied with the medical care they receive. Research shows they often change physicians, citing communication problems. It's common for doctors to talk down to their female patients and minimize their symptoms, and many doctors also fail to provide crucial health information.

What exactly do we want from medical professionals? "Women are looking for a partnership with their physicians," says Patricia Carney, a registered nurse and researcher at the University of Washington in Seattle. "The old model of doctor as authority figure is dead."

Despite the problems, there are plenty of doctors who are good for women. McCall's asked medical experts and patients to help us identify the traits of these doctors — whether family physicians, obstetrician-gynecologists or other specialists. The essential qualities fall into these categories: 1) a nonsexist attitude; 2) an up-to-date knowledge of women's-health issues; 3) good communication skills; 4) a willingness to provide information; and 5) a considerate approach to care. This report looks at today's problems and tells you how to find a doctor who's woman-friendly.

HOW DOCTORS FEEL ABOUT WOMEN

Experts acknowledge that a woman's gender can hamper the care she gets. For one thing, men have been the subjects of more medical studies than women; doctors simply don't know as much about women's risk factors, symptoms and how they respond to treatment. But experts also say another part of the problem is that some doctors view women as overly emotional and anxious about their health.

"When a doctor dismisses chest pains in a female patient as 'nerves,' or abdominal pain as 'stress,' this is not only bad medicine but sexist medicine, and it happens all the time," says Lila Wallis, M.D., a clinical professor of medicine at Cornell University Medical College and chair of the Task Force on Women's Health Curriculum for the American Medical Women's Association. "Blaming symptoms on nerves or stress can seriously delay an accurate diagnosis and treatment."

In fact, studies have found that with women, doctors are more likely to attribute health complaints to

From *McCall's* (June 1994), pp. 46-48, 50-54. Reprinted by permission of Rhoda Donkin Jones, health writer.

emotional causes than they are with men, according to a report on gender issues in medicine from the Council on Ethical and Judicial Affairs of the American Medical Association (AMA). The report cited a study of 390 patients who underwent exercise radionuclide scans, a test to determine the heart's ability to pump blood. Of those with abnormal results, 40 percent of the men, compared with 4 percent of the women, were referred for further testing. Women were more than twice as likely to have their symptoms attributed to psychiatric or other non heart-related causes — a fact that could have hurt their care, said the report.

The AMA council found gender discrepancies in other areas of medical care as well. Women were less likely than men to receive diagnostic tests for lung cancer or to receive kidney transplants if they had kidney disease. Commenting on why men on kidney dialysis might have been more likely to receive a kidney transplant the researchers wrote: "Men's financial contribution to the family may be considered more critical than women's. A kidney transplant is much less cumbersome than dialysis."

COMMON MISTAKES

Some doctors may miss medical clues in women because the symptoms don't jibe with what those doctors learned in medical school. "When women describe their problems, they may not fit so-called normal diagnosis patterns, so doctors stop listening," says Carolyn Clancy, M.D., director of primary care at the Federal Agency for Health Care Policy and Research in Rockville, Maryland. "Historically, male physicians have dominated the profession, and medical training has been based on the male body as the norm."

Beware of doctors who talk down to you, use terms like honey, *or withhold information from you.*

It's an issue of both not knowing what to listen for and an inadequate knowledge base."

It's unfortunate that medical practices are based on men's physiology, says Wallis, because sex differences affect all the body's functions and organs, including digestion, resistance to infection, the heart and circulation. Women's hormones can shape the course of illnesses. Women also respond differently than men to many medications; for example, women metabolize alcohol in medications at a much slower rate than men do.

More information about women's health is expected. The National Institutes of Health now require that the scientists they fund include women in clinical studies or, if they don't, provide a valid reason why not.

In the field of women's health especially, doctors can't rely on what they learned in school; they must take the initiative by keeping up with the latest research on women's health. That's no small task, says Catherine Curran, M.D., a family-practice physician in Seattle. To keep up with this rapidly changing area, doctors must read journals and interact with their peers at meetings and seminars, she says.

A FAILURE TO COMMUNICATE

When doctors write off women's symptoms, communication breaks down. Women seem to have a harder time than men in communicating with physicians.

Consider the findings of a 1993 survey of 2,500 women and 1,000 men by Louis Harris and Associates for The Commonwealth Fund, a New York City philanthropy. The survey found that 41 percent of women said they've changed their physicians because they were dissatisfied with their care; only 27 percent of men said this. The major reason women gave for changing doctors was communication problems. For example, 25 percent of women said they'd been talked down to, compared with about 12 percent of men. And 17 percent of women, compared with 7 percent of men, had been told that a medical condition was "all in their head."

Many women also report that their doctors don't listen to them and don't encourage dialogue, says Peter Franks, M.D., an associate professor of family medicine at the University of Rochester. Take Jane Pollen,* a 40-year-old attorney and mother of two from Philadelphia. "My doctor listens to me for about 30 seconds, then interrupts and starts in with his own conclusions," she says. "I feel like I should apologize for asking questions."

Look for these 6 key signs:

1 Timely health information is available.

2 The staff is accessible to answer questions by phone.

3 The doctor uses his or her office, not the exam room, to discuss treatment options.

4 The doctor clearly explains your condition, using a model if appropriate.

5 The gown is comfortable and the exam room is warm.

6 The speculum used for the pelvic exam is warmed.

Some evidence suggests women who cannot talk to their male physicians may do better with female doctors. After studying videotapes of clinical interactions, Debra Roter, a professor in the department of health policy and management at the Johns Hopkins School of Hygiene and Public Health, concluded that female doctors generally devote more time to an office visit, ask more questions and tend to encourage their patients to talk more about themselves.

But experts stress that having a female doctor doesn't guarantee good communication. "The trick is for patients to find the physician — male or female — who engages them," says Franks. "When patients are engaged in a meaningful dialogue with their physician, they end up with better medical care. Doctors who don't listen miss the raw data that patients bring to the diagnosis," he says. "There is no textbook that replaces what people report about themselves."

INFORMATION, PLEASE

Another aspect of good communication is a doctor's providing his or her patients with health information. This includes knowing and explaining all your options when you need medical treatment.

If a doctor is your primary-care physician, it's crucial that he or she inform you about prevention. Cervical cancer can be averted if you have timely Pap exams. Breast cancer that's caught early through mammograms and breast self-exams has a better cure rate. And the risk of osteoporosis and heart disease may be reduced with the right diet and exercise.

Doctors should base prevention advice on a woman's age, lifestyle, and personal and family medical history, says nurse Patricia Carney. Unfortunately, this isn't happening in many doctor's offices, according to a recent study led by Carney and Allen J. Dietrich, M.D., of Dartmouth-Hitchcock Medical Center

Finding the Right M.D.

To find a good physician, gather names and then check out prospective doctors until you find one you're satisfied with. Ask friends or colleagues for suggestions. You can also call the referral service of a reputable hospital. Most will provide the names of doctors who have the specifications — such as specialty, gender and location — you're seeking. To find out if a doctor is board certified, call the American Board of Medical Specialties at 800-776-2378. And to check if there are any complaints registered against a doctor, call your state medical board.

When you go in for an appointment, look for these clues that suggest a doctor is woman-friendly.

- **A nonsexist attitude:** The doctor should treat you like a mature human being. Beware the doctor who uses terms of endearment, like *honey* and *dear*, when addressing you, or who speaks to you as if you were a child. Also, you shouldn't sense that you're talked down to, which is evidenced by comments such as "I'll make that decision."

- **An up-to-date knowledge of women's-health issues:** Ask physician questions about an area of women's health you know something about, or take in an article you've read. Then see if his or her answers indicate knowledge of and interest in the subject. Another tip-off that a physician is well-informed about women's health is doing careful breast and pelvic exams. "The doctor should describe everything she's doing during the procedures to make you a partner in the process," says Wallis.

- **Good communication skills:** A good communicator will listen carefully to what you say, ask questions and encourage discussion. Other signs that you have a good rapport with the physician: You feel comfortable talking openly; you're not interrupted; and the doctor uses what you say as a point of reference when discussing your problem.

- **A willingness to provide health information:** This means thoroughly explaining procedures and medical treatments, including the success rates, side effects and alternatives to the treatment. Primary-care physicians should also inform you about important prevention strategies such as taking in enough calcium and fiber, limiting fat intake, exercising and scheduling screening tests at the right time.

- **A considerate approach to care:** Take notice of the attention paid to your physical and emotional comfort, advises Caryl Mussenden, M.D., an obstetrician-gynecologist in Washington, D.C. Are you ushered into an exam room only to be left alone for half an hour without any explanation? Do consultations take place while you're wearing a gown in the examination room? These are clues that the doctor may not be concerned enough with your feelings. The attitude of the staff also influences how you feel. "These people have the first contact with patients, so they must care about each patient and convey that in every way," says Mussenden.

Ten Top Hospitals For Women

Just as there are woman-friendly doctors, there are also woman-friendly hospitals. McCall's consulted with doctors across the country to identify hospitals that stand out for their special interest and expertise in women's health. The ten listed below were most often named as being outstanding in a specific area of major concern to women. Some have initiated cutting-edge research that applies specifically to women; others offer a unique approach to treating — as well as preventing illness.

But there are many other fine hospitals, and by no means is it necessary to travel a long distance to receive excellent care. A woman can often do just as well close to home, where she has the benefit of support from her family and friends. Wherever you go, It's up to you to be sure you get state-of-the-art care.

UCLA MEDICAL CENTER, LOS ANGELES
Outstanding In: Breast Cancer

At the University of California, Los Angeles, Breast Center, patients are seen by a team of specialists that may include a surgeon, a radiation therapist, an oncologist, a plastic surgeon and a psychologist. The center also offers a special program for women who are at high risk of developing breast cancer and counsels them in genetics, nutrition and stress reduction.

EMORY UNIVERSITY SCHOOL OF MEDICINE, ATLANTA
Outstanding in: Heart Disease

Heart attack is the leading cause of death in American women. Emory has done pioneering research in female heart disease, including one of the largest studies to examine the outcome of coronary angioplasty and heart surgery in women. Overall, the study found, the women who underwent these procedures were older than the men and suffered more complications. This points out that women need to be diagnosed earlier for heart disease.

MEMORIAL-SLOAN KETTERING CANCER CENTER, NEW YORK CITY
Outstanding in: Lung and Colon Cancers

Sloan Kettering is one of the most innovative centers for treating lung cancer, the number-one cancer killer of women. The center offers a variety of options for patients who cannot be treated by surgery alone, including new kinds of radiation therapy, immunotherapy and treatments with plant-derived drugs such as Taxol.

Sloan Kettering has also started a multidisciplinary program to prevent colon cancer, the third largest cancer killer in women (after breast cancer). The center provides genetic counseling and dietary guidance. For colon cancer, doctors stress conservation surgery to preserve bowel function.

BRIGHAM AND WOMEN'S HOSPITAL, BOSTON
Outstanding in: Prenatal and Birthing; Rheumatology

Brigham and Women's, equipped with the most advanced technology, is known for caring for high-risk mothers. It has now added a Center for Women and Newborns to allow a woman to go through labor, delivery and recovery in her own private room.

Brigham and Women's also provides comprehensive care for a wide range of rheumatologic concerns facing women, including arthritis, rheumatism, multiple sclerosis and lupus. In addition to diagnostic services and treatment, the hospital offers ongoing management of these illnesses.

THE NEW YORK HOSPITAL–CORNELL MEDICAL CENTER, NEW YORK CITY
Outstanding in: Infertility

The hospital's Center for Reproductive Medicine and Infertility has one of the highest in-vitro fertilization success rates in the country. It offers the latest approaches to treating infertility, including intra-cytoplasmic sperm injection (ICSI), a new procedure for male infertility.

MAYO CLINIC, ROCHESTER, MINNESOTA
Outstanding In: Osteoporosis

Mayo, one of the world's largest referral centers for osteoporosis, is also one of the most active research centers on causes, diagnosis and treatment of the disease.

THE UNIVERSITY OF TEXAS M.D. ANDERSON CANCER CENTER, HOUSTON
Outstanding in: Gynecological Cancer

Since the 1950s M.D. Anderson has offered care for women with ovarian, uterine, cervical and endometrial cancer. The hospital stresses conservation surgery to preserve organ function and fertility.

THE MENNINGER CLINIC, TOPEKA, KANSAS
Outstanding in: Depression

Menninger offers special cognitive-therapy sessions in women-only groups as well as extensive services for designing individual treatment plans for depression.

(Continued)

Top Ten Hospitals For Women (continued)

MAGEE-WOMENS HOSPITAL, PITTSBURGH
Outstanding in: Gynecology

Magee has established a research facility dedicated exclusively to women's heath issues. It has opened a new Menopause Center, which specializes in "complex cases" — that is, women who, in addition to going through menopause, may also suffer from other conditions, such as osteoporosis.

UCSF MEDICAL CENTER, SAN FRANCISCO
Outstanding in: AIDS

The University of California, San Francisco, Women's HIV Clinic was founded to meet the special needs of women. Besides offering quality primary and gynecological care, the clinic works closely with UCSF's Pediatrics AIDS program, since many patients have children who are HIV-positive.

---

in Lebanon, New Hampshire. The researchers sent women posing as 55-year old patients to more than 50 community practice physicians. The women were instructed to say that they had high-fat, low-fiber diets and family histories of colon and breast cancers. Despite the obvious red flags thrown up by these statements, only one in five physicians gave dietary advice, and 35 percent failed to perform a breast examination unless it was specifically requested.

Research also suggests that doctors aren't doing a good job of counseling their patients about disease-prevention strategies during menopause. A recent Gallup survey polled 833 women between ages 45 and 60 about their experience with menopause. Results: Even though the women were most concerned with emotional well-being and the risk of osteoporosis and heart disease, their doctors were more likely to focus on how to cope with short-term physical symptoms, such as hot flashes and night sweats.

THE COURTESY FACTOR

A respectful attitude is a final quality that may influence your satisfaction with a doctor. Some doctors make an effort not to keep patients waiting long and try to make their exams as comfortable as possible, says Wallis. This may include steps like warming the speculum before a pelvic exam.

This sensitivity matters most when you feel vulnerable or threatened. Patty Murphy,* a 30-year-old teacher, recalled her clinicians' behavior during her breast surgery at the Breast Clinic at Faulkner Hospital in Boston. "They had classical music playing when I came into the operating room," says Murphy. "During the surgery one woman held my hand, while the surgeon explained the procedure so I didn't feel helpless."

Rhoda Donkin Jones is a freelance writer in Seattle, Washington.

Trace Your Family Tree

Charting your relatives' medical history can save your life

By Ruth Papazian

When it comes to health, the apple doesn't fall far from the family tree: Research suggests that an astonishing number of diseases — from rare to common — have some sort of hereditary link.

That is why constructing a family health tree can offer life-saving glimpses into your future. If you're at risk of inheriting a serious disease, you can get regular checkups to spot early symptoms and increase the chances for a cure. You may also want genetic counseling, to learn the risk of passing a disease on to your children.

Aside from health problems caused by accident or infectious disease, you can assume that most every disease in your family's background has some sort of genetic basis. These can be divided into two classes: *susceptibility diseases*, in which genes don't cause the problem but influence your risk of becoming ill; and *purely genetic diseases*, which people almost invariably develop if they inherit the requisite genes.

Susceptibility diseases typically occur later in life and include major ailments such as heart disease, diabetes (especially the non-insulin-dependent type) and several types of cancer, including breast, lung, colorectal (colon and rectal), prostate, ovarian and skin. The inherited tendency to develop a disease probably results from complex interactions among several genes. Also on the list of disorders with a genetic component: rheumatoid arthritis, allergies, asthma, glaucoma, Alzheimer's disease, osteoporosis, glaucoma and behavioral and emotional problems including schizophrenia, alcoholism and depression.

Although genes set the stage for these disorders, the actual illness is usually caused in part by some environmental factor — cigarette smoke in the case of lung cancer, for example, or high-fat diets in heart disease and non-insulin-dependent diabetes, as well as prostate, colorectal and perhaps ovarian cancer. Luckily, people who know that a susceptibility disease lurks in their family tree may be able to control those nongenetic risk factors, or at least be on the alert for early symptoms.

For example, if your mother or sister developed breast cancer before menopause, your lifetime risk would be as great as one in three, vs. one in nine for other women. (Early onset of any disease increases the probability that heredity played a role.) A family history of breast cancer means you should get annual mammograms beginning at age 35, plus frequent professional exams.

As for purely genetic diseases, there are more than 4,000 — most of them rare — that result from defects in single genes. If you have such a disorder in your family tree, your chance of inheriting it depends on the nature of the gene responsible.

For instance, if one of your parents died of a heart attack before age 60, there's a one-in-five chance that he or she had familial hypercholesterolemia (an inherited extremely high cholesterol level); if so, there's a

From *American Health* (May 1994), pp. 80-84. Reprinted by permission of *American Health*. © 1994 by Ruth Papazian.

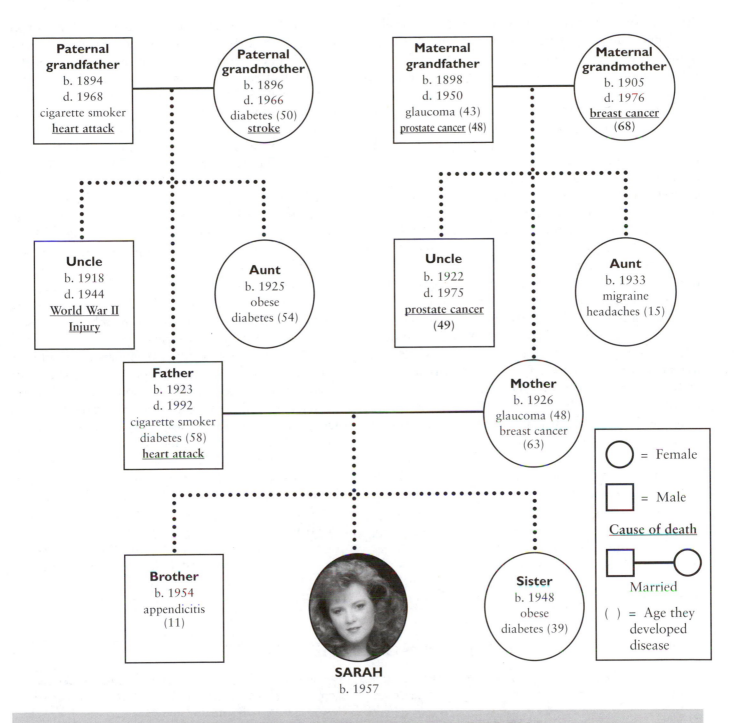

Paternal grandfather
b. 1894
d. 1968
cigarette smoker
<u>heart attack</u>

Paternal grandmother
b. 1896
d. 1966
diabetes (50)
<u>stroke</u>

Maternal grandfather
b. 1898
d. 1950
glaucoma (43)
<u>prostate cancer</u> (48)

Maternal grandmother
b. 1905
d. 1976
<u>breast cancer</u> (68)

Uncle
b. 1918
d. 1944
<u>World War II Injury</u>

Aunt
b. 1925
obese
diabetes (54)

Uncle
b. 1922
d. 1975
<u>prostate cancer</u> (49)

Aunt
b. 1933
migraine headaches (15)

Father
b. 1923
d. 1992
cigarette smoker
diabetes (58)
<u>heart attack</u>

Mother
b. 1926
glaucoma (48)
breast cancer (63)

Brother
b. 1954
appendicitis (11)

SARAH
b. 1957

Sister
b. 1948
obese
diabetes (39)

○ = Female

□ = Male

<u>Cause of death</u>

□—○ Married

( ) = Age they developed disease

SARAH'S FAMILY MEDICAL HISTORY

Sarah risks inheriting non-insulin-dependent diabetes from her father's side of the family and breast cancer and glaucoma from her mother's side. But the two fatal heart attacks on her father's side shouldn't cause concern; both occurred relatively late in life and probably stemmed from major risk factors — smoking (her grandfather) and both smoking and diabetes (her father).

Diabetes: Sarah's sister already has it. Sarah and her brother should have their blood sugar monitored regularly; they can help ward off the disease by exercising and adopting a prudent diet.

Glaucoma: Sarah and her two siblings should have yearly eye exams to detect glaucoma at its early stages.

Breast cancer: Sarah and her sister face a higher than normal risk, since their mother and maternal grandmother developed it. Both sisters should have a baseline mammogram between the ages of 30 and 35, and yearly mammograms after 35; her sister should lose weight, since obesity adds to her risk.

Finally, Sarah should alert her brother to the fact that he's at increased risk for *prostate cancer.* His maternal grandfather and uncle both developed it early in life. He needs regular screening: each year, a digital rectal exam, plus a PSA (prostate-specific antigen) test.

50-50 chance you have it too. The gene responsible for familial hypercholesterolemia is "dominant": Inherit a defective version from one parent and you'll get the disease, even if your other parent gave you a normal copy.

Familial hypercholesterolemia, which affects one in every 500 people, can clog arteries and lead to a heart attack at an early age. If you have a family history of heart disease, be sure to get your cholesterol level measured. Once detected, an abnormally high cholesterol level can often be controlled with a lowfat diet and cholesterol-lowering drugs.

Familial adenomatous polyposis, another inherited disorder, afflicts one in 8,000 people and almost always results in intestinal cancer. ("Surviving a Family Curse," below, describes a family coping with this dominant-gene problem.) Other dominant diseases include Huntington's disease (the degenerative nervous-system disorder that killed singer Woody Guthrie), adult polycystic renal disease (a kidney disorder) and Marfan's syndrome (characterized by abnormally long limbs and heart problems). Diseases controlled by a dominant gene rarely skip a generation, so you've probably been spared if neither of your parents had the disease, even if a grandparent did.

Fortunately, most purely hereditary diseases are "recessive"; that is, they afflict only those unlucky enough to inherit two copies of a defective gene — one from each parent. The most common of these recessive diseases seem to target certain ethnic groups.

For example, about one in 25 white Americans carries the gene for cystic fibrosis (CF), one of the most common lethal hereditary diseases (for those of northern European descent the risk is somewhat higher). The gene defect in CF results in a thick, sticky mucus in the lungs; the mucus encourages severe respiratory infections that usually prove fatal by age 30.

A CF carrier — with one abnormal and one normal gene — will be healthy. But if someone with the gene marries another carrier, their offspring will have a one-in-four chance of inheriting two defective copies of the gene and being born with CF. Following the discovery in 1989 of the gene that causes CF, a blood test became available that can tell whether a person is a carrier and whether a couple's fetus will develop the disease.

Purely hereditary diseases (or disorders) that usually affect only men are called X-linked recessive diseases. The best known are hemophilia, color blindness and Duchenne muscular dystrophy. An X-linked disorder is transmitted from mother to son by a gene on one of her two X chromosomes. Each son has a 50-50 chance of getting the disease, from inheriting just a single copy of the recessive gene.

Mom may be a healthy carrier, since her other X chromosome carries a normal copy of the gene, which masks the defective one. But her son, with his X chromosome paired with a Y from his father, isn't as lucky. A woman should suspect she may be a carrier of an X-linked disorder if the disease has shown up in a male relative.

Virtually every month, researchers identify a gene linked to yet another hereditary disease; these findings are leading to increasing numbers of blood tests to identify people who carry these genes or who are destined to develop the diseases. To take advantage of these advances, you must first learn whether you or other family members are at risk.

Gathering information about illnesses that run

SURVIVING A FAMILY CURSE

Larry Howard* had considered his family's medical history a curse, but knowing about it probably saved his life.

Larry's mother, three brothers and a sister all had been diagnosed with familial adenomatous polyposis, a disease in which thousands of polyps — tiny wartlike growths — sprout from the lining of the large intestine (colon). People with this condition (about one in 8,000) almost always develop colon cancer from polyps that turn malignant.

Larry's mother and his four affected siblings had to have their colons removed to prevent cancer from taking hold — the treatment reserved for severe cases. But Larry and his other sister, Mary, thought they had been spared.

Since early adolescence, when the polyps generally arise, Larry and Mary had taken part in the Johns Hopkins University familial polyposis study, undergoing annual sigmoidoscopies (visual examination of the lower third of the colon) and receiving clean bills of health. Ten years ago, when Larry was 32, he was told he didn't need any more checkups, since his risk of having inherited the disease seemed minimal.

Then last year he and Mary were given a new blood test, developed at Johns Hopkins, that identifies the gene that causes familial polyposis. The test determined that Mary did not carry the defective gene, but Larry did. Sure enough, a subsequent exam revealed sprouting polyps.

Larry plans to have his colon removed later this year. His three children have taken the blood test too: One of the three has tested positive.

*Not his real name

in your family is not as daunting as it may seem — especially if you ask relatives for help. Here is a guide for constructing your medical family tree:

1. **Make a list** of your first-degree relatives (parents, siblings and children) and second-degree relatives (grandparents, aunts and uncles). Adding more peripheral branches to your tree usually isn't worthwhile: The more distant the relative, the less relevant his medical fate is to you (you and your second cousin, for example, inherit only about 3% of the same genes). A possible exception: when you need more evidence to confirm a pattern involving a serious health problem such as cancer or heart disease.

2. **Construct your family tree,** using the sample as a guide. Your name and the names of your siblings go on the bottom row. On the row above, put the names of your parents, along with the names of their brothers and sisters. The names of all four grandparents go on the top line. It's customary to put male relatives in squares and female ones in circles and to indicate marriages by connecting relatives with horizontal lines.

3. **Record the following information for each relative:**

   • *Date of birth, date of death, and cause of death.* If necessary, you can usually obtain this information from the death certificate. To get a copy, contact the department of vital records in the state where the relative lived. (Be sure to check the family Bible first — birth and death certificates are often tucked inside the covers.)

   • *All known illnesses and major surgeries including the age when they occurred.* This information could be more relevant than the cause of death — if an uncle had a heart attack at age 40 but died 20 years later from an automobile accident, for example. Medical records are the most reliable sources for this information.

   Ask relatives who are still living either to give you copies of their medical records or to sign a consent form allowing their doctors to give you this information. To obtain a deceased relative's records, contact the doctor or hospital that treated him; those names should be on the death certificate. You may have to provide a letter of consent from your relative's next of kin, as well as a copy of the death certificate.

   • *Lifestyle factors that may have contributed to illness.* For instance, heart disease would be less of a genetic threat if you found that the uncle who suffered the heart attack at age 40 was a chain smoker. Most every family has a self-appointed

"historian" who is the repository of family lore. You may be able to learn about relatives' lifestyles by talking to that person.

   • *Occupation (optional).* This information may be important if there were job-related factors (such as exposure to toxic chemicals) that may have contributed to illness, miscarriage or birth defects.

   • *Unusual physical characteristics.* Prominent features or chronic skin rashes could hint at certain medical conditions or birth defects (but you'll want to corroborate your hunches with medical records or other documents). Again, the family historian may be a good source. Family photo albums can also be revealing: A grandmother's "dowager's hump," for example, probably indicates that she had osteoporosis.

As you research your family medical tree, be prepared for difficulties. Information may be unavailable (some family members may not cooperate, for example), or it may not exist (as when a child died and no diagnosis was ever made) or it may not be accurate (family legend, for example, may attribute an aunt's pregnancy loss to a miscarriage when in fact she had an abortion).

A little tact goes a long way. Family members may not want to talk about sad events or what they consider to be the family's dirty laundry. A good approach: "My doctor is interested in Cousin Bobby's condition because it could affect the children I may have. Can you tell me about his problem so that we can calculate the risks?" Offer to share your completed tree with relatives, along with the opinions of medical or genetic experts you consult.

Now that you've constructed your family tree, here are some tips on interpreting it:

- Your tree's two most important "branches" are your mother and father: Each gave you half your genetic inheritance, so their diseases will be most relevant to you and your siblings.

- The earlier a disease develops, the more likely that heredity played a role in it (except for ailments with obvious nongenetic causes such as infections).

- A disease that strikes two or more relatives at the same age is likely to be strongly influenced by heredity.

- A clustering of cases of the same disease on one side of the tree is more likely to suggest that genes play a strong role in causing it than a similar number of cases scattered on both sides. On the other hand, your risk of inheriting a purely hereditary disease like cystic fibrosis would actually be greater when it's present on both your mother's and father's side.

If you have questions about your family tree, you should show it to your doctor. If the doctor suspects a genetic problem, you will probably be referred to a genetic counselor, who can assess your risk of developing the diseases you're worried about, and of passing them on to a child. A counselor can also tell prospective parents if a fetus can be tested for conditions of concern.

Genetic counselors typically have a master of science degree in genetics and are certified by the American Board of Medical Genetics. Your family doctor, obstetrician or pediatrician can probably refer you to one, or you can contact a major hospital or medical school in your area or your local chapter of the March of Dimes for referrals (for further information, see "For More Help").

Your medical family tree should be a living, growing document. As you and your brothers and sisters get married and have children, keep adding to it: It can contribute to your health today and to the health of future generations.

Ruth Papazian, a New York City-based writer specializing in health and medicine, is constructing a family

A Reading for Critical Thinking

Now that researchers are addressing the inequities in clinical research on women, what's the next step? Undoubtedly, any new information must be integrated into the care we receive. Is developing a new women's health specialty the best way to accomplish that goal?

Women's Health Care: A Specialty of Our Own?

When it comes to women's health, who sees the whole picture of the whole woman? For too many women, the answer to that question is "no one."

Even if tomorrow — by some miracle — researchers uncovered the remainder of the information we need about our bodies and the diseases that concern us the most, another pressing problem would remain: Who would pull it all together?

Women's health care tends to be divided between "reproductive care" and "everything else." Thus, even currently available information is parceled out among medical specialties, with different physicians applying what "fits" their area of expertise.

The result is often fragmented and uneven — and potentially dangerous — medical care, says Karen Johnson, M.D., a clinical scholar in women's health at Stanford University. "It means that a woman often has to see more than one physician just to have her basic health care needs met — but that no one physician is following the overall picture of her health."

The solution is clear, she asserts: "If we're going to receive the full benefit of American health care and research, it's imperative that we have a medical discipline of our own, a discipline in which the study of women's health is not only encouraged but valued."

ONE-STOP SHOPPING?

Proponents of a women's health specialty argue that women's health care currently resembles a jigsaw puzzle that's missing some critical pieces — and has unneeded duplicates of others.

Creating a specialty would provide women with "one-stop shopping" for health care, they argue. Under this scenario, a woman could trust that her physician is truly coordinating her care, filling in any gaps, clearing up problems with overlapping care, and eliminating miscommunications among physicians.

Moreover, they say, women could expect their women's health specialist to be trained to:

- diagnose and treat diseases that disproportionately affect women (such as lupus, diabetes, rheumatoid arthritis, and thyroid disease);

- diagnose and treat conditions that manifest themselves differently in women (such as heart disease and AIDS); and

- recognize that a woman's hormonal and metabolic characteristics can affect a drug's action, necessitate "non-standard" drug dosages, or lead to drug interactions.

And Dr. Johnson, who's also a psychiatrist, argues that women's health specialists should be trained in the psychosocial aspects of women's health. Women are disproportionately affected by depression, domestic abuse, and poverty, she points out; thus, we need a multidisciplinary approach that treats not only the physical but also the emotional and socioeconomic facts of our often complex lives.

REINVENTING THE WHEEL?

But opponents argue that establishing a women's health specialty is nothing more than reinventing the

From *Women's Health Advocate* (March 1995), pp. 4-6. Reprinted with permission from *Women's Health Advocate Newsletter*. For subscriptions call 1-800-829-5876 and ask for the introductory price of $16 per year, a 33% discount.

wheel, assuaging women's frustrations by recreating what already exists.

"We already have a specialty that deals with women's reproductive issues, namely obstetrics and gynecology. And internists and family physicians are trained as well in women's health," says Nancy Dickey, M.D., a family physician in Richmond, Texas, who's also vice-chair of the American Medical Association's Board of Trustees.

Other critics argue that women and men are more alike than different, that much of our physiology is identical. Moreover, even in areas where there are differences, those differences aren't enough to mandate a completely new specialty, they say. As an extreme example, they note that even though heart disease may manifest itself differently in men and women, that doesn't mean we need one cardiologist for men and another for women.

In musing over the question of whether there's enough information about women's health to warrant a new specialty, even Silvia Wassertheil-Smoller, Ph.D., head of the Women's Health Initiative trial at Albert Einstein College of Medicine in New York, notes, "That's a tough question. While it's true that women's health problems may not be recognized as such by traditional health care providers, it isn't clear that the solution is to create yet another specialty that might further fragment care."

THE PEDIATRICS PATTERN

The debate is hardly an esoteric one: Several medical schools are now incorporating women's health into their courses, and certain medical specialties are battling for their piece of the women's health pie (see "Beyond the 160-Pound Male"). In California, the debate has even spilled over into health maintenance organizations.

Dr. Johnson applauds this new awareness of women's health care. However, she adds that it represents "a developmental step" toward the final goal rather than a goal in and of itself.

She draws a parallel with pediatrics: Earlier this century, when the idea of establishing pediatrics as a standalone medical discipline was first proposed, "First, we saw a single clinic established for children, then a hospital, then specialized tracks in established medical school programs. Finally, it became clear that a separate pediatric specialty made sense."

HOW TO FIND CARE

In the meantime, how can you find someone who's knowledgeable about women's health?

As it stands now, any physician in the U.S. who wants to call himself or herself a "women's specialist" can do so regardless of his or her training. (The only certified women's care specialists are graduates of advanced nursing programs in women's health care.)

Beyond the 160-Pound Male

The call for a separate women's health specialty is beginning to make the medical world sit up and take notice.

Several medical schools, medical centers, and organizations now hold seminars aimed at "retraining" practicing physicians in areas of women's health. Among existing medical specialties, a turf war has broken out: Both the American College of Obstetricians and Gynecologists and the American Academy of Family Physicians claim women's health as their own domain and are working hard to justify their positions.

What about current medical students? At present, only a handful of medical schools offer training in women's health care as part of their curriculum.

Most medical students are taught only how a particular disease affects a 160-pound male, says Karen Johnson, M.D., a clinical scholar in

women's health at Stanford University.

But that may change, thanks to Congress. Last year, the Health Resources and Services Administration (HRSA) was directed to work with the National Institutes of Health and the U.S. Public Health Service to evaluate the gaps in medical education and propose a model curriculum on women's health for medical schools.

The report is expected to be presented to Congress next month. "No one will be required to adopt our curriculum," says Betty Hambleton, chief of planning, evaluation, and legislation at HRSA's Bureau of Health Professions. "But it should serve as a framework or model that could be used to guide a medical school in developing its own curriculum on women's health."

A few medical schools have already developed quasi-specialist

training in women's health. The medical schools at Brown and Tufts universities offer two-year fellowship programs in women's health for physicians who have completed their residency training in primary care.

Albert Einstein College of Medicine and the University of Pittsburgh School of Medicine have set up special tracks on women's health care as part of their existing internal medicine residency programs for new internists. And women's health programs have popped up at several other medical schools as well.

The new approaches to teaching medicine require students to consider examples of women in all their subjects, not just during ob-gyn lectures. Thus, if a lecture focuses on cholesterol levels, the interplay between estrogen and cholesterol must be covered, along with such standard topics as dietary intake.

Moreover, many hospitals and physicians have realized that they can bring in more patients simply by adding the word "women" to their title.

Thus, it's up to you to ask some pertinent questions:

• If you see only one physician, ask about additional training or areas of expertise. For example, does your internist or family physician have broad training in obstetrics and gynecology? Conversely, is your obstetrician-gynecologist trained in areas other than reproductive care? How will your doctor ensure that you don't miss out on important tests, such as mammograms or cholesterol tests?

• If you see more than one physician, does each realize that the other exists, that you're being treated for more than one condition? Is each physician aware of your different medications? Is one physician coordinating your care?

• If you're considering a "woman's health center," what services does the center offer? Is it focused primarily on one area (such as reproductive care or menopause), or is it more broad-based? Does the center exist primarily as a marketing ploy, or does it represent a genuine attempt to offer integrated health care? Will one physician coordinate your care? If you need to be referred to another physician, where does that physician practice?

Most of all, do you have a good working relationship with your physician?

"The most important thing is to feel comfortable with your physician so that you can be honest about your health and ask questions about any recommendation," Dr. Dickey points out. "The best care comes when a doctor and patient have formed a partnership and complement one another."

The HMO Angle

Now that managed care plays such a large role in the lives of many Americans, one California development is generating a great deal of attention: As of Jan. 1, 1995, some obstetrician-gynecologists can be considered primary care providers by health maintenance organizations, if they have the appropriate training.

The law was sparked by women's discontent: "I heard from several women who were frustrated that their HMO wouldn't allow them to go directly to their ob-gyns," says California Assemblywoman Jacqueline Speier, who pushed the legislation through. Instead, patients — male or female — saw a family physician internist in the HMO first. Women were then referred for a second appointment with an ob-gyn, if needed. Now, says Ms. Speier, every California health plan has to allow qualified ob-gyns — defined as those who've had training in primary care — to be listed as primary care providers.

Women's Health Watch

Information for Enlightened Choices from Harvard Medical School

Women Doctors

According to statistics released by the American Medical Association recently, it is increasingly likely that the doctor you see for routine care will be a woman. The AMA data indicate that while about only 20% of physicians are currently women, female students make up 40% of enrollment in medical schools. Moreover, a higher proportion of women than men are entering internal medicine, the principal primary-care specialty. This trend, along with interest in quality of care, has prompted research into the effects of gender on the doctor/patient relationship. While no investigations have indicated that either men or women do a better job of keeping their patients alive and in good health, a few studies have turned up subtle differences in the way male and female primary-care doctors respond to female patients.

These studies, most of which have been conducted in the last 10–15 years, are generally small, and their findings can in no way be extrapolated to every doctor — either male or female. As we all know well, interpersonal relationships are so complex that many of the contributing factors can't be adequately measured or even described. Yet, this research to date has produced several interesting observations, which seem to bode well for the relationship between women patients and their female physicians.

- *Tests prescribed.* A 1993 study from the University of Minnesota of almost 25,000 women in a large health plan determined that those who had a female primary-care physician were twice as likely to have an annual Pap smear as those whose internists were men. They were also 41% more likely to have a mammogram than those with male doctors. However, there is no evidence that male *gynecologists* order fewer such tests.

- *Length of visit.* As a rule, female doctors seem to spend more time with their patients during office visits. In one of the latest studies, which involved 25 male and 25 female physicians at Massachusetts General Hospital in Boston, researchers videotaped office visits of both male and female patients. They found that the male doctors spent an average of 22.4 minutes with women patients, and women doctors spent an average of 29.9 minutes.

- *Interpersonal dynamics.* Many studies have hinted that female doctors are more likely to treat patients as equals. The Boston study bore this out, finding that conversations were most balanced when both doctor and patient were female. On average, female doctors made 261 utterances (defined as meaningful strings of words) during a visit, and women patients spoke 254 times. In comparison male doctors spoke 208 times and their female patients, 175.

  The tenor of the conversations between doctor and patient more frequently indicated a partnership, rather than a paternalistic relationship, when both parties were women. The Boston group found that the word "we" was exchanged most frequently between female patients and doctors, and that supportive gestures, including nods, smiles, and responses of agreement, were also the most frequent in this setting.

- *Information exchange.* Most studies have found that women patients volunteer more information to women doctors. However, the Boston researchers noted that women provided — and received — the same amount of information from physicians of both sexes.

THE PATIENT'S RESPONSIBILITY

If there's a message in these studies, it may be that many of us feel more comfortable discussing the most intimate details of our lives with another woman. However, we can't expect any doctor — male or female — to be a mind reader. To ease the flow of information during your next visit, do some advance preparation. Jot down your symptoms and the drugs you are taking. If you're seeing a new doctor, bring your medical history, as well as your concerns and questions.

Primary Care of Lesbian Patients

By Jocelyn White, M.D., and Wendy Levinson, M.D.

During the last decade the recognition of AIDS has led to a marked increase in the education of physicians about the care of gay men. This knowledge has resulted in a better understanding of HIV-related concerns and the general health needs of these patients. In the "pre-AIDS" era the medical literature rarely discussed the health needs of gay men. As a result few health care providers felt competent or comfortable providing them with service. Similarly, the care of lesbians has received little attention, and medical literature rarely addresses the needs of this group.[1–3] Lesbians constitute approximately 10% of the female population.[4] They represent a large group of patients with unique medical, psychological, and social needs.

The dictionary definition of a lesbian is "a female homosexual," meaning a woman who is sexually attracted to other women. For practical purposes this definition is too narrow because lesbianism is not only a sexual orientation but also an identity. A lesbian identity is based on emotions and psychological responses,[4, 5] societal expectations,[5, 6] and the individual's own choices in identity formation.[5, 7] Therefore, some women are sexually active with women but do not identify themselves as lesbians. Most lesbians prefer the term lesbian as opposed to gay or homosexual because it also refers to emotions, behavior, and a cultural system.[5]

Lesbians are a diverse group in terms of sexual practices. They may be celibate or sexually active with women, men, or both. Most lesbians either are currently sexually active with women exclusively or are celibate[8] although, in one study, 77% of lesbians had at some point participated in heterosexual coitus.[1] The specific sexual practices of an individual patient determine her risks of particular diseases. In this review the authors make an effort to base recommendations on the sexual-practice histories of individual patients.

SEXUALLY TRANSMITTED DISEASES

Sexually transmitted diseases (STDs) in lesbian patients are less common than either in heterosexual women or in gay men. This may be due in part to the lack of penile–vaginal intercourse among lesbians. Lesbian sexual practices include kissing, breast stimulation, manual and oral stimulation of the genitals and anus, friction of the clitoris against the partner's body, and penetration of the vagina and anus with fingers and devices.[1, 9] There are no gynecologic problems unique to lesbians and none that occur more often in lesbians than in bisexual or heterosexual women. Therefore, lesbian sexual practices are unlikely to increase risks for gynecologic problems, including STDs.[1] Lower risk for STDs is also likely to be due to the relative epidemiologic isolation of this population from men.

Most of the information about STDs in lesbians comes from three studies. Robertson and Schacter[10] screened 148 symptomatic and asymptomatic women for syphilis, cervical gonorrhea, infection with herpes simplex virus, and *Chlamydia trachomatis* infection. These women had responded to an advertisement for the study and had been sexually active exclusively

Received from the Good Samaritan Hospital and Medical Center, Oregon Health Sciences University, Portland, Oregon.

Address correspondence and reprint requests to Dr. White: Department of Medicine-R200, Good Samaritan Hospital and Medical Center, 1015 NW 22nd Avenue, Portland, OR 97210.

with women for six months. Johnson et al.[1] conducted a written survey of the past medical histories and health care attitudes of 1,921 self-identified lesbians attending music festivals. Degen and Waitkevicz[9] reviewed the charts of women presenting to a lesbian health clinic, collecting information about the incidence of STDs. The results of these studies may not be generalizable to all lesbians because of sample bias. The changing rates of syphilis and gonorrhea in the general population since these studies were performed also may limit the usefulness of these results.

Lesbians appear to have a lower incidence of syphilis and gonorrhea than does any other population except those who have never been sexually active at all.[9] Robertson and Schacter[10] found no case of syphilis or gonorrhea in 148 sexually active lesbians. Degen and Waitkevic[9] found one positive VDRL among 120 women tested. This woman was a health care worker whose sexual partner tested negative for syphilis, and the investigators postulated an occupational source of this infection. The survey by Johnson et al.[1] found no reported case of syphilis or gonorrhea in women who had been sexually active exclusively with other women. Based on these data, routine screening for gonorrhea or syphilis in lesbians does not appear to be cost-effective. Testing is appropriate only in the setting of other risk factors, especially recent heterosexual exposure.[11]

Other STDs common among heterosexual women rarely have been reported in the lesbian population. Chlamydia and herpes virus rarely are cultured from lesbians who have been sexually active exclusively with women.[1, 9, 10] Herpes can be transmitted between women but the prevalence in the lesbian population seems to be low. Pelvic inflammatory disease (PID) also appears to be rare among lesbians, although two unconfirmed cases have been reported.[10] Venereal warts caused by human papillomavirus (HPV) are uncommon unless the patient has had heterosexual contact.[1, 9] Since women who have venereal warts may theoretically transmit them, their female partners should be evaluated. Unlike in the gay male population, enteric infections due to hepatitis A, amoeba, shigella, and helminths have low prevalences in lesbians. The lack of penile–anal transmission may play a role in this. Hepatitis B does not occur unless other risk factors are present.[8, 12, 13]

While many STDs are uncommon in lesbians, vaginitis frequently occurs. In one study of 229 lesbians with genital symptoms undefined by the authors, 38% had nonspecific vaginitis, 24% vaginal candidiasis, 23% cervicitis (organisms not specified), and 14% Trichomonas vaginitis.[9] Nonspecific vaginitis, more recently called bacterial vaginosis, is due to multiple organisms, including *Garnerella vaginalis*, Peptostreptococcus, Bacteroides species, Mobiluncus, and genital strains of mycoplasma. Little is known about the pathogenesis of bacterial vaginosis, including whether it may be transmitted between women. Physicians should inquire about vaginal discharge in partners and evaluate partners with symptoms.

Vaginal candidiasis occurs in lesbians. Because bisexual women report it more often than do lesbians, it is probably related to heterosexual contact,[1] but transmission between women is possible.[9, 14] Partners of lesbians with vaginal candidiasis should be treated. *Trichomonas vaginalis* has been found in women who are sexually active exclusively with women, women with no sexual contact at all,[1] and lesbians who have sexual contact with bisexual women.[15] Among 53 lesbians sexually active exclusively with other women, three had Trichomonas.[9] Trichomonas may be transmitted by fomites such as damp towels and underwear or possibly had hand–genital contact.[1, 9] Based on this information, clinicians should include trichomoniasis in the differential diagnosis of vaginal discharge in lesbians. Sexual partners of lesbians should be treated for trichomoniasis as well.

In review, syphilis, gonorrhea, infection with chlamydia, and PID are unusual in women who are sexually active exclusively with other women. Routine screening for syphilis, gonorrhea, and chlamydia infection is probably not necessary. Herpes and infection with HPV also are uncommon but transmission between women may occur. Because all three common forms of vaginitis have been reported in lesbians, physicians should consider these infections in lesbians presenting with vaginal discharge.

HIV AND AIDS

The most recent data from the Centers for Disease Control (CDC) concerning AIDS in lesbians reported 164 cases as of June 30, 1991. Ninety-three percent of these women were intravenous drug users (SY Chu, personal communication, January 16, 1991).[16] Transmission of HIV between women may have occurred in two cases.[17, 18] Menstrual and traumatic bleeding were probably the source of transmission. However, HIV has since been cultured from cervical and vaginal secretions and cervical biopsies taken throughout the menstrual cycle.[19] Therefore, HIV theoretically may be transmitted by infected women who are not bleeding. Nonetheless, the low rate of transmission from infected women to men[20, 21] implies a low rate of transmission between women.

Although the prevalence of HIV infection is low in lesbians without risk factors, physicians should counsel lesbians to avoid any contact with cervical and vaginal secretions, menstrual blood, and blood from vaginal and rectal trauma in partners who have not tested negative for the virus. Barriers believed to be effective for oral–genital contact include latex squares, known as dental dams, and latex condoms or gloves cut open and laid flat. For vaginal penetration latex gloves used on hands and condoms on sexual toys may be appropriate. The efficacy of these barrier methods has not been tested.

Besides sexual transmission, artificial insemination with either fresh semen from donors in the community or frozen semen from sperm banks[22, 23] may infect lesbians with HIV. Sperm banks routinely test donors for HIV infection at the time of donation and six months later before releasing the sample for use. Donors of fresh semen should be HIV-negative and free of HIV risk factors. However, because of delays in seroconversion,[24] it is possible for lesbians to be exposed to HIV with fresh semen from a seronegative donor. Lesbians should avoid fresh semen, especially fresh semen from donors with unknown HIV status.

In review, being a lesbian does not confer any additional risk of HIV infection. A decision to test lesbians for HIV infection should, therefore, be based on individual risk factors. Physicians should recommend safer sex practices with partners whose HIV status is unknown and screening of all sperm donors.

CANCER

There is no population-based study of cancer risk in lesbians. As a result, physicians should screen lesbians for cancer based on individual risk factors. Until research on cancer risk in women without a history of heterosexual contact exists, standard screening guidelines for women should apply.

Cervical cancer appears less common among lesbians than among heterosexual women. Risk factors for cervical cancer include early age of first coitus with a man, infection with HPV, and possibly infection with herpes simplex II virus.[25-28] Many lesbians have had heterosexual contact. Human papillomavirus and herpes virus can be transmitted by genital–genital and oral–genital routes. Therefore, lesbians theoretically are at risk for cervical cancer, but it is probably rare in lesbians with no heterosexual contact.

Current American Cancer Society (ACS) recommendations and other preventive health guidelines[29] give no information for cervical cancer screening in women who are celibate or who are sexually active with women only. One study found that abnormal Pap smears were present for less than 3% of the lesbians tested,[10] as compared with 12% for a planned parenthood population.[30] A survey study reported history of abnormal Pap smears for 12% and 16% of lesbians and bisexual women, respectively.[1] In each study, abnormal tests were associated with a higher number of heterosexual contacts. In the absence of data defining the appropriate Pap smear frequency in women who are sexually active exclusively with women, we recommend screening these women every three years, similar to the ACS maintenance screening interval.[29] Women with a history of significant heterosexual contact or another known risk factor should be screened according to guidelines.

There is similarly no specific information about breast cancer, endometrial cancer, or ovarian cancer in lesbians. Epidemiological studies suggest an increased risk of breast cancer among nulliparous women, women who are older when they give birth for the first time, and women who have never breast fed.[31, 32] Many lesbians fall into these categories and their physicians should adhere to current guidelines for breast examination and mammography.

Ovarian cancer has been reported to occur more frequently in women who have not used oral contraception and those who have not given birth.[33, 34] Endometrial cancer is also more common in nulliparous women. This may, however, be due to its apparent association with infertility and with polycystic ovary disease.[35] Some lesbians may be at a slightly higher risk for ovarian and endometrial cancers. Therefore, physicians should follow current guidelines on screening for these cancers where available.[29]

PARENTING AND REPRODUCTIVE ISSUES

Parenting plays a role in the lives of many lesbians, and the decision to parent is usually a deliberate and carefully weighed one. Lesbians may have children from previous heterosexual relationships,[36] adoption, artificial insemination, heterosexual intercourse, or being foster parents.[37, 38] Some members of society oppose motherhood for lesbians due to concerns about the sexual development and sexual orientation of the children.[38–41] Studies have not demonstrated differences between children raised by lesbians and those raised by heterosexuals.[41–45] Open communication with children about parents' lesbianism appears important in family function.[43]

Most lesbians find artificial insemination, also called alternative insemination or alternative fertilization, the preferred method of conception.[37] Legal statutes regarding artificial insemination vary from state to state, but most refer only to married women and assume a physician will do the procedure. The law is unclear regarding a physician's responsibility and liability toward a lesbian who has been inseminated. Some physicians feel uncomfortable performing artificial insemination for lesbians. We and others believe it is ethically justifiable but not obligatory for physicians to inseminate lesbians.[39–41, 46, 47] A physician who feels unable to comply with a patient's wishes should refer the patient to another provider for the service.

A pregnant lesbian may find it more difficult than other women to gather support for her pregnancy. The development of her identity as a mother may also be more complex.[38] Primary care physicians can support the pregnant lesbian by demonstrating nonjudgmental attitudes and encouraging acceptance of lesbian motherhood among members of the obstetric team and childbearing classes.[38, 48] Physicians should encourage patients' partners to participate in fertility assessment, semen selection and insemination, prenatal care, and delivery.[38] Partners may need emotional support after delivery as well.

PSYCHOSOCIAL AND PSYCHOLOGICAL ISSUES

The American Psychiatric Association removed homosexuality from its list of mental illnesses in 1973.[49] Overall, psychological illness is no more common in lesbians than in heterosexual women,[50, 51] but lesbians have unique psychosocial issues and often limited social support to help them cope. The issues most relevant for primary care physicians include homophobia, "coming out," adolescence, alcohol abuse, suicide, lesbian battery, and hate crimes.

Stress experienced by lesbians may be a result of a conflict between who they really are and the identity they express to the outside world.[49] Although lesbians' self-esteem is similar to that of heterosexual women,[52] lesbians often find it difficult to act in accordance with their identity because of society's negative attitudes, known as homophobia.[53] Societal attitudes may be combined with the lesbian's own internal homophobia developed from years of living in an intolerant society, thus compounding the stress.

Lesbians may not have the same degree of social support as their heterosexual counterparts have from family, coworkers, or religious organizations. Lesbians derive support most often from partners, friends, and lesbian and gay community organizations.[49, 54, 55] The quality of the relationship with a partner can be particularly important to a lesbian's psychological well-being.[56] Discord in a lesbian couple can be even more stressful than it is for a married heterosexual couple because of a lack of social support. Evaluation of a lesbian patient's support network is necessary to determine the patient's ability to cope with stressful life events.[57]

A second psychosocial issue for lesbians is the process of discovering one's sexual orientation and revealing it to others. This process is known as "coming out" and may occur at any age. Stage theories for coming out have been well described.[58–61] One critical examination of six theories delineates four stages: 1) awareness of homosexual feelings; 2) testing and exploration; 3) identity acceptance; and 4) identity integration and self-disclosure.[62] The process involves a shift in core identity that can be associated with significant emotional distress,[63] especially if family and peers respond negatively. Prevailing social attitudes influence the experience of coming out.[62, 64] Internalized homophobia and societal homophobia cause the lesbian to perform a sophisticated and fatiguing "cost–benefit" analysis for each situation in which she considers coming out.[63] If the costs are high, she may ultimately become socially isolated or deny the identity.[48, 63] Lesbian adolescents are particularly vulnerable to the emotional distress of coming out and this distress often confounds their developmental tasks.[58] Parental acceptance during this process, especially maternal, may be the primary determinant of the development of healthy self-esteem in adolescent lesbians.[65, 66] Signs of sexual orientation confusion in adolescents may include depression, diminished school performance, alcohol and substance abuse, acting out, and suicidal ideation.[67] In fact, gay and lesbian youth are two to three times more likely to attempt suicide and may account for 30% of completed youth suicides.[68] It is important for the primary care provider to screen adolescents for these signs and to consider sexual orientation confusion in the differential diagnosis of depression and substance abuse.

Third, alcohol abuse may be more common in lesbians than in heterosexual women. Reports of alcohol abuse rates in lesbians range from 7% to 35%,[9, 69–72] up to three times higher than those for heterosexual women.[73] These figures may be artificially elevated because the lesbians surveyed may not be representative of the population and rates of alcohol abuse may have changed since these studies were conducted. Recently a national mail survey[49] from a lesbian population mailing list with 37,500 entries showed that 59% of the subjects had used alcohol to cope with stress and 42% had considered suicide. Some reports have suggested that lesbians are at significantly higher risk than heterosexual women for suicidal ideation and suicide attempts.[49, 74] Such studies should be repeated to confirm and update this information with regard to changes in prevailing societal attitudes toward lesbians. As part of a comprehensive clinical evaluation, primary care providers should screen all women, including their lesbian patients, for alcohol abuse and depression. Treatment for these conditions should be nonjudgmental of the lesbian identity and sensitive to the needs of lesbians.

Battery of lesbians by their female partners has been recognized. One study reports that 39 of 104 self-identified lesbians 22 to 52 years old have experienced battery by a partner.[75] Alcohol or drug use appears to have been involved in 64% of these incidents. In other reports, lesbians perceived that interpersonal power imbalances contributed to battery[76] and that women's shelters were not responsive to the needs of lesbians.[77] These studies are limited by sample size and selection and so may not be generalizable. However, physicians should be alert to the possibility of battery in evaluating all women, including lesbians.

A final area of concern, hate crimes, or bias crimes, are words or actions directed at an individual because of membership in a minority group.[78] According to a study for the U.S. Department of Justice, lesbians and gay men may be the most victimized group in the nation.[79] Many recent studies report that hate crimes against lesbians, including verbal abuse, threats of violence, property damage, physical violence, and murder,[80, 81] are increasing each year.[82, 83] Also, lesbians at universities report being victims of sexual assault twice as frequently as do heterosexual women.[84]

Perpetrators of hate crimes often include family members and community authorities. Twenty-five percent of lesbians in a Philadelphia study reported being the victim of a crime committed by a family member.[83] Also, many gay and lesbian adolescents may leave home because of abuse related to their sexual orientations. The primary care provider should be aware of the possibility that a patient has been a victim of violence, particularly when patients present with symptoms of depression or anxiety.

THE DOCTOR–PATIENT INTERACTION

Many lesbians are reluctant to share their sexual orientation with physicians for fear of negative judgments and homophobic responses.[14, 37, 85–94] Some lesbians do not share this information even when asked.[94] Bad experiences with health care professionals make lesbian patients more likely to terminate care and avoid routine screening.[87, 89] On the other hand, physicians may feel inexperienced in dealing with lesbian health issues or uncomfortable deciding what language to use to elicit information sensitively. Because of both patient and doctor discomfort, important information is often not shared.

An effective doctor–patient interaction has three functions: information gathering, rapport building, and patient education.[95] This framework also applies

to the interaction between a physician and a lesbian. The physician should ask questions of all women that will elicit the information needed to identify lesbian patients and provide appropriate medical care; develop a nonjudgmental attitude that conveys a sense of acceptance; and provide educational information, resources, and referrals sensitive to the needs of lesbians.

Gathering information from female patients about the lesbian lifestyle and sexual practices is the first stumbling block encountered by practitioners. The most commonly used patient interview questions often lead to inaccurate or incomplete information with regard to lesbians.[37] They set up barriers for the lesbian patient because they assume she is heterosexual: "What form of birth control do you use?", "Are you married?", and "When was the last time you had intercourse?" are examples of common barrier-forming questions. Examples of questions that facilitate communication include: "Have you ever had sex with men, women, or both?"; "Are you in an intimate relationship with a man or a woman?"; "Whom do you include in your immediate family?"; "Do you have a lover or life partner?"; "Do you need contraception?"; and "If you become ill, is there someone important to you whom I should involve in your care?".

Physicians should ask these questions of all women from adolescence through old age. Not uncommonly physicians have the misperception that the sexual history is important only for patients in their middle years. It is important to recognize elderly lesbians because of their risk of social isolation. Physicians may be a significant source of support to these patients.[52, 96–101]

Once a physician has provided a nonjudgmental approach and asked questions sensitively, a trusting relationship is more likely to develop. Sensitivity to important concerns of the lesbian patient improves rapport.[14, 37, 49, 57, 67, 86, 92, 102] For example, offering to include a partner in the discussion and ensuring that the partner be able to enter the delivery room or intensive care unit demonstrate acceptance. The physician also builds rapport by discussing the stress of homophobia and exploring perceptions of the health care system.

Physicians may also show acceptance by ensuring that office and hospital forms include options such as "living with a partner" or "living as a couple," in addition to standard choices. These forms also should refer to a "spouse" or "partner." Physicians can ensure that all next-of-kin policies and discussions of advance directives include the possibility of a lesbian partner. Brochures on lesbian health issues displayed in waiting areas also demonstrate acceptance and understanding.

Providing education for lesbian patients involves physician self-education and compilation of reference materials and brochures on medical topics of interest to lesbians, such as safer sex for lesbians, STDs in lesbians, and parenting issues for lesbians. Instruction in preventing the transmission of STDs, including HIV infection, should be clear and specific to lesbian sexual practices. Physicians should be able to educate lesbians about risk for cervical cancer based on sexual history. They should also be able to counsel patients or refer patients for counseling about such issues as parenting, coming out, battery, and hate crimes.

Referrals should include other providers and community-based resources sensitive to the needs of lesbians.[5, 57, 90, 92, 103] Hotlines, bookstores, and bibliographies can help educate. Youth groups and senior groups, community centers, lesbian and gay religious organizations and retirement centers, and counselors who deal with lesbian issues provide support. Gay and lesbian 12-step programs and substance abuse support groups are also available.

Finally, it is important for physicians to discuss explicitly with lesbians the documentation of sexual orientation in the chart. The issue of confidentiality is complex and beyond the scope of this article. However, we suggest that when a patient does not want her lesbian identity documented, the physician may consider using a coded entry in the chart. This provides the physician with a record to remind him or her about the patient's sexual orientation but prevents inadvertent breaches of confidentiality through use of the chart.

CONCLUSION

Many primary care providers are presently caring for lesbian patients without recognizing their sexual orientation or their unique medical and psychological needs. Enhanced knowledge and skills will allow these physicians to provide optimal and sensitive patient care for lesbians. Clearly, much more research on this group is needed to provide appropriate guidelines for clinicians.

REFERENCES

1. Johnson SR, Smith SM, Guenther SM. Comparison of gynecological health care problems between lesbians and bisexual women. *J Reprod Med.* 1987;32(11);805–11.
2. Council on Scientific Affairs. Health care needs of a homosexual population. JAMA. 1982;248:736–9.
3. Good RS. The gynecologist and the lesbian. Clin Obstet Gynecol. 1976;19(2):473–82.
4. Kinsey AC, Pomeroy W, Martin CE, Gebhard PE. Sexual behavior in the human female. New York: W. B. Saunders, 1953.
5. Lockard D. The lesbian community: an anthropological approach. J Homosex. 1986;11(3-4):83–95.
6. Blumstein PW, Schwartz P. Lesbianism and bisexuality. In: Goode E, Troiden RR (eds). Sexual deviance and sexual deviants. New York: William Morrow, 1974;278–95.
7. Ponse B. Identities in the lesbian world: the social construction of self. Westport, CT: Greenwood Press, 1978.
8. Ryan C., Bradford J. The National Lesbian Health Care Survey: an overview. In: Shernoff M, Scott WA, (eds). The sourcebook of lesbian/gay health care, 2nd ed. Washington, DC: National Lesbian/Gay Health Foundation, 1988;30–40.
9. Degan K, Waitkevicz HJ. Lesbian health issues. Br J Sex Med. 1982;May:40–7.
10. Robertson P, Schacter J. Failure to identify venereal disease in a lesbian population. Sex Transm Dis. 1981; 8(2):75–6.
11. Ernst RS, Houts PS. Characteristics of gay persons with sexually transmitted disease. Sex Transm Dis. 1985; 12(2):59–63.
12. Walters MH, Rector WG. Sexual transmission of hepatitis A in lesbians [letter]. JAMA. 1986;256:594.
13. William DC. Hepatitis and other sexually transmitted diseases in gay men and lesbians. Sex Transm Dis. 1981;8(4):330–2.
14. Johnson SR, Palermo JL. Gynecologic care for the lesbian. Clin Obstet Gynecol. 1984;27(3):724–30.
15. Sivakumar K, De Silva AH, Basu RR. *Trichomonas vaginalis* infection in a lesbian. Genitourin Med. 1989;65: 399–400.
16. Chu SY, Buehler JW, Fleming PL, Berkleman RL. Epidemiology of reported cases of AIDS in lesbians, United States 1980–89. Am J Public Health. 1990;80(11): 1380–1.
17. Sabatini MT, Patel K, Hirschman R. Kaposi's sarcoma and T-cell lymphoma in an immunodeficient woman: a case report. AIDS Res. 1984;1(2):135–7.
18. Marmor M, Weiss LR, Lyden M, et al. Possible female-to-female transmission of human immunodeficiency virus [letter]. Ann Intern Med. 1986;105–969.
19. Poole L. HIV infection in women. In: Cohen PT, sande MA, Volberding PA (eds). The AIDS knowledge base. Waltham, MA: The Medical Publishing Group, 1990; 4.2.9:1–10.
20. Redfield RR, Markham PD, Salahuddin SZ, et al. Heterosexuality acquired HTLV-III/LAV disease (AIDS-related complex and AIDS): epidemiologic evidence for female-to-male transmission. JAMA. 1985;254:2094–6.
21. Schultz S, Milberg JA, Kristal AR, Stoneburner RI. Female-to-male transmission of HTLV-III [letter]. JAMA. 1986;255:1703–4.
22. Chiasson MA, Stoneburner RL, Joseph. SC. Human immunodeficiency virus transmission through artificial insemination. J Acquir Immune Defic Syndr. 1990;3: 69–72.
23. Eskenazi B, Pies C, Newsletter A, Shepard C, Pearson K. HIV serology in artificially inseminated lesbians. J Acquir Immune Defic Syndr. 1989;2:187–93.
24. Imagawa DT, Lee MH, Wolinsky SM, et al. Human immunodeficiency virus type 1 infection in homosexual men who remain seronegative for prolonged periods of time. N Engl J Med. 1089;320:1458–62.
25. Campion MJ. Clinical manifestations and natural history of genital human papillomavirus infection. Obstet Gynecol Clin North Am. 1987;14(2):363–88.
26. Mitchell H, Drake M, Medley G. Prospective evaluation of risk of cervical cancer after cytological evidence of human papillomavirus infection. Lancet. 1986;i:573–5.

27. Reid R, Stanhope CR, Herschman BR, Booth E, Phibbs GD, Smith JP. Genital warts and cervical cancer: I. Evidence of an association between subclinical papillomavirus infection and cervical malignancy. Cancer. 1982; 50:377–87.

28. Reid R, Crum Cp, Herschman BR, et al. Genital warts and cervical cancer: III. Subclinical papillomavial infection and cervical neoplasia are linked by a spectrum of continuous morphologic and biologic change. Cancer. 1984;53:943–53.

29. Hayward RSA, Steinberg EP, Ford DE, Roizen MF, Roach KW. Preventive care guidelines: 1991. Ann Int Med. 1991;114:758–83.

30. Sadeghi SB, Sadeghi A, Cosby M, Olincy A, Robboy SJ. Human papillomavirus infection: frequency and association with cervical neoplasia in a young population. Acta Cytol. 1989;33(3):319–23.

31. Kelsey JL. A review of the epidemiology of human breast cancer. Epidemiol Rev. 1979;1:74–109.

32. Byers T, Graham S, Rzepka T, Marshall J. Lactation and breast cancer. Evidence for a negative association in premenopausal women. Am J Epidemiol. 1985;121(5): 664–74.

33. The Cancer and Steroid Hormone Study of the Centers for Disease Control and the National Institute of Child Health and Human Development. The reduction in risk of ovarian cancer associated with oral-contraceptive use. N Engl J Med. 1987;316:650–5.

34. Cramer DW, Hutchison GB, Welch WR, et al. Determinants of ovarian cancer risk: I. Reproductive experiences and family history. J Natl Cancer Inst. 1983;71:711.

35. Jackson RL, Dorherty MB. The Stein-Leventhal syndrome: analysis of 43 cases with special reference to association with endometrial cancer. Am J Obstet Gynecol. 1957;73:161.

36. Kirkpatrick M. Clinical implications of lesbian mother studies. J Homosex. 1987;14(1–2):201–11.

37. Zeidenstein L. Gynecological and childbearing needs of lesbians. J Nurse Midwifery. 1990;35(1):10–8.

38. Wismount JM, Reame NE. The lesbian childbearing experience: assessing development tasks. Image: J Nurs Schol. 1989;21(3):137–41.

39. DiLapi EM. Lesbian mothers and the motherhood hierarchy. J Homosex. 1989;18(1–2):101–21.

40. Freedman B, Taylor PJ, Wonnacott T, Brown S. Nonmedical selection criteria for artificial insemination and adoption. Clin Reprod Fertil. 1987;5:55–66.

41. Strong C, Schinfeld JS. The single woman and artificial insemination by donor. J Reprod Med. 1984;29(5): 293–9.

42. Green R. The best interests of the child with a lesbian mother. Bull Am Acad Psychiatry Law. 1982:10(1):7–15.

43. Brewaeys A, Olbrechts H, Devroey P, Van Steirteghem AC. Counselling and selection of homosexual couples in fertility treatment. Hum Reprod. 1989;4(7):850–3.

44. Hanscombe G. The right to lesbian parenthood. J Med Ethics. 1983;9:133–5.

45. Golombok S, Rust J. The Warnock Report and single women: what about the children? J Med Ethics. 1986; 12:182–6.

46. Kottow M. The right to lesbian parenthood [letter]. J Med Ethics. 1984;1:54.

47. Fletcher JC, Magnuson WG. Artificial insemination in lesbians, ethical considerations. Arch Intern Med. 1985; 145:419–20.

48. Stevens PE, Hall JM. Stigma, health beliefs and experiences with health care in lesbian women. Image: J Nurs Schol. 1988;20(2):69–73.

49. Gillow KE, Davis LL. Lesbian stress and coping methods. J Psychosoc Nurs. 1987;25(9):28–32.

50. Weinberg MS, Williams CJ. Male homosexuals; their problems and adaptations. New York: Penguin Books, 1974;198–203.

51. Freedman M. Homosexuality and psychological functioning. Pacific Grove, CA: Brooks-Cole (Division of Wadsworth), 1971;88–90.

52. Christie D, Young M. Self-concept of lesbian and heterosexual women. Psychol Rep. 1986;59:1279–82.

53. Herek GM. Beyond "homophobia": a social psycological perspective on attitudes toward lesbians and gay men. J Homosex. 1984;10(1–2):1–21.

54. Kurdek LA. Perceived social support in gays and lesbians in cohabiting relationships. J Pers Soc Psychol. 1988; 54(3):504–9.

55. Albro JC, Tully C. A study of lesbian lifestyles in the homosexual micro-culture and the heterosexual macroculture. J Homosex. 1979;4(4):331–44.

56. Kurdek LA, Schmitt JP. Perceived emotional support from family and friends in members of homosexual, married, and heterosexual cohabiting couples. J Homsex. 1987;14(3–4):57–68.

57. Whyte J, Capaldini L. Treating the lesbian or gay patient. Dei Med J. 1980;52(5):271–80.

58. Schneider M. Sappho was a right-on adolescent: growing up lesbian. J Homosex. 1989;17(1–2):111–30.

59. Raphael SM. "Coming out": the emergence of the movement lesbian. Dissertation Abstracts International, 1974;35:5536A. (University Microfilms No. 75–5084).

60. Minton HC, McDonald GJ. Homosexual identity formation as a developmental process. J Homosex. 1984; 9(2–3):91–104.

61. Spaulding EC. The formation of lesbian identity during the "coming out" process. Dissertation Abstracts International, 1982;43:2106A. (University Microfilms No. 82–26834).

62. Sophie J. A critical examination of stage theories of lesbian identity development. J Homosex. 1986;12(2): 39–51.

63. Gonsiorek JC. Mental health issues of gay and lesbian adolescents. J Adol Health Care. 1988;9:114–22.

64. Faderman L. The "new gay" lesbians. J Homosex. 1985; 10(3–4):85–95.

65. Savin-Williams RC. Coming out to parents and self-esteem among gay and lesbian youths. J Homosex. 1989;18(1–2):1–35.

66. Savin-Williams RC. Parental influences on the self-esteem of gay and lesbian youths: a reflected appraisals model. J Homosex. 1989;18(1–2):93–109.

67. Anstett R, Kiernan M, Brown R. The gay–lesbian patient and the family physician. J Fam Pract. 1987;25(4): 339–44.

68. Feinleib MR. Report of the Secretary's Task Force on Youth

A Reading for Critical Thinking

Is managed care good for women's health?

By Leslie Laurence

In June 1991, two months after her fourth son was born, Donna Encheff started feeling depressed. She was tired from the birth, but after three previous deliveries, she knew these weren't normal blues. Encheff, then 33, visited the Bakersfield, California, family physician she'd been seeing for several years, who diagnosed her with postpartum depression and prescribed the antidepressant Prozac.

Despite the medication, Encheff's depression persisted, and soon she developed a potpourri of new symptoms, including chronic headaches on the right side of her head. Her doctor, a member of a managed care plan that is part of Clinicians Health Network, finally referred her to a psychiatrist, Darell Shaffer, M.D., who was new to the network's roster. Dr. Shaffer knew that neurological problems could trigger symptoms like Encheff's, so he requested a magnetic resonance imaging (MRI) scan of her brain to rule out a brain tumor. Clinicians denied his request for the $1,000-plus test because, they said, her condition had already been documented as psychological. "It was one of those managed care shocks," says Dr. Shaffer.

As the months passed and Encheff's condition worsened, her husband, Dana, began an exhausting

Affordable, quality care and an emphasis on prevention — that's the promise. The reality: Hassles getting to the gynecologist, new barriers against abortion and a slowdown in research crucial to women.

battle to get Donna the care he was sure she needed. After an appeal and a four-month wait, Encheff finally got her MRI, which revealed a lesion in her brain. When a specialist on Clinician's list dismissed the lesion as nothing out of the ordinary, Dana questioned the diagnosis and filed a request to see a specialist outside the network. The request was denied. In November 1993 Encheff was briefly admitted to a psychiatric hospital after she started hallucinating and hearing voices. When the plan refused to cover the hospital stay, Dana fought them on that too.

In the summer of 1994, Dana finally drove his wife to Los Angeles for a consultation with Keith Black, M.D., a renowned neurosurgeon at the University of California at Los Angeles School of Medicine. Dr. Black suspected that the lesion Encheff's doctors had written off was in fact a precancerous tumor. After a second MRI, which the Encheffs paid for themselves, he strongly recommended surgery.

A week later, after a call from Encheffs' lawyer, the health plan agreed to let Dr. Black perform the operation. When he did, he found a venous angioma, a mass of twisted blood vessels that had been pressing on Donna's right temporal lobe. Once it was removed,

From *Glamour* (August 1996), pp. 202-205, 237-240. Reprinted by permission of Leslie Laurence, co-author, with Beth Weinhouse, of *Outrageous Practices: How Gender Bias Threaten's Women's Health*, (Rutgers University Press, 1997). She also writes a nationally syndicated women's health column for Universal Press Syndicate.

Donna's psychotic and depressive symptoms immediately disappeared. Had the angioma ruptured, Donna could have died or suffered paralyzing brain damage.

Donna's psychiatrist, who describes her as "the sanest sick person I've ever met," says he wishes he had fought harder for his patient. "I probably should have contacted the HMO myself," Dr. Shaffer told the Encheff's lawyer. "But I really didn't want to jeopardize my relationship with them because I'm dependent on them for referrals."

"I put too much trust in the doctors," Donna Encheff says of her three-year ordeal. "If it hadn't been for my husband, I'd probably be dead."

Jeanne Manning, of Summit, New Jersey, has a different story to tell about managed care. The 32-year-old was pregnant with triplets, the result of in vitro fertilization. Although she had an obstetrician-gynecologist through Oxford Health Plans, she wanted to be cared for by a doctor who specialized in high-risk pregnancies. After some finagling — her ob-gyn wasn't allowed to refer her to another specialist, so she had to find and sign up with a primary care doctor who could — she had her first visit with an Oxford perinatologist in October 1995.

At about the same time, Manning received a call from Dodi Girard, a high risk maternity nurse employed by Oxford. Girard told Manning that she would be her case manager, available 24 hours a day to answer her questions. Girard would also be Manning's go-between with Oxford, advocating for coverage of whatever her doctor said was necessary.

"Jeanne was in high danger of delivering prematurely," says Girard. "We wanted her to have all the services she needed to have a healthy pregnancy."

Although the two never met, Manning spoke to Girard on the phone every two to three weeks for the rest of her pregnancy. Says Manning, "I didn't have to keep explaining my story over and over again to different people. I could throw questions at her. It gave me great peace of mind."

Manning visited her perinatologist at least every three weeks and had ultrasounds every other visit. In December, 20 weeks into her pregnancy, Manning's doctor wanted her to go on bed rest. Girard arranged for a nurse to set up a home uterine monitor for Manning.

In her twenty-fourth week of pregnancy, Manning started to dilate and had to be hospitalized for 12 days. Before she was discharged, a nurse taught her how to inject herself with a drug to prevent contractions. Manning was briefly hospitalized twice during her eighth month, but she made it to term: On the afternoon of April 14, 1996, Manning's three healthy babies were delivered via C-section. First came Kaitlyn, at six pounds, three ounces; followed by Patrick, five pounds, 11 ounces; and Mary, five pounds, three ounces. Four days later, the babies accompanied their mother home — a rarity for multiple births.

HMOs offer generous coverage for contraception . . . but fewer than half cover all five major methods.

Over the nine months Manning received about $50,000 worth of care but paid only $10 per doctor visit. The savings to Oxford were even greater. Had the triplets been born prematurely and needed a lengthy stay in the intensive care unit, the cost easily could have exceeded $1 million.

"Oxford did a good job," says Manning. "And I loved the fact that I was assigned a caseworker who knew what I was going through."

Donna Encheff and Jeanne Manning represent the two faces of managed care: in Encheff's case, a corporate entity seemingly more interested in containing costs than in protecting the patient; in Manning's, a system apparently dedicated to giving members the care they need to prevent more serious illnesses down the road.

This Jekyll-and-Hyde split makes it all the more difficult to sort out the true effect of managed care on women's health. On one side are severely ill women who complain about having essential care delayed or denied — a trend beginning to be documented by research studies, not just scary anecdotes. On the other side are stories of women receiving generous coverage for conditions neglected by traditional insurers — stories that are also bolstered by research.

86 percent of HMOs cover mammograms . . . but they routinely deny full coverage for breast reconstruction after a mastectomy.

In fact, for every study that suggests managed care doesn't hurt members' health, there's another study that says it does. Depending on which survey you choose to believe, people covered by the various forms of managed care are more — or less — satisfied with their medical treatments than people with traditional insurance. "We know a lot about how services worked under the old system," noted Commonwealth Fund president Karen Davis and research director Cathy Schoen in a recent paper. "We know very little about this new system."

But one thing is clear: Our doctors are operating under a whole new set of rules.

To stay in business, physicians are surrendering their ability to make their own decisions. While managed care promises that one physician will coordinate all our medical needs, in fact it's often a corporate executive — or even a clerk — who decides who gets which treatment, when and for how long. Doctors are being encouraged to provide services outside their areas of expertise — and many are bending to the pressure. And because managed care plans hold the purse strings, our physicians, who say they live by the rule "first, do no harm," cannot always afford to be our advocates.

In interviews with nearly 100 doctors, patients. industry analysts and managed care executives, *Glamour* has learned that the bedrock practices of managed care — the gatekeeper system that coordinates care through primary doctors, restrictions on visits to specialists and subspecialists and limits on hospital stays — are hitting women hardest.

This is largely because women *need* more health care than men. Women suffer from more cancers at younger ages than men do, so they need regular screening for breast, endometrial, ovarian and cervical cancers. Young women need maternity care, contraceptives and sometimes abortions. Women are twice as likely as men to be treated for depression and a have a much higher percentage of eating disorders. They get endometriosis and pelvic inflammatory disease. In all, women account for two thirds of doctor visits and more than half of the nation's spending on health care.

New computer rechecks of Pap smears will save lives — but so far not a single managed care plan has agreed to cover the improved tests' cost.

Because women make more demands on the system, they also stand to benefit most from managed care's lower costs and emphasis on prevention. In some areas, they already do benefit: Women in managed care get more generous coverage for contraceptives and prenatal care and are more likely to receive Pap smears, pelvic exams and mammograms than women with traditional insurance. Some HMOs are making sure that breast-cancer patients are offered breast-sparing lumpectomies and are not pushed into having inappropriate mastectomies. Many plans are working hard to reduce cesarean births and unnecessary hysterectomies.

But the promise of *quality* care for women is so far unfulfilled. Unnecessary surgeries are being reduced but so are necessary ones. The emphasis on prevention looks good on paper but is too often a "very inexpensive way to try to show that you provide quality when you don't," says Seth Spotnitz, M.D., a neurologist in Gadsden, Alabama, and president of

Physicians Who Care, a 3,500-member group that opposes managed care. The reality for most women in such plans today: narrowed choices and less say than ever in decisions about their health.

HOW GATEKEEPERS HURT WOMEN'S HEALTH

The guiding principle of managed care is to keep costs down by having generalists handle the basics, from routine gynecology and dermatology to some neurological problems. It's only fair to ask, then, How qualified are primary care doctors to provide the basics to women?

There's no doubt that for some conditions, primary care providers do a fine job. A recent study of patients with high blood pressure and non-insulin-dependent diabetes found no difference between those treated by primary care doctors and those treated by specialists, whether in an HMO or the traditional fee-for-service system. But good grades in two subjects don't add up to an A in women's health for primary care doctors.

In fact, while hard data is scarce, there are strong hints that in many other basics these doctors are flunking. A study at Chicago's Cook County Hospital found that more than 40 percent of internists and family practice residents would not think to counsel a healthy woman about family planning and German measles immunization (important for preventing birth defects). They were also remiss in talking about sexually transmitted diseases and safer sex. Other studies have found that although generalists are the biggest prescribers of antidepressants, they are less likely than psychiatrists to diagnose and correctly treat depression. A 1996 Institute of Medicine report concluded that primary care doctors lack the training they need to function the way managed care companies expect them to.

For instance, in most plans a primary care doctor is supposed to take care of unusual gynecological symptoms, such as vaginal bleeding, says Jane Orient, M.D., an internist and executive director of the Association of American Physicians and Surgeons. "If an older woman is having unusual bleeding, she needs to have a sample taken from the uterus to rule out endometrial cancer," she says. "General internists are simply not trained to do that; I'm an internist and I haven't got a clue how to do it. General internists aren't even that good at doing a pelvic examination."

It's in these obstacles to getting quality reproductive health care that women really feel the pinch of managed care. Women tend to think of ob-gyns as their primary doctors — after all, these are the physicians they need most often. Many managed care plans, however, look at obstetrics and gynecology as special services to be carefully parceled out. The resulting problems range from the petty hassles of getting referrals to new barriers to abortion.

Patricia Partridge's ordeal is a common experience for women in the new system. The 49-year-old Tampa, Florida, woman visited her ob-gyn for her annual checkup. A Pap smear showed an abnormality in her cervical cells. If she'd had traditional insurance, Partridge could have immediately gone back to the ob-gyn for a colposcopy (a look at the cervix under magnification) and biopsy of cervical tissue. But her Humana plan required her to call her primary care doctor first for an ob-gyn referral — in plain English, for permission to see her ob-gyn a second time. That took more than a week.

Now she needs to see the ob-gyn a third time to make sure the problem is gone — but it's been ten days and the second referral still hasn't come. "I don't know how many people I've talked to, telling them I really need that referral," says Partridge. "I'll probably end up going to my primary doctor's office to get it, but I ought to be able to do all this over the phone. It takes me an hour round-trip to get to my primary doctor, plus the hour I might have to spend there. Here I could be going straight to my ob-gyn and getting well."

Seventy-three percent of women oppose going through a gatekeeper to see their ob-gyns, according to a Gallup Poll conducted for the American College of Obstetricians and Gynecologists (ACOG). A few plans are getting the message: Harvard Pilgrim Health Care in Brookline, Massachusetts, allows a woman to visit her ob-gyn anytime for any reason; Kaiser Permanente often allows women to designate an ob-gyn as their primary care provider; U.S. Healthcare allows ob-gyns to treat certain problems that come up during an exam without a primary doctor's OK. But a 1994 survey of 236 HMOs found that half limited women to one ob-gyn visit without a referral per year. This is more than just a hassle: If a woman is less than aggressive about working the system, she could lose crucial weeks or months before a serious problem is properly diagnosed and treated.

Forcing women to get permission from gatekeepers for reproductive services has a particularly troublesome impact on abortion access. Take the case of Rhona Dennis. The 33-year-old child-care worker in Rhinebeck, New York, went to her health plan's clinic in January 1994 to find out what was causing her debilitating cramps. She was surprised to learn that she was six weeks pregnant — and that she had multiple fibroids, at least one of which was the size of a grapefruit. Told she was likely to miscarry or suffer a life-threatening hemorrhage if she attempted to carry the baby to term, she and her husband decided on an abortion.

Dennis wanted an ob-gyn to perform the abortion, but she was required to go to a primary care doctor for a referral to yet another clinic. When she did, the primary care doctor noticed the cross around Dennis' neck. "Are you religious?" he asked. "Not particularly," she replied. He went on to tell her that many women feel guilty after having an abortion. Then he sent Dennis to his nurse, who gave her antiabortion religious pamphlets and told Dennis to consider carrying the pregnancy to term and giving up the baby for adoption.

"She wanted to make me feel like a baby killer," says Dennis. "If I could have kept this child I would have, but it might have cost me my life." She demanded and got her referral — to a clinic an hour and a half away.

"Managed care is not making abortion access easy for women," says Shirley Gordon, a director at the Center for Reproductive Law and Policy, who found widespread problems with delayed referrals and biased counseling in a survey of women and family-planning providers in New York state. "Reproductive health services are so time sensitive. It's crucial that women have direct access to providers."

WHY OB-GYNS CAN'T FIX MANAGED CARE

Ease of access to ob-gyns is obviously crucial for women. But many ob-gyns go further, arguing that women's problems with managed care would largely be solved if gynecologists could become primary care providers. Can these doctors, who train as surgeons, truly function as generalists?

The 1993 Gallup Poll for ACOG found that ob-gyns are as likely as other primary doctors to provide blood pressure checks and counseling about smoking, alcohol and drug use. And while a study for the Council on Graduate Medical Education found ob-gyn training deficient in almost half of 60 essential primary care components, this is changing: As of January, all ob-gyn residents must now complete a four-month rotation in internal medicine and one month each in emergency and geriatric medicine.

Women in managed care start prenatal care early . . . but they're usually required to leave the hospital a day after giving birth.

Some ob-gyns, however, question whether this approach is really in the best interest of patients. "Where does the time spent training in primary care come from? Gynecologic specialty training," says Jan Seski, M.D., a gynecologic oncologist at Allegheny General Hospital in Pittsburgh. "You can't eat your cake and have it too."

There's another reason that advocating for ob-gyn gatekeepers may be wrong-headed. Managed care is fast becoming a system that pits doctor against doctor; anyone placed in the role of gatekeeper will feel pressure to overstep the bounds of his or her competence.

Here's how that pressure works: An increasing number of plans pay doctors a fixed monthly "capitation" fee for each patient. (About 70 percent of HMOs pay some of their doctors this way.) To discourage pricey procedures and referrals to specialists, plans also withhold 10 to 30 percent of a doctor's total capitation until the end of the year. Each referral costs the gatekeeper a percentage of the money withheld. Doctors who rarely refer will get most of their withheld money. Those who frequently refer may not only get nothing back but also face being fired from the plan, thereby losing dozens or hundreds of patients.

So just as generalists have strong financial incentives to limit referrals to ob-gyns — even if that requires them to perform procedures they weren't trained for — ob-gyn gatekeepers may be loath to send women to subspecialists if the referral is going to cost them. In particular, ob-gyns may be slow to refer women to infertility experts, perinatologists and oncologists who specialize in reproductive cancers.

"There's a tremendous competition among physicians to maintain their level of income," says Dr. Seski. A recent survey by the American Medical Association found that ob-gyns' income dropped 9 percent in 1994, to a median of $182,000. Some ob-gyns say managed care has forced them to take 30 percent pay cuts. There's no reason for women to feel sorry for doctors who pull down this kind of money. But the squeeze on ob-gyns' pocketbooks may be affecting women's care.

Managed care companies are refusing to pay for research . . . and often won't let their members participate in studies.

Take infertility: Richard Buyalos, M.D., assistant professor in reproductive endocrinology and infertility at the UCLA School of Medicine, says he's seeing more gynecologists treating patients with fertility problems, rather than referring them to specialists. Crunched for time and with no experience in fertility treatments, gynecologists, he says, are more apt to do incomplete workups — for instance, failing to check sperm for problems or fallopian tubes for blockage.

Specialists say ob-gyns also tend to continue too long with treatments that aren't working, for example, keeping women on the ovary-stimulating drug Clomid or doing intrauterine inseminations for 12 or more months (instead of the recommended three to four months). "I see patients in their late thirties and early forties who have been mismanaged for a year," says Dr. Buyalos. "By the time they come to see me, they've exhausted whatever potential to conceive that they had."

Delaying infertility treatment isn't going to shorten a woman's life expectancy, but delaying an ovarian cancer diagnosis might. There is little hard data, but at conferences and seminars, oncologists are trading horror stories about a trend: "I'm seeing more women coming in with masses in their ovaries — advanced stage disease — who had first been operated on by ob-gyn doctors," says Michael Berman, M.D., a gynecologic oncologist and professor at the University of California-Irvine Medical Center. Gynecologic oncologist Beth Y. Karlan, M.D., an associate professor at the UCLA School of Medicine, says ob-gyns too often fail to remove the entire tumor. She calls these inappropriate surgeries "peek and shriek" operations.

Despite gynecologic oncologists' intensive training in the biology and surgical removal of reproductive cancers, managed care plans don't always recognize these specialists, hindering doctors' ability to make proper referrals. "I'm listed in many of these HMO books as an ob-gyn," says Dr. Seski. "They don't even have a category for gynecologic oncology."

MANAGED CARE IS AN OBSTACLE TO HEALTH RESEARCH

Experts agree that if you're seriously ill, your best option may be to enroll in a clinical trial, where promising cutting edge treatments are compared to the current state of the art. Research does more than help individual patients. Current clinical trials, such as the Women's Health Initiative, will provide crucial information about long-neglected women's health issues, such as how hormone replacement therapy and low-fat diets affect breast and colon cancer, osteoporosis and heart disease risk.

But except for a few large plans — including Kaiser Permanente, some of whose patients are enrolled in the Women's Health Initiative — managed care companies have not been willing to either invest in research *or* allow their members to participate. David Alberts, M.D., deputy director of the Arizona Cancer Center at the University of Arizona in Tucson, recently saw three women who wanted to enroll in a trial of a new ovarian cancer drug. "The diagnostic tests, blood work, X rays, CAT scans and my own time were free," he says. "But all the managed care companies said no." The reason? According to Dr. Alberts, "The women might experience a side effect that would require hospitalization, and the companies would not take responsibility for such a charge."

This wasn't his first rebuff. Two years ago Dr. Alberts conducted a small study showing that retinoic acid (the active ingredient in the acne medicine Retin-A) could increase the cure rate of moderate cervical dysplasia, a precancerous condition, by 50 percent. Because of resistance from managed care plans in the area, however, Dr. Alberts has not been able to enroll enough women to conduct a follow-up study — even though the treatment could help women avoid surgery and ultimately save the plans money. "The word *research* is anathema to managed care," he laments. In fact, at the nation's top cancer centers, clinical trial enrollment is down 10 to 15 percent.

Cost cutting could put the squeeze on new cancer-screening tests, too. Last year, two rescreening systems designed to make Pap smears more accurate were approved by the FDA for use by labs. One of them, Papnet, displays suspicious cells on a high-resolution monitor, making abnormalities easier to catch. The other, AutoPap, rescreens all normal slides and identifies the least normal 10 percent for reexamining, thus significantly decreasing the number of slides mistakenly read as negative.

The AutoPap recheck costs labs an extra $5 to $7 per slide to perform, however, and Papnet costs an additional $18 per slide. At press time, both tests were being used in a few labs — but not a single HMO had made a decision to cover the extra cost.

REDEFINING MEDICAL NECESSITY: THE PLUSES AND MINUSES

In the old days, doctors decided what treatments were medically necessary for their patients. Now, managed care executives — who sometimes get bonuses for denying coverage — decide whether an expensive procedure is called for.

There's a plus side to this for women: By establishing criteria for surgical procedures and refusing to authorize unnecessary or inappropriate operations, managed care is protecting women from overtreatment. Most HMOs use "utilization review" to deny hysterectomies for benign conditions, for instance. One study suggests that managed care plans are already under the national average of six hysterectomies per 1,000 women ages 15 to 44. U.S. Healthcare,

among other plans, has tackled the boom in cesarean births by paying doctors more when a patient who's had a previous C-section gives birth vaginally.

But as with most things in managed care, there's another side to the story. Barbara Del Carlo, a case manager who has worked with a variety of managed care plans nationwide, says she too often finds herself defending requests for care to clerks who base decisions on a rigid recipe of symptoms. "I believe in clinical guidelines," Del Carlo says. "When someone requests a home uterine monitor, for instance, it's fair to ask, 'Has she had preterm labor before? Is she having contractions?' "But, she asks, what about the woman who answers no to these questions, but who is experiencing spotting or is pregnant with triplets? "You need someone handling the calls who can say, 'Maybe it doesn't fit into the recipe I see in the book, but she needs to be on a monitor,'" says Del Carlo. "What frightens me is there aren't enough people thinking these things through."

Managed care companies keep a tight rein on expensive treatments by defining medical necessity to their own advantage. Linda Peeno, M.D., a medical ethicist in Louisville, Kentucky, who worked as a medical director at a number of managed care plans, says, "We'd never tell patients the criteria for medical necessity. Unless it was almost an emergency, we went through a phase of saying we did not cover it."

Many expensive treatments are excluded because they are dubbed "experimental." This has been a particular problem with autologous bone marrow transplants for advanced breast and ovarian cancers, for which few treatments exist. Another tactic is to define surgeries as primarily cosmetic, a ploy that hits women especially hard. Among the operations some companies refuse to authorize: varicose vein removal after pregnancy, breast reduction surgery for pain, and reconstructive surgery after mastectomy.

A survey of 1,558 plastic surgeons conducted by the American Society of Plastic and Reconstructive Surgeons found that almost 30 percent had had patients denied coverage for breast reconstruction after mastectomy. Christine Horner-Taylor, M.D., a plastic and reconstructive surgeon in the Midwest, finds it especially galling that the same HMOs that deny breast reconstruction will cover penile implant surgery. One Ohio HMO, she says, paid 100 percent of the costs of any reconstructive surgery *except* when it had to do with a woman's breasts, for which it paid only 80 percent.

"This is outrageously sexist," says Dr. Horner-Taylor, who has helped draft legislation — so far passed in 12 states — requiring insurers to cover the full cost of reconstructions after mastectomy.

The charge of sexism rings true for at least some insiders. Dr. Peeno says that at the companies she worked for, "There was a real sense of prejudice against women. In meetings the attitude was that many complaints affecting women were psychological, that if we could get a handle on the hysterical components of women's needs, we wouldn't have to pay."

And though the goal of limiting overused surgeries like hysterectomies is a worthy one, the feminist rhetoric used by savvy companies rings hollow when a woman and her doctor decide hysterectomy is the best treatment and the HMO says no. Gordon M. Goldman, M.D., a St. Louis ob-gyn, says that a woman with fibroids may have heavy, flooding, week-long periods that cause her to miss a week of work each month. "A hysterectomy will take care of it," he says. "But many managed care plans say. 'Give her pain medication.'"

"A patient in one of the managed care groups I work with, in order to have a hysterectomy for pain, has to have a gastrointestinal workup, a urologic workup and a psychological evaluation," says John C. Nelson, M.D., a Salt Lake City ob-gyn and deputy director of the Utah Department of Health. "I think all that is a barrier between the patient and her physician, and I think it's sexist. You don't make a man have a psychological evaluation when he wants a vasectomy."

Managed care's cost cutting extends to pressuring doctors to reduce the time their patients spend in the hospital when they do have surgery. This has particular relevance to women: 25.5 million women had surgery in 1993, compared with 16.1 million men.

One important example is childbirth: These days, many women covered by managed care plans can't remain in the hospital more than one day after a normal delivery and two days after a cesarean section, down from a norm of 3.9 and 7.8 days respectively in 1970. Says Michael Mennuti, M.D., former chair of ACOG's obstetrics practices committee, "We're hustling mothers out of the hospital with a set of instructions."

"Drive-through deliveries" appear to be resulting in an increase in the number of infants being sent home with undetected jaundice and dehydration, requiring a subsequent hospitalization. In some cases, dehydrated or jaundiced infants sent home by managed care doctors have suffered brain damage and death. While many plans send nurses to check on newly discharged mothers and their babies — an approach that can make quick discharges work well — ACOG says that the quality of home care varies widely around the country, making early discharge equivalent to "a large, uncontrolled, uninformed experiment."

Managed care companies contend that they don't tell doctors when to discharge women. Insiders tell a different story. "We would do reviews of every patient who was in the hospital," says Dr. Peeno of her work as a managed care medical director. "Our job was to call and talk directly to the physicians because they would have to interrupt patient care and that hassles them the most. If you created enough difficulty you could get the physician to the point where he wouldn't even ask for an authorization [to hospitalize a patient longer]."

Doctors who advocate too hard for their patients face "deselection," a fancy way of saying they're being fired. Holly Roberts, D.O., a Red Bank, New Jersey, ob-gyn, often let exhausted maternity patients stay in the hospital longer than 24 hours. Then a representative from the plan that about 20 percent of her patients were enrolled in came calling, armed with graphs plotting her patients' hospital stays against those of other physicians in the plan. "I was above the median," she says. "He said that the only thing keeping me in the system was that I had a low C-section rate. The message was clear: If I didn't get my patients out sooner, I'd be taken out of the HMO. I realized it was my neck or my patients'." She started discharging all new mothers without medical complications earlier.

WHY MANAGED CARE ISN'T COORDINATED

Managed care has long claimed that its real forte is in the streamlined coordination of care by one team leader: the primary care doctor. These doctors are charged with getting to know their patients well and with monitoring the quality of every service the patient receives. It's a determinedly old-time image of the doctor-patient relationship, à la Marcus Welby — and in a system where doctors are denied control over some of the most basic elements of patient care, this image is a fantasy.

Take lab tests: Physicians once sent Pap smears and other tests to one or two labs whose pathologists they knew. Now many deal with ten or 20 different labs nationwide that have cut deals with managed care companies. "A lab may do a phenomenal job with Pap smears, but I don't know that," says Carolyn Runowicz, M.D., professor of ob-gyn at Albert Einstein College of Medicine-Montefiore Medical Center in New York City. "And I don't have time to call and ask, 'Who's reading my Paps today and what kind of experience do they have?'"

Few patients know that plans reap big profits by forcing doctors to prescribe from lists of preferred drugs. While doctors can ask to get drugs not on the list, most say it's too much trouble. What that means: Patients may not get the best drug, with the fewest side effects, for their condition. (Susan Horn, Ph.D., of the Institute for Clinical Outcomes Research in Salt Lake City, found that when a drug wasn't listed, doctors usually prescribed it less than 2 percent of the time.) Many plans also require pharmacists to replace brand-name drugs with cheaper generics, and some require "therapeutic substitution," which means a patient may get a different drug than the one prescribed.

Continuity of care is threatened by the new system as well. Managed care plans typically reserve the right to drop a doctor from their rosters for reasons that have nothing to do with skill or patient satisfaction, forcing pregnant women, people with cancer and AIDS, and others in the middle of complicated treatments to start over with a new practitioner. A three-city study by the Commonwealth Fund found that people already bounce among plans with alarming frequency: Nearly half of those surveyed had been forced to switch health plans and doctors at least once because of a job change, marriage, divorce or a change in employer benefits. The same study found that 67 percent of doctors had been asked to join a new managed care plan by a patient; 24 percent had been denied the chance to continue caring for these individuals.

One thing is clear: The new medicine is putting the onus on women to become advocates, not only for themselves but for their families.

"We're in a system that depends on your being assertive: challenging your doctor and going through appeals," says Timothy McCall, M.D., author of *Examining Your Doctor: A Patient's Guide to Avoiding Harmful Medical Care* (Citadel Press). "But do we really want a system that demands that people who are sick be more assertive in order to get the best health care?"

Leslie Laurençe is a syndicated health columnist and coauthor, with Beth Weinhouse, of *Outrageous Practices: The Alarming Truth About How Medicine Mistreats Women* (Fawcett Columbine).

The Life Savers

Medical Tests You Shouldn't Ignore

by Katherine Griffin

Judging from the efforts spent on preventive medicine, it would seem that my cats' health is more important to their veterinarian than mine is to my doctor. Every few months, the kitties get computerized reminder cards, letting me know that it's time to refill Willie's worm pills or bring Houckli in for her distemper shot. But if I had to wait for my doctor to remind me that it's time for a Pap smear or a skin exam, I might still be waiting.

It's not that I have a negligent doctor. It's just that, like most physicians, he's busy dealing with the sick folks who show up at his office every day. Once I do get in to see him, he's happy to talk about what I can do to keep myself healthy, and order any screening tests that I may need. But I have to take the initiative.

That's a position that lots of us are finding ourselves in these days when it comes to preventive health care. Doctors just aren't as good as they should be about keeping women up to date on the tests than can detect medical problems early. A 1995 report on preventive care from researchers at the University of California, Los Angeles, found that 40 percent of women over the age of 40 hadn't had a professional breast exam during the previous year — despite the fact that this low-tech, inexpensive procedure is just about universally recommended as a way of catching breast cancer in its early stages.

The UCLA researchers also found, not surprisingly, that women without health insurance were the most likely to go without preventive care. But even insured women sometimes had a hard time keeping up with widely recommended screening tests.

"Health insurance is getting so complicated that women aren't sure what they're covered for," says Roberta Wyn, of UCLA's Center for Health Policy Research, who coauthored the report. "As health plans become more competitive, people are switching plans more frequently. There is less continuity of care."

Under these circumstances, a woman needs to take her own preventive measures. What follows is a guide to the most important medical tests for women who are healthy and want to stay that way. There is broad consensus that the first five tests should be part of every woman's standard medical care; the last three are recommended for women with certain risk factors.

Sure, it can be time-consuming to make all those appointments to have yourself poked and prodded and scanned. And while most of the tests are covered by insurance plans, the total charge and the amount you'll pay out of pocket can vary, depending on your coverage and where you live.

If it all seems like too much trouble, remember that the point of getting these tests is to keep preventable diseases from stealing more of your time, your money, and your life. After all, you don't want your cats to outlive you.

CHOLESTEROL

Heart disease is the number one killer among women, and high levels of cholesterol, a fatty substance in the blood, raise the risk of stroke as well as heart disease. If you know your cholesterol is high, you can treat it by going on a low-fat diet or by taking cholesterol-lowering drugs.

What to expect: Total cholesterol can be estimated from a small drop of blood. If that reading is above 240 milligrams per deciliter, you'll need to have a larger blood sample taken to measure the levels of "bad" (low-density lipoprotein, or LDL) and "good" (high-density lipoprotein, or HDL) cholesterol, and triglycerides (other fats in the blood). Your HDL should account for at least 25 percent of your total cholesterol count. These measurements will help your doctor pinpoint your risk more precisely.

When to be tested: Experts differ on this one. The National Cholesterol Education Program recommends that all women be tested every five years from age 20 onward. Although these experts acknowledge that heart disease in young women is rare, they say that any young woman who learns that her cholesterol level is high will be more motivated to cut her long-term risk by exercising and eating a low-fat diet.

But recently the American College of Physicians and the U.S. Preventive Services Task Force reported that unless a woman has a family history of heart disease, she doesn't need to be tested until age 45, or until she's reached menopause. Their reasoning? A young woman who learns she has high cholesterol is likely to be advised to lower it by changing her diet. If that isn't effective, the next step is usually drug treatment. That's overkill, these experts say, because before menopause, most women's risk of heart disease is so low that high cholesterol does little to raise it. Since not much is known about the long-term effects of cholesterol-lowering drugs, it's better to hold off on them until later, when the likelihood of heart disease is greater and the possible risks of the drugs would be outweighed by greater benefits.

Women with a family history of high cholesterol or heart disease, however, need to consult their doctor about being tested earlier and more frequently. For women over 45, the recommendations converge: Most experts call for testing every five years.

Test tips: You'll need to fast for nine to 12 hours before getting the HDL/LDL/triglyceride test.

Cost and coverage: The cost ranges from $30 for a simple test to as much as $100 for one that measures HDL, LDL, and triglyceride levels. Most insurers will cover both tests.

MAMMOGRAM AND CLINICAL BREAST EXAM

For women over 50, numerous studies have shown that an annual mammogram, along with a clinical breast exam by a physician or nurse-practitioner, cuts the risk of dying of breast cancer by more than a third. When you're talking about a disease that kills one out of every 30 women, that's an important edge to have.

What to expect: During a clinical breast exam, a health care provider carefully feels all areas of your breasts, looking for any suspicious lumps. For a mammogram, your breasts are compressed between glass plates while X-rays are taken, which the radiologist will examine for early signs of cancer.

When to be tested: If you're over 50, you should have a clinical breast exam annually and a mammogram every one to two years. If you're between 40 and 49, an annual clinical breast exam is a good idea. However, many breast cancer specialists also recommend that women in their forties get regular mammograms. Although large-scale studies haven't yet provided conclusive evidence that annual tests can save lives in this age group, some research has suggested that they might.

Here's why: One-fifth of breast cancers occur in women younger than 50, and their tumors tend to grow more quickly than in older women, says Robert Smith, an epidemiologist and director of detection and treatment at the American Cancer Society. Since surviving breast cancer hinges so crucially on finding a tumor when it's still small, it's probably better to err on the side of caution, and go ahead and schedule an annual test. This strategy is most likely to benefit women whose first mammogram shows that their breasts are fatty, rather than dense, because abnormalities are easier to spot in fatty tissue.

Still, this more cautious approach is not without its own risks. Because breast cancer is less common among women in their forties, getting an annual mammogram is more likely to turn up an abnormality that turns out not to be cancer — a "false positive" — than it is to find a cancer. By one estimate, a woman who gets a mammogram every year between 40 and 49 has a 30 percent chance of a false positive result. Some of these suspicious lesions will need to be biopsied to make sure they're not cancerous; biopsies increase the risk of scarring, which can make later mammograms more difficult to read.

Women younger than 40 should get a clinical breast exam every three years beginning at age 20. A woman whose mother, grandmother, sister, or aunt has had breast cancer should begin getting mammograms five to ten years before the age at which her relatives were diagnosed.

Any woman who gets a mammogram will be reassured to know that the quality of the test has improved, thanks to new federal standards set in 1994 that require annual facility inspections and improved training of doctors and technicians.

Test tips: Squeezing the breasts between the mammography plates can be uncomfortable if breasts are tender, so it's best to avoid being tested the week before your period. Take an over-the-counter pain reliever an hour before. And don't use talcum powder or deodorant the day of the test; tiny flecks can show up as calcifications on the X-ray. Clinical breast exams are most effective when done slowly, sometimes taking as long as five minutes.

Cost and coverage: The average cost of a mammogram is around $85, though it can range from $35 to $300. Most states have now passed laws requiring that insurance policies cover mammograms, but women in their forties are likely to have difficulty getting coverage. A clinical breast exam can be done during any routine doctor visit, so the cost is negligible.

COLON CANCER

Colorectal cancer is one of the deadliest forms of cancer, killing some 40 percent of those who get it. The tests to detect it are no picnic, but they indisputably save lives in people over the age of 50, who are at greatest risk. A recent study of 46,000 Minnesotans over 50 found that those who were tested annually were 33 percent less likely to die of the disease than those who weren't screened at all.

What to expect: Colon cancer is detected by checking for blood in a stool sample — a test known as a fecal occult blood test — or by inspecting the interior of the colon for pre-cancerous polyps by way of a flexible device, called a sigmoidoscope, inserted into the rectum.

When to be tested: Since risk increases sharply with age, screening isn't recommended until after age 50. But past that point, experts agree that it's crucial to get the blood test every year. By the time this cancer can be picked up by the test, it's likely to be fairly far along and growing quickly. The Minnesota study found that those who had the blood test every other year were no better off than those who didn't have it at all.

Sigmoidoscopy is recommended every three to five years for people over 50. Those who are at high risk for colon cancer because a close family member has had it, or because they themselves have had polyps or inflammatory bowel disease, should substitute a more thorough visual examination of the colon, called a colonoscopy, for the sigmoidoscopy.

Test tips: For 72 hours before the fecal occult blood test, you'll need to eat a high fiber diet. But avoid red meat, aspirin, large amounts of vitamin C, and certain fruits and vegetables — get a complete list from your doctor — all of which can throw off the test. The colon will need to be emptied, by means of laxatives or an enema, before a sigmoidoscopy or colonoscopy.

Cost and coverage: A fecal occult blood test can cost from $20 to $30, while a sigmoidoscopy is in the range of $200 to $300. Medicare doesn't cover these tests, although increasing scientific evidence of their effectiveness is adding weight to physicians' arguments that it should. Many private health insurers do cover the tests.

PAP SMEAR

Since the test was introduced in the 1940s, deaths from cervical cancer have dropped by more than 50 percent. Women who are screened every year cut their risk of dying of this cancer by 93 percent.

What to expect: Your doctor will gently scrape cells from the surface of your cervix, which will be sent to a lab to be examined for subtle changes that might indicate cancer.

When to be tested: That depends on your risk, which is directly related to your sexual activity. Most women have at least two of the factors that put them at high risk for cervical cancer and mandate screening every year: sexual activity that began in their teens, smoking, having a partner who's had more than one sex partner in his life, and having more than one partner themselves.

Once a woman becomes sexually active, she should get three consecutive annual tests. If all three tests are negative, she can — if she and her partner are monogamous, or if she's no longer sexually active — schedule subsequent tests every two or three years. Her doctor, however, still might counsel yearly tests. While newly available computerized methods of reading Pap smears should help labs trim false negative rates, many physicians continue to recommend annual testing as a safeguard against lab error.

Test tips: A Pap test is most accurate when done 12 to 14 days after the first day of menstruation. Check with your physician to make sure that the lab meets accreditation standards set by the College of American Pathology, and ask whether the lab is using the new computerized methods for checking the smears.

Cost and coverage: From $10 to $20. Most insurers cover the test, with health maintenance organizations more likely to pay for it than traditional fee-for-service plans.

BLOOD PRESSURE

If you're a white woman, chances are one in five that you have high blood pressure; if you're African-American, your chances are one in three. The longer high blood pressure goes undetected and untreated, the higher your risk of heart attack, stroke, and liver and kidney damage. But a quick and simple test can detect it, and it can be easily treated by weight loss, diet, exercise, or drugs.

What to expect: An inflatable cuff is wrapped around your upper arm to measure the systolic pressure as your heart contracts, and the diastolic pressure as your heart relaxes.

When to be tested: People who have previously tested normal — 140/85 or below — should be checked at least every other year. You should be tested annually if you're African-American, moderately overweight, or have a family or personal history of hypertension.

Test tips: Don't panic if a single test turns up a high reading. Stress, some medications, and even the time of day can affect your results. In fact, as many as

25 percent of those whose pressure is mildly elevated when tested in the doctor's office have "white coat" hypertension, brought on by the stress of the doctor visit.

If your pressure is elevated, your doctor should take several readings, over the course of several weeks, before making a definitive diagnosis. To increase test accuracy, steer clear of caffeine, nicotine, nonsteroidal anti-inflammatory drugs, and cold medications in the hours before your appointment.

Cost and coverage: Because an office test is generally done as a matter of course when you see a doctor for some other reason, the charge is negligible.

BONE DENSITY

Knowing what shape your bones are in can help you decide whether you need hormone replacement therapy or bone building drugs. Doctors often recommend HRT for post-menopausal women who are worried about losing bone as they age, but many are reluctant to take it: While it strengthens bones, it also increases risk of uterine — and possibly breast — cancer. The new drugs offer another option for women who find that their bones are thin but don't want to take hormones.

What to expect: There are several different versions, but the most accurate is called dual X-ray absorptiometry, or DXA. It uses a very low radiation X-ray to measure the density of bone at the spine or hip, and is sensitive enough to detect bone loss down to one percent. You'll find out how much bone mass you have, compared both with an average woman of your age and body size, and with a hypothetical young woman at peak bone strength.

When to be tested: After menopause, when you're weighing the decision between hormone replacement therapy or bone-building drugs.

Cost and coverage: $150 to $250, with Medicare willing to pay in some states but many private insurers not.

HIV

Being tested for HIV is stressful, but early knowledge of infection allows a woman to take advantage of medications that can prolong her life and improve its quality. It can keep her from transmitting the virus to her partner. And, if she's pregnant, taking the antiviral drug AZT can reduce the likelihood that she'll transmit HIV to her unborn child.

What to expect: A sample of blood is taken, then run through two laboratory tests. If the initial test, called ELISA, shows that antibodies to the AIDS virus are present, then a confirmatory test called the Western blot is run on the same sample.

When to be tested: The Centers for Disease Control and Prevention recommends that women in the following categories take the test: pregnant women and those who intend to conceive, as well as anyone who's had unprotected sex with partners whose HIV status they aren't sure of, who have used intravenous drugs or had a partner who did, or who have another sexually transmitted disease.

Test tips: It takes from three to six months for antibodies to the virus to show up in the blood. If you've gotten a negative test result less than six months after engaging in risky behavior, you should be tested again after six months.

Cost and coverage: Cost is $75 for the ELISA and $30 to $100 for the Western blot. Insurers are likely to cover them, but if you're concerned about the confidentiality of your results, you can find an anonymous test site by calling the CDC's National AIDS Hotline, at 800/342-2437.

SKIN CANCER

The incidence of malignant melanoma is on the rise. So is the number of its fatalities. Unlike many other cancers, melanoma is likely to strike younger people; about a third of cases are found in those under 45. The only cure is to catch and treat it before it invades other parts of the body. (Other skin cancers, like basal and squamous, are less deadly but more common than melanoma.)

What to expect: A doctor will examine your skin from head to toe, including your scalp. She'll be looking for moles that are irregularly shaped; have variegated colors; are asymmetrical; are greater than the size of a pencil eraser; or have grown or changed since the previous visit.

When to be tested: The American Cancer Society recommends that people aged 20 to 39 get a skin exam every three years, and those over 40 be examined annually. An annual skin examination is most important for anyone with risk factors for melanoma: lots of moles, pale skin, a family history of the disease, and two or more blistering sunburns in childhood or adolescence.

Test tips: It's best to have a dermatologist do your skin exam. One study showed that dermatologists have a 97 percent chance of catching melanoma; the rate for primary care physicians is much lower.

Cost and coverage: The cost is usually the typical charge for a regular office visit, which may vary from $35 to $135, and most insurers will cover the exam. If you're part of a managed care plan or an HMO, you'll need a referral from your primary care physician.

Katherine Griffin is a staff writer.

PART 2

Emotional Health, Stress, and Self-Esteem

ealth is not determined by one factor alone. There are a variety of areas that impact health and well-being, and they are intertwined. Health is impacted by, and made up of, physical, spiritual, environmental, social, and emotional variables. Women's health can be affected differently than men's in all of these areas. For example, women are prescribed antidepressants more than men. Why is it that depression is diagnosed and treated at a higher rate in women than men? Is it that women with physical complaints or ailments may be treated as having emotional or psychological problems instead? For example, when a woman goes to the doctor to discuss menopausal symptoms or menstrual symptoms, does the physician diagnose and treat the presenting symptoms as physical in nature or as psychological or emotional? How would that influence the treatment prescribed?

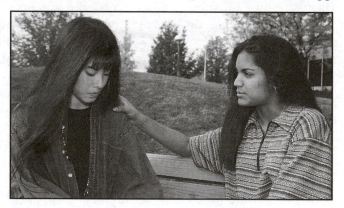

This section contains a variety of readings on a broad range of topics. What links them together is that each reading touches on issues of emotional health and self-esteem. Each of the readings address issues that have an impact not only on physical health but on emotional health and well-being as well. One controversial reading in this section discusses diet pills and the role they play in weight management. Not only are there questions about the safety of diet pills, even the newer kinds, there is also debate over whether or not they are in fact the best way to achieve long-term weight loss. Diet pills alone do not teach you how to eat. And will women who are not obese, but think that they are overweight, use and possibly abuse these pills? As with many issues, there are no easy answers. Diet pills may work for some women, but women also tend to see themselves as overweight when they are not. This reading should provide the basis for a discussion of women, weight, and self-esteem.

Another reading on a controversial issue is the reading on date rape. An alarming, new development in the date rape controversy is use of the drug Rohypnol (pronounced row-hip-nole), which has turned up in the last couple of years on some college campuses. This sedative-hypnotic, or sleeping pill, is not legally available in the United States, even for medicinal purposes, but it is an approved medicine in most other parts of the world, prescribed mainly for the short-term treatment of sleep disorders. It is inexpensive and has attracted young users. The DEA reports that high school students have used Rohypnol as a "cheap drunk," while college students mix it with beer to enhance the feeling of drunkenness. It has been linked to date rape because there have been reports that it has been given to females without their consent in order to produce disinhibition and amnesia. Tasteless and odorless when mixed with alcohol, the drug produces a feeling of drunkenness, with little or no recollection of events that happen while it takes effect. Street names include rophies, ropies, ruffies, roofies, roche, R-2, mexican valium, rib, and rope. (Please see the **Quick Reference Guide to Topics/Readings/WWW Sites** and **Appendix A: WebLinks: A Directory of Annotated World Wide Web Sites** to select WWW sites that coordinate with the readings in this part.) FYI, at the site *Web of Addictions*, No. 93, http://www.well.com/user/woa, you can find up-to-date information on Rohypnol.)

Medical Report

BY PAUL RAEBURN

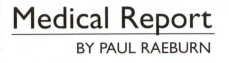

A Reading for Critical Thinking

Diet Pills

They're back. Are they any better?

The U.S. Food and Drug Administration opened a new war on fat this spring when it approved Redux, the first prescription diet drug to hit the market in more than 20 years. Obesity searchers greeted the news with enthusiasm. "It's a real breakthrough," says John Foreyt, Ph.D., a psychologist at Baylor College of Medicine in Houston.

Redux is a breakthrough — but not the one dieters have been seeking. Redux represents only a slight advance over pills long on the market. Foreyt and others are excited mainly because its approval signals a more kindly attitude toward diet drugs at the FDA. Two experimental obesity drugs, which could prove to be true innovations, are expected to be approved soon. "We're on the threshold," says Foreyt. "There will be many more drugs."

In the meantime, the Redux marketing machine is swinging into action. Wyeth-Ayerst Laboratories moved quickly to make Redux available in June, only weeks after its approval. Publisher William Morrow is rushing out a book for September called *The Redux Revolution* by Sheldon Levine, M.D. People are already flooding doctors offices with calls about the drug. "I think it is going to sell like crazy," says Richard Atkinson, M.D., an obesity specialist at the University of Wisconsin Medical School in Madison.

But questions about the value of diet drugs remain. Though designed for people with health problems caused by excess weight, there's nothing to stop doctors from prescribing Redux to people interested in its cosmetic effects. "That's what I'm afraid of,"
says Foreyt. "There are always some people who overuse these medications."

Are diet drugs safe? Are they the best way to lower the risks of obesity-related aliments, such as heart disease and diabetes? Will they produce long-term weight loss? Before you burn your low-fat cookbooks and running shoes, here's what you need to know.

Redux, known generically as dexfenfluramine, has been used in 65 countries, in some cases for as long as ten years. Dexfenfluramine is an improved form of another diet drug, fenfluramine, or Pondimin, which has been on the market since 1973. Unlike amphetamines, the dangerous and highly addictive diet drugs of the past, Redux and Pondimin curb appetite by acting in complex ways on a chemical messenger in the brain called serotonin.

Although these drugs are not addictive or even energizing, they do have side effects. They have been linked to a very small risk of primary pulmonary hypertension, in which the heart has trouble pumping blood through the lungs. (The condition can be fatal, but it is rare, occurring in about 18 cases per one million Redux users, compared with one or two cases per one million normally.) Other side effects are generally mild. "Some people feel drowsy and fatigued," says Dr. Atkinson. "Some have diarrhea. And some feel a little blue, or are not able to think quite as clearly." In one study, 28 percent of Redux users reported feeling tired, compared with 20 percent of control subjects. The other side effects were reported far less often.

Redux is no miracle cure. The evidence suggests that when combined with diet and exercise, Redux

From *Glamour* (August 1996), pp. 42, 45. Reprinted by permission of Paul Raeburn, the author of *The Last Harvest*, published by the University of Nebraska Press, and the science editor at *Business Week*.

can aid weight loss and thus cut the risk of heart disease and diabetes. But regular exercise can produce nearly the same benefits without any drawbacks. Adding Redux produces a little more weight loss, but not much. The FDA's approval was based largely on a yearlong European study of 822 men and women who were more than 20 percent overweight. All embarked on a diet and exercise program: half also took Redux. After a year, one half of the Redux users had lost at least 5 percent of their initial weight. One in five lost at least 15 percent.

That sounds impressive until you look at actual pounds shed: Redux users had a mean weight loss of 22 pounds. The control subjects, who followed the same diet and exercise regimen, lost nearly 16 pounds. Researchers suspect that using Redux without dieting or exercising would be unlikely to produce much weight loss at all. That's partly because the drug works by suppressing hunger pangs, explains Foreyt, and hunger is just one of the reasons people eat. "People eat for emotional reasons too — depression, stress, boredom and loneliness," he says. "If there's ice cream in the freezer and you're bored, you can easily override the drug."

Studies also show that once the drugs are stopped, patients gain the weight right back. Most researchers agree that Redux and its successors will be like medications for high blood pressure or diabetes: They must be taken for life. Yet Redux has been proven to be safe for only one year, long-term studies have not been done. There's also the cost to think of: Redux costs $70 to $75 a month.

Given the drugs' modest effects, and the fact that they may need to be used for life, why are researchers so thrilled? Part of the answer lies in their frustration with other methods of weight loss.

More than 33 percent of Americans are carrying enough extra weight to contribute to high blood pressure, heart disease or diabetes. That's up from 25 percent in 1980. Once women hit age 30, their rate of obesity is higher than that of men. At any given time, one of three women and one of five men say they are trying to lose weight. Initially, dieters are often successful. Many lose 10 percent of their body weight, but nearly all of them regain the weight within five years. For people whose health is at risk because of excess pounds, a safe, modestly effective drug that helps them make other changes is better than nothing.

"Losing even 5 percent of overall body weight and maintaining that loss can improve a patient's health and well-being," says JoAnn E. Manson, M.D. of Harvard Medical School. That is particularly true, she says, for very obese people, for whom "losing weight and maintaining that weight loss has been perceived as an unattainable goal."

"With weight losses of even 5 percent," agrees Dr. Atkinson. "you get beneficial changes in blood pressure, in diabetes and in blood fats like cholesterol."

In the long run, Redux will probably prove most effective for a small group of overweight people. In the European study, 32 percent of users lost one third of their excess weight; only 17 percent of controls lost that much. For now, however, there's no way to tell who will benefit most from the drugs, says Rena Wing, Ph.D., a psychologist at the University of Pittsburgh Medical Center who studies obesity treatments. Furthermore, she says, "we don't know whether there are certain diet and exercise interventions that will be most helpful to people when used along with the drug."

Wayne Callaway, M.D., of George Washington University Medical Center in Washington, D.C., says there is one clue that could help identify those most likely to benefit from Redux. Evidence suggests that the drug may work particularly well in people with a condition called insulin resistance, a precursor of diabetes. Redux may delay the onset of diabetes in such people, says Dr. Callaway, in addition to producing weight loss.

But cosmetic effects are likely to prove disappointing to people who expect dramatic changes in their

Who Are the Best Candidates for Diet Drugs?

Redux is being recommended for people with a body-mass index (BMI) of 30 or more. For a woman 5'6" tall, that translates into a weight of about 185 pounds. For people with obesity-related conditions like high blood pressure, diabetes or high cholesterol, Redux is recommended at lower weights (a BMI of more than 27, or about 165 for a 5'6" woman).

Do I have to exercise and watch what I eat while taking the drug?

Yes. By stemming hunger pangs, Redux modestly boosts the effects of exercising and eating healthily. Researchers expect the drug to have little effect if taken alone.

Do the drugs produce long-term weight loss?

Apparently not. In studies, patients who stopped taking the drugs gained the weight back.

Is there any other way to get the health benefits associated with Redux?

Yes. Eating healthily and exercising regularly lowers blood pressure, improves cholesterol and reduces the risk of diabetes and heart disease.

looks. "People lose 30 pounds, and they're really pleased for a year," says Dr. Atkinson. "And then they say, 'I'd like to lose another 30 pounds,' but they've gone beyond the drugs."

Meanwhile, research on drug treatments for obesity continues. One drug being investigated, called sibutramine (Meridia), acts on serotonin, as does Redux. But it also acts on another neurotransmitter, suggesting it might be more effective. Another experimental drug, called Orlistat, interferes with enzymes needed to digest fat, blocking fat absorption. Even more sophisticated drugs are being developed that could target particular sites in the brain, possibly revving up metabolism without adverse effects.

At the very least, researchers hope that the effectiveness of Redux and its successors will help counter the widespread belief that obesity is due simply to a lack of self-control. Obese people shouldn't get drugs, the theory goes, they should get their hands out of the refrigerator.

It's an attitude that makes Dr. Atkinson cringe. "When people say that all a fat person has to do is eat normally" he says, "that's probably not so. I think everybody agrees there is a physiological component to obesity. The number of people who are fat simply because of a psychological problem is vanishingly small."

Paul Raeburn has written extensively about health and science. He is the author of The Last Harvest (Simon & Schuster).

HARVARD WOMEN'S HEALTH WATCH

We're Not Like Men

Like most other human activities, work can be harmful to our health. While women aren't immune to the types of stresses that contribute to strokes and heart attacks in men, these stresses seem to affect us differently.

Although research into the physiological effects on women of holding a job is scanty, early studies seem to indicate that as our professional lives begin to mimic those of the men around us, our blood pressure and cholesterol readings rise accordingly. Yet these investigations also hint that we may still be somewhat protected from developing heart disease, partially because we handle pressure differently.

Response to stress. Whenever humans perceive a situation as challenging or threatening, our brains transmit signals to the adrenal glands, ordering the release of two substances, epinephrine and norepinephrine, which were once collectively known as "adrenalin"and are now referred to as catecholamines or "stress hormones."

Catecholamines stimulate heart rate, raise blood pressure, and ready the body to perform at a higher than normal level. Like other stimulants, they are very helpful in small doses. However, sustained high levels of stress hormones can lead to hypertension and heart disease.

Physiological studies have indicated that although this response is essentially the same in men and women, the situations that trigger it vary according to gender. Men's catecholamine levels generally rise more sharply in response to competitive and intellectual challenges, while women's increase more dramatically during stressful personal situations.

Researchers at the Karolinska Institute in Stockholm, Sweden, who are conducting an ongoing study of Volvo employees, have found that women in managerial positions or in traditionally "male" occupations like law and engineering experience catecholamine influxes almost as great as those of men while taking tests of mental acuity. Yet men tend to wind down rapidly after office hours. According to the Volvo study, the catecholamine levels of male executives began to drop at the stroke of five o'clock. In contrast, those of their wives (who were also managers) continued to rise during the evening, partly in response to the family responsibilities they faced.

Blood pressure. A team from Cornell Medical Center in New York City found much the same situation: Men's blood pressure tended to fall as soon as they walked through their front doors, while women's pressure, particularly that of working mothers, experienced no such decline.

The Swedish investigators also found that men's and women's blood pressures varied with their emotions. The men's tended to rise most sharply when they were angry; the women's when they were anxious. Although some studies have indicated that anger rather than competitiveness or time urgency is the "toxic" component of Type-A behavior that increases men's risk for heart attack, there is no evidence that either anger or anxiety raises women's risk of coronary heart disease.

Serum cholesterol. In the Volvo study, men, on average, had higher levels of LDL-cholesterol (the "bad" one) and lower levels of HDL-cholesterol (the "good" one) than did women. However, when the participants were classified by job ranking, female managers had LDL readings that were almost as high as those of their male counterparts. Nonetheless, women who were identified as Type A according to their scores on psychological tests had LDL levels that were the same as those of less competitive Type B women and significantly lower than those of Type A males. HDL levels remained higher in women regardless of job ranking or personality type.

WHAT DOES IT MEAN?

At present it appears that entering the labor force or even assuming a high-pressure job and running a household won't raise our risk for heart disease up to the same level as men's. It is also likely that the protective effect of estrogen, which we enjoy during most of our working years, is sufficient to keep LDL and HDL in balance.

Some scientists have also postulated that women may not suffer the cardiac consequences of stress as severely as men because they are more adept at identifying the causes of discomfort and dealing with them. A recent study by researchers at the University of Tennessee indicated that women are less vulnerable to stress than men because we employ approaches such as exercise, rational discussion, and contemplation to dispel it. Until we have the word from more definitive studies, the best way to avoid coronary heart disease isn't to quit your job, but to get sufficient aerobic exercise, follow a low-fat diet rich in fruits and vegetables, avoid becoming over weight, and refrain from smoking.

Depression

Way Beyond the Blues

by Sandra Arbetter

Maria hasn't smiled in a month. Not even when her terrier rushes around in circles trying to bite his tail. Not even when her boyfriend lip-syncs to the Spin Doctors. Either of those things used to set her to howling, but lately she just wants to stay in her room and sleep, and it's a struggle for her to get up in the morning and go to school.

Andy, on the other hand, is always smiling. He talks nonstop, and his energy is endless. He jumps into things without a second thought — he drives too fast, drinks alcohol, and can't wait to bungee jump. At night his mind races over the next day's activities, until he finally falls into a restless sleep.

Which of these two may be depressed? If you say Maria, you're right. And if you say Andy, you're right, too. Even though they act very differently, they both are in the midst of a long period of depression. If you say that's confusing, you're right again. Depression is a murky pool of feelings and actions that scientists have been trying to plumb since the days of Hippocrates, who called it a "black bile."

To further muddy the waters, feelings of depression come and go in most of us from time to time. But short periods of sadness or hyperactivity don't mean clinical depression.

Clinical depression is severe enough to require treatment. It lasts a longer time than the blues — at least two weeks — and it interferes with daily life — school, friends, family. It's considered a medical disorder and can affect thoughts, feelings, physical health, and behaviors. Here's what it's not: It's NOT a personality weakness or a moral lapse. And it's NOT the fault of the person who is depressed.

Science Whips Up a Moral Dilemma

Ron was a pleasant, quiet boy who liked to spend time by himself, mostly with his computer. His mother said he "moved at his own pace," which was a bit slower than the rest of the family.

When Ron was 17, he withdrew further from others, stopped showering and shampooing, and even lost his interest in computers. His parents arranged for him to see a psychiatrist, who prescribed an antidepressant medication.

To say he responded well would be an understatement. He was peppier than ever before, moved faster, laughed more readily, liked being with people, went from being a B to an A student, and got a girlfriend.

His doctor was pleased — but puzzled. Now that Ron was no longer depressed, should he go off medication and return to his former quiet self? Or should he stay on medication and retain his livelier, more confident personality? Did the medication uncover the "real" Ron who had lived a lifetime beneath a cover of chronic, mild depression? Or did it create a false self?

Antidepressants are designed to relieve the symptoms of depression. But is it OK to use them as what one doctor called "mood brighteners"? That's the question posed by author Peter Kramer, M.D.

Mental health experts express the concern that we will look to a pill to make us feel better and we'll ignore the external problems in our world. Some fear that antidepressants interfere with reality by making things look more positive. Or could it be that depression distorts reality by making things look more grim?

Diagnosing depression in a teenager is not easy, says Dr. Richard Marohn, past president of the American Society of Adolescent Psychiatry. That's because it's normal for teens to have mood swings — within limits.

It's a confusing time of life, says Marohn. For one thing, the teen's body is changing. Teenagers have little control over those changes. Secondly, their relationship with parents is changing, and teens are pulled between the security of home and the challenge of testing out their own beliefs.

So how do you tell if it's depression? Time tells, says Marohn. If your feelings affect your schoolwork, your activities, your relationship with family and friends, then it's beyond normal.

Suicidal urges and plans are also a warning sign. But even that's not surefire, because lots of teens have transient thoughts of suicide.

Finally, adolescent depression is difficult to diagnose because adolescents don't necessarily look sad and depressed. To be a teen means to externalize feelings and deal with the world through action. So depression may show up as truancy, running away, violent behavior, or substance abuse. Teens may self-medicate with alcohol or other drugs to try to feel better.

WHAT IS DEPRESSION?

Lots of people assume they know what depression is because they've had at least a touch of it. It's natural to feel sad when you're hit by one of life's inevitable losses. It's a loss when you start kindergarten and give up the safety of home. It's a loss when you move to a new house and leave the old one behind. It's a loss to break up with a boyfriend or girlfriend, and it's even worse when he or she is doing the breaking up.

The sadness that comes with events like these can be intense at first, but usually mellows in a short while. If you get back to a relatively normal state in a week or so, there's nothing to worry about. But if

CHECK THESE SYMPTOMS

Changes in habits and personality are clues to depression. Here are some specifics:

1. There's no interest in school and grades fall.
2. Being with friends holds absolutely no appeal.
3. Sleep problems are common — either not being able to fall asleep at night or wanting to sleep all day.
4. Appetite is out of whack. There's either no desire for food, or the person seems to be eating all the time.
5. The person is obsessed with thoughts of death, maybe suicide. It's estimated that 15 percent of people with major depression commit suicide, and many more attempt it. There are 6,000 suicides by adolescents each year, and depression is the biggest risk factor.
6. Everything seems hopeless, and there's the feeling it will never get better.
7. Headaches, stomachaches, or other aches and pains appear.
8. It's impossible to concentrate or make a decision.

feelings of great sadness or agitation last for much more than two weeks, it may be depression.

Depressed feelings after a major loss, such as the death of a loved one, last much longer, and no one expects recovery in a week or two. Experts won't make a diagnosis of depression (at least, not right away) if a person has had a recent major loss. They'll also hold off if a person is taking certain medications or has certain illnesses that bring on depression-like symptoms.

WHAT IT FEELS LIKE

Anyone who's ever felt sad has only the barest clue as to what major depression is like, according to one 16-year old who recently spent three weeks in a hospital after taking an overdose of pills.

"I had this buzzing in my head all the time," says Emmy, a small, dark-haired girl with large brown eyes. "And I felt tired. I didn't want to do anything except lie on my bed and listen to tapes. When my friends called, I didn't feel like talking to them. I knew they were getting mad, and sometimes I'd try to talk on the phone, but I couldn't push the words up out of my throat."

Emmy had always been a good student and had managed a B+ average while holding a job at a discount store and swimming in competition. Her father was a building contractor, and her mother was a secretary.

How Antidepressants Work

Antidepressants help people feel better by affecting neurotransmitters and, in turn, brain function. Neurotransmitters are brain chemicals that help nerve cells communicate with each other. Certain ones are thought to control feelings of security and alertness.

Although the specific effects have not been worked out, it is though that antidepressants work by helping to regulate the dysfunction in the brain that is causing a person to feel depressed.

"My mother never liked her job, and she kept telling me that I needed to get into a good college so I could be a lawyer and have a happier life than she had. I know now that she was struggling with her own problems, but I used to worry all the time that I was disappointing her. I wanted so badly to be an A student, but no matter how hard I studied, I couldn't pull it off.

"Then I just started not caring. Nothing special happened; I just shut down. I felt so alone, like I was living in a bubble and couldn't punch my way out. I felt like screaming so someone would notice me.

"And I was so tired all the time. Nobody can understand that. I wasn't tired physically like after a swim meet or staying up late. I was tired in every cell of my body, so that I couldn't think straight, and it was too much of an effort to eat. Finally, one day I decided it was too much of an effort to live. That's when I took the pills."

The doctor prescribed an antidepressant drug for Emmy for about six months, and she and her parents were in family therapy for more than a year. She's a junior now and planning to go to college to study environmental sciences. Her mother is in law school.

DEPRESSION IS A MIXED BAG

For a long time, people who were feeling depressed were told to "snap out of it," and, if they didn't, people said they had a flaw in their personality. That's simply not true and only added guilt to the heavy burden these people were already carrying.

Research in the last decade or two has shown, first of all, that there are several kinds of depression and a multitude of causes.

- Major depression: More than one episode of clinical depression is considered major depression, an illness marked by hopeless feelings, inability to feel pleasure, physical changes or complaints, thoughts of death and suicide. The Public Health Service estimates that 11 million people in this country have episodes of major depression, women outnumbering men more than 2 to 1.

- Bipolar disorder (also known as manic-depressive disorder): A person with this illness alternates between periods of high activity, or mania, and periods of hopelessness or depression.

In the manic phase, people may talk a lot — and fast. They have feelings of greatness and think nothing is beyond them. They've been known to go days without sleeping. They've got lots of thoughts racing through their mind at once. They often act on these thoughts and get into trouble because of their behaviors. So, if you have a friend who is in the manic

phase of this illness, don't be surprised if you get a call at three in the morning about his or her plans to save the earth.

Bipolar disorder occurs in about 1 percent of the population, or about 2 million people, equally in men and women. Bipolar disorder can take years to develop into its classic form. When a bipolar disorder emerges during adolescence, it's sometimes hard to distinguish it from the normal emotional ups and downs associated with that age.

- Seasonal Affective Disorder, or SAD: It's not exactly a news flash that most people feel better when the weather is sunny and bright than when it's gloomy. But for some people, wintry weather brings on feelings of depression. Here's one explanation: Many of the body's functions operate on circadian cycles, which are about 24 hours in length. Lack of light puts these cycles out of whack. One treatment is to have patients sit under bright lights for a few hours each day.

- Dysthymia: This is low-level chronic depression. It's usually not severe enough to put someone in the hospital, or to prompt suicide, but it robs a person of the capacity to take pleasure in living.

WHY, OH, WHY?

Experts don't completely understand the causes of depression, but there seems to be an important interplay of two factors: environmental and biological.

Environmental factors include such events as death of a parent, parents' divorce, physical or emotional abuse, family violence, and other difficult family relationships. A depressive episode can be triggered by moving, graduating, losing a job, winning an award, or a hundred other life changes. It can be related to emotional conflicts within the person, such as a past experience that was not resolved. It's been described as "anger turned inward." Or it can come on for no apparent reason.

Biological factors, primarily changes in brain function, are an important aspect of depression. It is not known whether the observed changes in the function cause depression, or whether depression from some other cause accounts for the changes in brain function.

There seems to be a genetic factor involved, too. A child whose parent has suffered from depression has a greater chance of developing the illness than a child with no family history of depression.

TREATMENT

Major approaches to helping depression are medication and psychotherapy, or counseling. Experts say upward of 80 percent of people with depression can be helped.

Medications affect brain function and reduce the symptoms of depression but do not provide a cure. All antidepressants have side effects. Experts worry that people will think of them as magic potions and not accept responsibility for their own behaviors. (See "Science Whips Up a Moral Dilemma".) Finally, parents are cautious about allowing medications for their children.

Psychiatrist Richard Marohn says that many experts view adolescent depression as short-lived and say treatment should deal with underlying issues rather than the symptoms themselves. Therefore, "talk therapy" is preferable and "most of us working with adolescents tend to stay away from medication." Exceptions are suicidal behaviors and depression that's been going on since childhood.

Dr. Marohn says he is concerned about the increasing lack of mental health services. "Kids wind up in prison," he says, rather than in hospitals where treatment is available and they may get some help.

TALKING IT OUT

Some experts say the most effective treatment for severe depression is a combination of medication and counseling. Counseling can help by making people aware of negative thought patterns, such as: "If I'm not perfect, people will think less of me." Or, "If I fail this test, it means I'll always be a failure." It can improve a person's ability to get along with others and to understand him- or herself better. It can bolster self-esteem.

What's more, there are lots of things people can do on their own to help themselves feel better. Michael Maloney and Rachel Kranz, authors of *Straight Talk About Anxiety and Depression*, suggest these:

- Try to focus on the positives about yourself rather than the negatives.
- Accept the fact that others aren't perfect. Then you won't be disappointed when they act human.
- Accept that you aren't perfect, either.
- Enjoy the present moment. Stop regretting the past and worrying about the future.
- Take care of yourself physically. Eat well, exercise, get plenty of sleep.
- Do something nice for yourself.
- Improve your surroundings. Clean your closet. Get a new poster. Surround yourself with things you like to look at.
- Talk to someone. Call up a friend you trust, or start a conversation with a neighbor to prove you can connect.
- Indulge your feelings. Let yourself cry and and wallow in sad songs. But only for a little while.

Depression is one of the most common mental illnesses of our era and responds well to treatment. So while people don't do anything to make themselves feel bad, they *can* do something to make themselves feel better. A generation ago, there was a comic strip character named Arthur, who walked everywhere with a cloud over his head. If he knew then what you know now, he'd reach up and pull out a silver lining.

FOR MORE INFORMATION

American Psychiatric Association
1400 K St. NW
Washington, DC 20005
Pamphlets: "Depression," Manic-Depressive Disorder." "Teen Suicide," single copy of each free. Booklet: "Let's Talk About It," $1 per copy. Also available in Spanish.

S. James
Consumer Information Center-3C
P.O. Box 100
Pueblo, CO 81002
Pamphlets: #564z "What To Do When A Friend Is Depressed — A Guide For Teenagers." #566z "You Are Not Alone," single copy of each free.

National Mental Health Association
1021 Prince St.
Alexandria, VA 22314-2971
Pamphlets: "Adolescent Depression," "Adolescent Suicide," single copy of each free with self-addressed, stamped business-size envelope.

American Academy of Pediatrics
Dept. C-Depression
P.O. Box 927
Elk Grove Village, IL 60009-0927
Pamphlet: "Surviving: Coping With Adolescent Depression/Suicide," single copy free with self-addressed, stamped business-size envelope.

Body Mania

*After a lifetime of work on the body-image front,
one of the country's leading experts reveals her insights
into the dilemma — and offers a way out.*

By Judith Rodin, Ph.D.

Judith Rodin, a professor of psychology, medicine, and psychiatry at Yale University is the author of more than 200 articles and papers as well as *Breaking the Body Traps* (William Morrow, 1992). She is codirector of the Yale Center for Eating and Weight Disorders and past president of the Society for Behavioral Medicine.

If *Pygmalion* were written today it would not be a story about changing Eliza Doolittle's speech, clothing, or manners, but rather about changing her face and body. Using methods from face-lifts to miracle diet to liposuction, women in increasing numbers are striving — with a degree of panic and, more often than not, to their own detriment — to match the ultimate template of beauty.

Has the situation worsened in the past few decades? The answer is undeniably yes. Since beginning this research 20 years ago, I have witnessed growing concern with appearance, body, and weight among women of all ages. Men, too, no longer seem immune.

In 1987, *Psychology Today* published the results of a survey of readers' feelings about appearance and weight. Only 12 percent of those polled indicated little concern about their appearance and said they didn't do much to improve it. The results of this survey are similar to those of many studies where the participants are selected at random: People feel intense pressure to look good.

An earlier survey on body image was published in *Psychology Today* in 1972. The 1970s respondents were considerably more satisfied with their bodies than were the 1980s respondents. The pressure to look good has intensified for both sexes in the last two decades. As the table below shows, our dissatisfaction has grown for every area of our bodies.

UNHAPPY BODIES

The survey also shows how important weight has become to body image; it is the focus of dissatisfaction in both studies and the area showing the greatest increase. I recently evaluated a survey for *USA Today* which also showed identical results. People today are far more critical of themselves for not attaining the right weight and look.

Body preoccupation has become a societal mania. We've become a nation of appearance junkies and fitness zealots, pioneers driven to think, talk, strategize, and worry about our bodies with the same fanatical devotion we applied to putting a man on the moon. Abroad, we strive for global peace. At home, we have declared war on our bodies.

It is a mistake to think that concern with appearance and weight is simply an aberration of contemporary Western culture. Generations of ancient Chinese women hobbled themselves by binding their feet in order to match the beauty ideal of the time. And we all remember Scarlett O'Hara in search of the 17-inch waist. What *Gone With The Wind* did not show us was that tight corseting induced shortness of breath, constipation, and, occasionally, uterine prolapse. But if we moderns are following a tradition hallowed by our forebears, the industrialization of fitness and

People Dissatisfied with Body Areas or Dimensions

1972	Men	Women	1987	Men	Women
Height	13%	13%	Height	20%	17%
Weight	35	48	Weight	41	55
Muscle Tone	25	30	Muscle Tone	32	45
Overall Face	8	11	Face	20	20
Breast/Chest	18	26	Upper Torso	28	32
Abdomen	36	50	Mid Torso	50	57
Hips and Upper thighs	12	49	Lower Torso	21	50
Overall	15	25	"Looks As They Are"	34	38

beauty is conspiring with other trends to raise the stakes to their highest point in history.

Of all the industrial achievements of the 20th century that influence how we feel about our bodies, none has had a more profound effect than the rise of the mass media. Through movies, magazines, and TV, we see beautiful people as often as we see our own family members; the net effect is to make exceptional beauty appear real and attainable. Narcissus was lucky: He had only to find a lake. The modern woman has television, in which she doesn't see herself reflected.

In my experience as a researcher and clinician, I have found that many women avoid the mirror altogether; those who do look may scrutinize, yet still fail to see themselves objectively. Most of us see only painful flaws in exquisite detail. Others still see the fat and blemishes that used to be there in the teenage years, even if they're no longer there.

Like a perverse Narcissus, a woman today looks at her reflection in a mirror and finds it wanting — and then is consumed by a quest to make herself fit the reflection the media has conditioned her to expect is possible. She works harder and harder to attain what is, as I will explain, most likely impossible. Ignoring the hours movie stars spend on makeup and hair, forgetting how easily and well the camera can lie, she aspires to a synthetic composite of what she thinks her reflection should be.

It is also likely that she is unaware of what other research shows: Such detailed attention has a negative influence on self-esteem. It makes us feel that many features of ourself are flawed, even those having little to do with weight or appearance.

Many of us have traveled through the looking glass with Alice into a world where what is and what might be blur and confuse us. We may be thin and

think we are not. We may be heavy and think that life isn't worth living because we do not match our culture's physical ideal. Our self-image has become far too plastic, too malleable. It depends too much on transitory moods, on what we feel is expected of us and how we feel we are lacking. It is not dependent enough upon a stable internal sense of ourself. We grow larger or smaller, in our mind's eye, in response to the image of woman modern society has encouraged us to idealize.

Unlike Alice, however, we have not returned. We are stuck there in a world of obsessional self-criticism, where what we see is not at all what we really are. The mirror is woman's modern nemesis.

Some call such obsession with appearance vanity — but that misses the point. We are responding to the deep psychological significance of the body. Appearance does indeed affect our sense of self and how people respond to us; it always has, always will. What's different today is that the body and how it looks has become a significant component of our self-worth.

WHY NOW?

Why do weight and appearance matter so much? And why now? What is occurring at this particular moment in time?

Our society has changed dramatically in this century. There are few remaining hierarchies or social structures based on religion, parentage, money, or education. Society has become more egalitarian, but intrinsic to human nature is the desire to judge, evaluate, and compare ourselves to others. If class and lineage no longer provide the tools for measuring ourselves against our neighbors, what are the new social standards? It is my premise that they are the more visible, tangible, observable aspects — first among these, the physical self.

Our bodies have become the premier coin of the realm. Appearance, good looks, and fitness are now the measure of one's social worth. How closely we can approximate a perfect body has also unfortunately become a sign of how well we're doing in life.

Not only is how we look suddenly of the utmost importance, but we have also come to accept and idealize a single image of beauty — slim but fit. The media now expose us to this single "right" look, and the beauty industry promises it is attainable by all. When the prescription for how we should look is so well-defined, deviations are all the more noticeable.

What's more, our culture holds out the lure of an easy fix for all corporeal dissatisfactions. The goal of looking good is attainable by anyone, as long as he or she works out hard enough, exercises long enough, and eats little enough. Beauty, health, diet, and fitness have become very big businesses. But they weren't always. During the late 1950s and early '60s — when models and Miss Americas wore girdles, did a little exercise just for their thighs and hips, and wore a size 10 — only overweight women dieted. A survey of *Ladies Home Journal* issues from the 1960s showed an average of only one diet article every six months. But by the mid-'70s almost every woman in America had tried some kind of diet, and losing weight was a national obsession.

Because we sincerely believe that the perfect body is attainable by anyone, Americans spend more on beauty and fitness aids than they do on social services or education. Such distribution of a primary resource is a shocking revelation of our true priorities.

Yet another reason appearance is everything today hinges on the blurring of traditional definitions of female and male. Our view of the differences between the sexes is in flux, as women move into such traditionally male domains as the office and men become more involved in the household. In many ways our bodies remain our most visible means of expressing the differences between the sexes. Having the right body may be a way for women who have moved into male occupations to declare their feminine identity without compromising their professional persona.

Asked to make it in a man's world, they are, like the rest of society, still confused about women's roles. Internalizing society's ambivalence, they succeed in one domain and fall back in the other, reverting to the traditionally feminine arena of competition over thinness and beauty.

In addition, the fitness movement, taken to extremes, has fostered the notion that a "good" physique not only equals a healthy body but a healthy soul. Getting in shape has become the new moral imperative — an alluring substitute for altruism and good work, the desire to look good replacing the desire to do good. In this new secular morality, values and ideals of beauty and appearance supplement moral and religious standards.

Today's moral transgressions involve eating something we feel we shouldn't have or feeling we don't look good enough or haven't tried hard enough to look good.

If our current self-absorption has its reasons, it also has its comforts. The quest for physical perfection is the up-to-date way we barter with the uncertainty of life. Like a set of worry beads, we always have our calories to count, our minutes of aerobics to execute. If everything else in our lives seems out of control, we at least have our diet and exercise regimens. In the chaos called modern life, ordering the body to do what we want it to may give us a much-needed illusion of control.

Where we differ, too, from our forebears is that the body today is no longer considered a finished product, a fait accompli. It is strictly a work in progress. And we devote ourselves to perfecting it with the dedication of the true artist. According to the American Society of Plastic and Reconstructive Surgeons, "aesthetic" surgeries are up 61 percent over the past decade. A marketing research firm in New York calculates that Americans spent $33 billion on diets and diet-related services in 1990, up from $29 billion in 1989. By the turn of the century we will be spending $77 billion to lose weight — just slightly less than the entire gross national product of Belgium.

THE LIMITS OF THE BODY

There is an overriding fallacy in this view of ourselves. The body is not infinitely malleable in the way that advertisers with a product to sell would have us believe. Despite wide dissemination of news about great advances in science and medicine, the individual American remains virtually unaware of the role that physiology plays in body weight, in determining how quickly we lose or gain weight and in how our general health and appearance respond to exercise and diet. Most of us are exposed to and accept a staggering amount of misinformation.

Genes play a major role in setting metabolism as well as body shape and size; they determine how much fat we burn, how much we can store easily, and where it's distributed on our bodies. One of our clinic patients came from a family where everyone had thick, solid legs and big thighs. For years she tried every diet that became popular. No matter how much she lost, no matter how thin she became, she couldn't change the size of her legs and thighs nearly as much as the rest of her body. "My greatest goal in life," she admitted, "is to have thin legs. . . . I know why women have liposuction. It's the ultimate solution. I used to dream about a big vacuum cleaner sucking out the fat — it was my constant childhood wish — but I just can't afford it yet."

THE PURSUIT IS COSTLY

The quest for the perfect body is, like most wars, a costly one — emotionally and physically, to say nothing of financially. It leaves most of us feeling frustrated, ashamed, and defeated. Yet we keep at it, wearing down our bodies and our optimism while narrowing the focus of our lives.

In addition, as a society obsessed with a set standard of beauty, we have become intolerant of and sometimes cruel to those who do not meet it, especially the overweight. We learn early in life that there is something shameful about obesity. And the obese are painfully stigmatized. Even children with a life-threatening chronic illness would rather be sick than fat.

Social Attitudes Scale

Please read the following statements and indicate how strongly you agree or disagree with each.

1. A man would always prefer to go out with a thin woman than one who is heavy.

Strongly Agree	Agree Somewhat	Agree	Neither Agree nor Disagree	Disagree	Disagree Somewhat	Strongly Disagree
❏	❏	❏	❏	❏	❏	❏

2. Clothes are made today so that only thin people can look good.

Strongly Agree	Agree Somewhat	Agree	Neither Agree nor Disagree	Disagree	Disagree Somewhat	Strongly Disagree
❏	❏	❏	❏	❏	❏	❏

3. Fat people are often unhappy.

Strongly Agree	Agree Somewhat	Agree	Neither Agree nor Disagree	Disagree	Disagree Somewhat	Strongly Disagree
❏	❏	❏	❏	❏	❏	❏

4. It is not true that attractive people are more interesting, poised, and socially outgoing than unattractive people.

Strongly Agree	Agree Somewhat	Agree	Neither Agree nor Disagree	Disagree	Disagree Somewhat	Strongly Disagree
❏	❏	❏	❏	❏	❏	❏

5. A pretty face will not get you very far without a slim body.

Strongly Agree	Agree Somewhat	Agree	Neither Agree nor Disagree	Disagree	Disagree Somewhat	Strongly Disagree
❏	❏	❏	❏	❏	❏	❏

6. It is more important that a woman be attractive than a man.

Strongly Agree	Agree Somewhat	Agree	Neither Agree nor Disagree	Disagree	Disagree Somewhat	Strongly Disagree
❏	❏	❏	❏	❏	❏	❏

7. Attractive people lead more fulfilling lives than unattractive people.

Strongly Agree	Agree Somewhat	Agree	Neither Agree nor Disagree	Disagree	Disagree Somewhat	Strongly Disagree
❏	❏	❏	❏	❏	❏	❏

8. The thinner a woman is, the more attractive she is.

Strongly Agree	Agree Somewhat	Agree	Neither Agree nor Disagree	Disagree	Disagree Somewhat	Strongly Disagree
❏	❏	❏	❏	❏	❏	❏

9. Attractiveness decreases the likelihood of professional success.

Strongly Agree	Agree Somewhat	Agree	Neither Agree nor Disagree	Disagree	Disagree Somewhat	Strongly Disagree
❏	❏	❏	❏	❏	❏	❏

These items test how much you believe that appearance matters. Score your responses as follows:
For items 1, 2, 3, 5, 7 and 8, give yourself a zero if you said "strongly disagree"; a 2 for "disagree"; up to a 6 for "strongly agree."
Items 4, 6, and 9, are scored in reverse. In other words, give yourself a zero for "strongly agree" and a 6 for "strongly disagree."
Add together your points for all nine questions. A score of 46 or higher means that you are vulnerable to being influenced by the great importance that current society places on appearance.

We learn these antifat attitudes in childhood, and they figure strongly into why normal-weight people greatly fear becoming overweight. In our research, we hear many people state that they would kill themselves if they were fat. While this is just a figure of speech, some overweight people are so unhappy about their appearance that they *do* contemplate suicide. A few follow through.

The accompanying test will give you an idea of how much you subscribe to society's standards of beauty.

The vast majority of American women have accepted at face value the message we have been continually exposed to: that beauty and physical perfection are merely a matter of personal effort and that failure to attain those goals is the result of not doing enough. Consequently, we are now subjecting ourselves and even our children to an ever more complicated regimen of diet, exercise, and beauty. We have come to believe in what I see as the "techno-body," shaped by dieting and surgical techniques.

Humans appear to be the only animals who decline to eat when hungry, who willingly starve the body. Occasionally they do it to feed the soul. Many religions have institutionalized fasting as a way of asking for redemption. But in the more modern version of these self-denial rituals, people fast and starve, purge and renew in search of a better self.

It has become fashionable, even politically correct, to worry about the environment. We rally to plant trees to save the Earth without even realizing that at the very same moment in history we are defacing and dehumanizing our bodies by using chemical peels, dermabrasion, hair dye, synthetic diet foods, and fake fats and sweeteners. Where is our concern for the human part of our environment?

WHAT IS THE PROBLEM?

My studies show that surgery, diet, and exercise are only symptoms of the real problem: body preoccupation and an obsessive concern with body image. In accepting the quick fix as a solution, we are overlooking the depth and complexity of the problem we are facing. Shedding pounds, counting calories, and pumping iron — manifestations of body preoccupation — are only a reflection of the fact that we now believe the body is the window to the self, perhaps even the soul.

The psychological self is fundamental to our preoccupation with the physical self. Of all the ways we

In an era of acid rain, AIDS, nuclear disaster, and poverty, we are embarrassed by our body preoccupation — but that, of course, does not stop it.

experience ourselves, none is so primal as the sense of our own bodies. Our body image is at the very core of our identity. Our feelings about our bodies are woven into practically every aspect of our behavior. Our bodies shape our identity because they are the form and substance of our persona to the outside world. Appearance will always be important because we are social beings. How we look sends messages, whether we want it to or not, and people respond to us accordingly.

The old saw cites death and taxes, but in fact we have one other nonnegotiable contract in life: to live in and with our bodies for the duration. People must learn to treat the issue of body image seriously and validate their concerns about their bodies. In my clinical experience, people find that hard to do because admitting how deeply we anguish about our bodies often leads to a profound sense of shame.

In an era of acid rain, AIDS, nuclear disaster, and poverty, we are embarrassed by our body preoccupation — but that, of course, does not stop it.

GETTING OUT OF THE BODY TRAP

Recognizing the problem is the first step to solving it. Our work has shown that people do better when they are nonjudgmental about their concerns with body, diet, and exercise patterns. These are not trivial worries and complaints, but painful experiences and issues deserving attention. It is crucial to acknowledge the scope and depth of what you are feeling. No one is alone in their body concerns. All women share them to some extent — as do many men these days, as well.

If you treat your body with more respect, you will like it better. What your body really needs is moderate exercise, healthy foods, sensual pleasures, and relaxation. Give it those, and it will respond by treating you better. Not everyone can afford expensive trinkets or clothes, but everyone can afford small indulgences — a long, warm bath, a half-hour of time off, a new haircut. Some of you will be amazed at how hard it is to do something nice for yourself. But treating your body better will make you feel better about yourself.

To break the body-image barrier, we must bring self-image into focus. When people worry about how they look, they are worrying about who they are. That's not necessarily good, but we need to acknowledge that there is a deep connection between the two. In my work with patients, I strive to help them overcome the feeling that their happiness rises or falls depending on what the scale said that morning.

We must also look at what we really want and need from our lives and pursue those goals; it is not wise to continue expending so much of our creative energy on thinness and appearance. Since our bodies are not infinitely plastic, it may be easier to add other joys to life than to subtract pounds. Increasing and nurturing self-complexity by expanding the number of roles we value may boost health in many ways. Current research suggests that multiple roles are typically health enhancing. Varying our routines and adding new interests to our lives will help broaden our horizons so that how we look is not the sum of what we are.

As a character in Henry Jaglom's movie *Eating* says, "Twenty or thirty years ago, sex was the secret subject of women. Now it's food." In fact, sex and food have become interchangeable. "I like the feel of food. I don't like knives and forks because I like to touch it all over," says one woman. Another: "I think it is erotic. It's the safest sex you can have, eating." Food. It is comfort, balm for a trying day in a trying world, sometimes even more. Moderation is the best advice. It is the key to body sanity.

Whether we want to value, accept, or change our bodies, we need first to change our minds. We have to relearn how we observe ourselves. Instead of searching for flaws, we must attempt to see ourselves objectively. We must scrutinize our appearance less.

Caring about our bodies is normal, but how we look has become far too significant. Women have become martyrs to their appearance, slaves of that impossible master, perfection. Men go through life judged mostly on their achievements; women bear the burden of society's image. Although the effort is exhausting and painful, the deep, psychological significance of the body has made it seem worthwhile.

The burden of maintaining a perfect body image is far too costly. Women are coupled by a tragic degree of self-consciousness that limits other aspects of their lives — friendships, careers, even families.

One of the most important steps toward changing your body image is to have compassion for the millions of women struggling with their own body-image problems — especially for yourself. It is time to face the person you see in the mirror with profound new insight: She hasn't been worrying about nothing. In fact, she hasn't been taking the real problem, body preoccupation, seriously enough. Neither has society. It's time to understand the price she has been paying and help her shed that burden.

Who's the
Healthiest
of Them
All?

By Laura Fraser

It's Saturday morning in Beverly Hills, just before class at the Slimmons fitness studio. Several women in tropically bright T-shirts and tights are taking their places on the dance floor, already tapping their aerobic shoes. Aside from the pink neon lights that zig-zag across the ceiling, this looks like a typical workout class, with one difference: Most of the participants weigh around 200 pounds.

Richard Simmons, the curly-haired fitness dynamo familiar to anyone who watches late-night TV, prances up to the front of the room, his fuchsia tank top and nylon shorts sparkling in the mirror. This is ground zero of America's weight loss culture, where Simmons inspires his followers to sweat their way to the nirvana of a thinner body. "The disco's open all night!" he yells, throwing a record onto the stereo. He leads the group in slow, stretching warm-ups before heating things up with grapevine steps, shuffles, and *Saturday Night Fever* moves.

In the back, I'm kick-stepping, shimmying, and sweating along with the rest. Simmons's routine is slower-paced than the aerobics classes I'm used to, which are geared toward sleek-bodied gym rats (at 5 foot 6 and 155 pounds, I'm usually the chubbiest one there). But it's still a good workout. It's surprising how well these large women move, throwing their bodies into steps with grace and gusto, and completing every set of stomach crunches, leg lifts, and bicycle kicks. Many seem to be in such good shape, with bulging calf muscles and confident dance posture, that I wonder: Is it possible to be fat and also fit?

Most members of the Slimmons class wouldn't say so. They're here to lose weight — and if they didn't think exercise would help them do just that, they might not show up for class. Between routines, Simmons keeps up a patter on the theme of weight loss. "If you have a problem, a baloney sandwich won't solve it," he says. At Slimmons, joining the ranks of the slender and healthy is the motivation and the fantasy. "Debbie lost 67 pounds," Simmons tells the group, pointing to a blond woman in her forties. "She had her belly button redone. She picked Cher's."

Simmons doesn't think it's possible to be fat and fit, either. "Fat kills," he says later, sitting on the lavender carpet of his *Gone With the Wind*-style mansion way up in the hills. "You go from being chubby, to fat, to obese, to morbidly obese. And then there's death." Only losing weight can save people from that fate, he believes. But try as he might, Simmons can't help everyone. His big brown eyes fill with tears. "I've lost so many people."

Most Americans agree with Simmons that fat kills. Why else would doctors always have us step on the scale first thing, or harp in public-health brochures about the risk of gaining weight? Why else would medical experts pen best-sellers with titles like *Fit or Fat* and *Lose Weight, Live Longer?* In the past two years, two highly publicized studies boiled every thing down to a simple dictum: If you want to duck heart disease, stroke, high blood pressure, diabetes, and even some cancers, you'd better not weigh too much. "Even mild to moderate overweight is associated with a substantial increase in risk of premature death," said Harvard epidemiologist JoAnn Manson, author of one of those studies.

Against this backdrop of medical certainty, however, late last year another study tracking weight's relationship to good health came to a different conclusion. Epidemiologist Steven Blair and colleagues at the Cooper Institute for Aerobics Research in Dallas followed 25,389 men who had checkups at the clinic since 1974. Yes, as a group fat men were more likely to get sick and die early than thinner ones, he found. But then Blair added the men's physical fitness to the equation. Among the fit men (those who exercised regularly), he found, the fat ones lived as long as the thinner ones. And the thinner men who were out of shape were nearly three times more likely to die young than the fat men who exercised regularly.

Think about it. The people who weighed average or below average lived no longer than the overweight ones — unless they exercised. And the chunky ones lived just as long — if they exercised. In other words, once Blair controlled for how much exercise the men did — and he's sure the same would go for women — their weight had no bearing on how long they lived.

What a bombshell, thought Steven Blair when he started seeing these results a few years back. It meant that the most influential obesity researchers in the land have spent the last few years beckoning us to fret and obsess about something that may be totally irrelevant: how much we weigh.

Worried, we certainly are. In a society where weight was already a daily concern for tens of millions of women, recent news from the health experts has been truly scary. C. Everett Koop, in his 1994 "Shape Up America" campaign report, called overweight "one of the most pervasive health threats affecting Americans today." Soon after, the Institute of Medicine declared war on the nation's "epidemic of obesity," which was followed by survey results showing that Americans had gained an average of eight pounds in the past decade. Fueling the alarm were the research findings of Manson and another Harvard epidemiologist, Walter Willett. Front-page headlines blared their message that being even 20 pounds overweight invites disease and poor health, and stories quoted the researchers as saying that the U.S. weight guidelines were far too lenient.

Both studies used as a measurement of weight something called Body Mass Index (weight in kilograms divided by height in meters squared). For point of reference, my BMI is 25. So is that of the average American woman, who is 5 foot 4 and weighs 144

If you're fit, Blair found, being 25 or even 75 pounds overweight is perfectly healthy. And if you aren't fit, being slim gives you no protection whatsoever.

pounds. Roseanne's BMI is probably well over 30, and someone like Kate Moss's is closer to 18. So here was what caught every one's eye: Manson found that anyone with a BMI of more than 21 — that's just 123 pounds for a 5 foot 4 woman — has a 30 percent higher risk of early death, unless she loses weight. Someone with a BMI of 25, Willett found, is twice as likely to keel over from heart disease as someone smaller.

Along comes Steven Blair with his message of hope for the chubby and alarm for the overconfident thin. As the author of stacks of articles on exercise published in prestigious medical journals. Blair has long been highly regarded by obesity researchers. But now he couldn't be more at odds with them. After all, he's found that as long as they get in good shape, someone who's overweight by 20, 30, or even 75 pounds is at no particular health risk. And, to the more than 100 million Americans credited with having healthy weights, Blair issues a grave warning. If you don't regularly work up a sweat — surveys show that two in three of us don't — being slim is no protection whatsoever.

To find his way to that conclusion, for the past ten years Blair has looked at results of checkups more than 100,000 people have taken at the Cooper Clinic, a colonial-style red brick building just down the jogging path from his institute. As part of that check-up, each subject climbed on the machine that's at the core of his research: the treadmill.

It's an innocent-looking gym machine, even when you're stepping up to it with electrodes attached to your chest to measure your heart rate. When I tried it, starting off, the pace seemed like an easy stroll; but, after several minutes, with the incline increasing, it became a hike up Mount Everest. The longer you can stay on the treadmill without crying uncle, the fitter you are, Blair says. Gasping for air, I kept it up for 21 minutes, just long enough to get a "superior" fitness rating for a woman my age, in her thirties. And to Blair, it's that number on the treadmill, not the one on the scale, that matters.

Blair follows a long line of epidemiologists who've analyzed large groups of people to try to figure out whether diet, fitness level, or weight is the real key to good health. But his conclusion that exercise (and also diet, though he doesn't study nutritional factors) is far more important than weight is based on more than his research. It's personal. Blair describes himself as "short, bald, and fat," and says there's not much he can do about any one of those traits. On the evidence of his own life, he says, "I am convinced that you can be fat and fit."

Indeed, Blair's BMI of over 30 puts him well into the supposed danger zone for disease and early death. Yet he exercises as regularly as he flosses his teeth, running several miles a day, and eats a diet loaded with vegetables and grains and low in fat. So even if he followed the advice to adopt an even lower-fat, lower-calorie diet, he doubts he'd get healthier or be able to keep the weight off. Study after study, he says, shows that obesity is mainly a matter of genetics, and that most dieters gain back what they lose.

Blair wonders if obesity researchers still focus on weight because of a bias against fatness. He points out that it would be almost impossible for him to get a study published in one of the leading medical journals that focused on the longevity benefits of exercise without taking weight into account. "Yet those journals publish papers on obesity that give very short shrift to physical activity and fitness." (His study was published in *International Journal of Obesity*, a specialty journal read mainly by doctors and researchers who study fatness.)

Many people who publish studies on the risks of obesity, he observes wryly, are themselves quite thin. "I may be biased, too, because I'm big," he says. "I'd just like to see someone collect data on activity and convince me I'm wrong."

So far, though, none of the studies credited with linking obesity to ill health — not Manson's, not Willett's, not any in the history of this field — factored in the subjects' fitness level. And that leads to mistaken results, Blair says, because though excess weight is associated with cardiovascular disease, high blood pressure, diabetes, and colon cancer, those are exactly the problems regular exercise can prevent.

"The kinds of diseases we see in overweight people are the same diseases we see in sedentary and unfit people of *every* weight," he says. Other researchers can always find a correlation between weight and early death because fewer heavy people than slender people exercise, he says. But that doesn't mean there are no fat exercisers (40 percent of the overweight people he's studied are reasonably fit), or thin people who haven't worked up a sweat in years.

"The challenge that I like to throw out to obesity researchers is, 'How can you be so sure it's weight that kills?'" Blair says, and chuckles. "Maybe it's just inactivity."

JoAnn Manson finds that hard to believe. "I'm the first to say that physical activity is tremendously important," she says. "But you can't go to the extreme of saying it's 100 percent physical activity,

and body weight means nothing." Manson, along with Walter Willett, doubts that fit, heavy people are as common as Blair suggests (she mentions football players as one exception) and thinks they are only a tiny subgroup of large people. "Overweight and inactivity are intimately linked," she says.

Manson, like most obesity researchers, argues that extra fatty tissue itself contributes to heart disease. In her scenario, fat cells — particularly those in the belly — release fatty acids directly into the liver, where they interfere with the liver's job of breaking down insulin, thereby increasing the amount of insulin circulating in the body. Thus ensues a vicious cycle known as insulin resistance, she says: With more insulin circulating, cells grow more resistant to what it does — metabolize fat — and so produce even more liver-damaging fatty acids. This can cause problems from high blood sugars, high blood pressure, and lower HDL (good) cholesterol to heart attacks. Some people, Manson says, can exercise so much that the effects of excess body fat are negligible. "But Steve Blair is the exception," she says "not the rule."

Blair agrees that belly fat itself can be dangerous, but says most anyone can fight off insulin resistance with regular exercise, which both burns off fat and tunes up the body's metabolism. In his view, that leaves only those with a 40-plus BMI (about a hundred points over average weight) — who in practical terms are too fat to get out and walk — actually *needing* to lose weight. That's 3 percent of us. Otherwise, the 35 percent of us who are categorized by the Institute of Medicine as "mildly" or "moderately" obese (BMI between 27 and 35) and even the additional 5 percent who are considered "severely" obese (between 35 and 40) are committing to crime against our health prospects, he says, We're just heavy.

"Across America, millions of women get on the scale every morning and have their day determined by the numbers they read," says Blair. "We need to forget about the scale and focus instead on regular activity."

A few researchers agree with him. "We've been far too hung up on weight," says C. Wayne Callaway, a George Washington University endocrinologist who's been waging a longtime campaign to loosen the U.S. Dietary Guidelines for weight. Though it's only one study, Callaway says, Blair's report begins to drive home the idea that weight is the crudest measurement of health. "I'd much rather see a heavy person who's been physically active in my office than a skinny person who's completely out of shape," he says. A couch potato is a couch potato, no matter what its size.

Callaway, like Blair, doesn't think fat is never a threat; if he sees a patient who exercises but still has a big belly and other risk factors for disease (high blood pressure or high cholesterol or blood sugar levels), he'll suggest the patient try to slowly trim down by exercising even more and cutting calories. But blanket advice that fat people need to lose weight makes no sense. "I see a lot of fit and fat people," he says, "especially women who have fat in their hips and thighs, which doesn't do them any harm."

To the average person who is worried about the size of her thighs, all this squabbling among researchers may just seem academic. After all, ask Blair, Callaway, Manson, or Willett and what you should *do* to improve your health, and you get exactly the same answer: Exercise regularly and eat a diet that is high in vegetables and grains and relatively low in fat. But to the person considering whether to lace up her walking shoes in the morning, thinking your health depends mostly on your weight encourages a certain mind-set. Let's say your weight meets the standards set by obesity researchers. Well, you'd logically ask, why work out? Or maybe you decide your weight puts you in the danger zone and do start working out. What then?

Unless you have someone like Richard Simmons telling you how wonderful you are, exercising solely to lose weight is usually a negative experience. "Many people are gung-ho in the beginning, but after three weeks, when they haven't lost a lot of weight, they stop coming," says Cinder Ernst, a personal trainer who teaches fitness classes for large women in San Francisco. "And then they've lost all the other benefits of exercise — flexibility, strength, mobility, stress reduction, and self-confidence."

People who exercise without expecting to thin down last much longer, Ernst says. Pay Lyons, the coauthor of *Great Shape: The Fitness Guide for Large Women*, agrees. She runs fitness classes for Kaiser Permanente in Oakland, California, and doesn't even encourage the women in her classes to lose weight.

"The big question with exercise, which is difficult to fit into your life, is, Why bother?" says Lyons, who, even at 5 foot 8 and 240 pounds (BMI of 37), looks like someone who hikes and swims regularly — which she does. "If your goal is to fit into size 8 jeans, you set yourself up for failure," she says. "But if you do it to improve the quality of your life, to get in shape, and to feel more coordinated, you'll feel satisfied with yourself."

In one of Lyons's Great Shape classes, in Vallejo, California, Judy Smith*, 50-something and perhaps 220 pounds, says she used to be afraid even to walk around the block for fear of ridicule. Now she not only dances twice a week, but seems on four other mornings. "I have more energy, mentally as well as physically," she says.

Is this woman — who lost a few pounds with exercise but will always be fat — as healthy as she would be if she somehow managed to lose 75 more pounds? Blair thinks so. But even if not, she has gotten into good enough shape to do well on his treadmill — a far more achievable goal than massive weight loss, and one that's made her a lot healthier. In a series of studies, he's found that for each minute longer you can huff and puff on his treadmill, your risk of early death declines by nearly 10 percent.

"Do I wish I was leaner?" Blair asks. "Yes, I do. But I don't have much control over that. I can control how much I exercise."

Many experts who focus on weight are themselves quite thin, Blair says. "I may be biased, too, because I'm big. I'd just like them to convince me I'm wrong.

In this culture, where thinness is not only associated with health, but with success, discipline, morality, and fantasies of a glamorous life, almost all of us long to be thin. Would I trade my size 12 body for a size 8? Sure, and if the Fairy Godmother wants to throw in an extra two inches of height and a photographic memory, I'm game. But this is real life here. Wishing, like dieting, won't give you a different body than the one you were born with.

In the privacy of his sherbet-hued living room, Richard Simmons must admit that for every one of his followers who loses lots of weight, many more find that their fat is very stubborn, Try as they might, he says, they're never going to wear thong-bottomed leotards or show their navels. Even he himself, he points out, exercise maniac that he is, has a little potbelly.

But even when his "ladies" don't lose a pound, he says, their blood pressure goes down, their cholesterol levels flatten out, they have more energy, and they feel better about themselves. "They're still fat," Simmons says. "But I see them blossom."

Thin or fat, *everyone* who exercises with him, Simmons must concede, gets healthy.

*This name has been changed

Laura Fraser is a contributing editor.

As researchers begin to understand the legacy of childhood sexual abuse, its long-term impact on women's physical and psychological health is becoming increasingly clear.

Sexual Abuse: The Longest Legacy

Childhood sexual abuse is a crime of the heart, a theft of innocence trust and self-esteem. And whether it's discovered immediately or revealed only decades later, it can have a long-term impact on a woman's health.

Only now is this damaging legacy being talked about openly, much less studied in any consistent way. Even so, it's becoming increasingly clear that abuse often has a hand in a diverse array of seemingly unrelated physical and psychological complaints including anxiety, depression, eating disorders, pelvic pain, gastrointestinal disorders, and chronic pain (see "A Common Thread").

Moreover sexual abuse isn't a rare phenomenon. Although firm numbers remain elusive, random interviews in the general population suggest that one in every five women has been abused, says psychiatrist Frank Putnam, M.D., chief of the Unit on Developmental Thaumatology at the National Institutes of Mental Health.

THE GREATEST PAIN

It's not hard to understand why sexual abuse is so damaging. A powerful and often deeply loved and trusted adult violates the physical, psychological and moral integrity of a dependent child. The acts are surrounded by shame, secrecy, fear, and often threats and physical pain. The violation can destroy a child's sense of trust, her feeling that the world is a good and safe place and even her sense of self.

Why some women manage to come through this trauma relatively intact and others break apart isn't well understood. Each individual's unique psychological makeup — perhaps an inborn hardiness or resilience — probably plays a role. But the circumstances of the abuse also appear to influence the outcome.

"It's hard to figure out what hurts the most" says Dr. Putnam. "We've looked at the age when the abuse first occurred, how long it continued, the type of abuse, the relationship of the perpetrator, and the reactions of the nonoffending parent — and they all appear to have some effect. But these factors are complicatedly connected in various ways," he says.

"We think that the relationship of the perpetrator is a very important variable," he continues. "The closer the relationship, the worse it is. A biological father and daughter, for example, appears worse than a step-father and stepdaughter."

Repressing Memories

Can a trauma be so unthinkable that the mind simply buries it and wipes out all memory of the event until some detail decades later brings it all back? That's one of the most hotly debated questions in the psychiatric community today.

Even critics of the "repressed memory movement" concede that about 18% of sexually abused women have some degree of amnesia.

The real controversy centers on charges that some therapists are using the phenomenon of repressed memory to find evidence of sexual abuse in nearly every woman who walks through the door.

Fortunately, most sexual abuse experts believe that such clinical situations are rare. More commonly, they say, women begin to recover memories in their daily lives and then seek therapy to help clarify the disturbing revelations.

The self-help movement, too, has come under some criticism. Many books have encouraged women to get needed help. But critics say that overly inclusive checklists of abuse symptoms and broad generalizations such as "If you think you may have been abused, then you were" ultimately do a disservice by eroding the legitimacy of a real and all-too-common crime against women.

From *Women's Health Advocate* (June 1996), pp. 4-5. Reprinted with permission from *Women's Health Advocate Newsletter*. For subscriptions call 1-800-829-5876 and ask for the introductory price of $16 per year, a 33% discount.

Earlier-onset abuse also seems to predict a worse outcome but it's also related to the length of time the abuse continues. Women who've had multiple abusers, Dr. Putnam notes, generally have more difficulty and may be more likely to develop dissociative symptoms, such as amnesia.

And disclosure of the abuse is another critical and complicated issue.

In a study recently submitted for publication, Dr. Putnam's group found that girls who disclose their

---

A Common Thread

Researchers now realize that a history of sexual abuse plays a role in several conditions:

- **Depression**. Women with a history of abuse are three to five times more likely to suffer from depression than women who weren't abused. Moreover, several studies have found that sexually abused women also are more refractory to treatment.

- **Anxiety disorders**. Childhood sexual abuse is believed to be a component of many cases of panic disorder, social phobia, and obsessive-compulsive disorder. A study reported in the February *American Journal of Psychiatry* found that 45% of a group of women with anxiety disorders had been abused, versus 15% of a control group. The link with panic disorder was particularly strong with 60% of those women reporting an abusive past.

- **Eating disorders**. The American Psychiatric Association estimates that 30% to 50% of women with eating disorders have a history of sexual abuse. Several studies have suggested high rates of sexual abuse among bulimic women in particular, but the true impact of abuse on eating disorders is a matter of continuing debate.

- **Substance abuse**. Among female substance abusers, 60% or more report sexual victimization in childhood. As with depression, sexual abuse both contributes to the development of the disorder and makes it harder to treat.

- **Gastrointestinal disorders**. In the April *Gastroenterology*, researchers reported that 60% of 239 women referred for treatment of gastrointestinal disorders had a history of sexual or physical abuse. The percentage varied according to diagnosis: 38% of 21 patients with ulcerative colitis reported a history of abuse, while 67% of 43 patients with irritable bowel syndrome and 84% of 19 patients with functional abdominal pain had been abused.

Like many studies on the health consequences of abuse, this investigation was flawed in that it didn't limit itself to sexual abuse. Hopefully upcoming studies will be able to shed more light on whether the long-term consequences of sexual abuse differ from those of physical or emotional abuse.

---

abuse have a harder time than girls who either don't disclose or are accidentally discovered. The researchers speculate that girls who tell feel more responsible for the devastating effects disclosure can have on a family.

How the disclosure is received appears crucial, as well. is the child believed? Does she have supportive people to help her? With children in particular, the response of the nonoffending parent is critical.

TELLING AND HEALING

When a woman seeks medical care, a history of sexual abuse will add another dimension to her treatment. The caregiver must treat the symptoms — the anxiety or unexplained pelvic pain, for example — but also work with the trauma history.

If a woman seeks therapy, its best to find a therapist who's sophisticated about the effects of post-traumatic stress disorder, Dr. Putnam says. That's because some of its symptoms, such as hallucinations and flashbacks are so unusual that a patient may be misdiagnosed as psychotic.

Most therapists believe that telling the story of the abuse is central to healing and that the victim can't resolve the experience until she tells and is heard not only by her therapist but by the people involved.

Though disclosure of sexual abuse is typically devastating for a family, many families do get beyond it, Dr. Putnam says. And the family members' responses are critical. "We find that the patient very much mirrors how well the family handles it," he reports. "If the family isn't doing well, the patient doesn't do well."

Concerning the long-term outcome for abused women, Dr. Putnam says, "Some women are relatively unaffected. They continue to have good social, educational, and occupational attainment. Then there are those who are really devastated, some of whom end up institutionalized. In between are the walking wounded — women who continue to have problems and never do as well as might have been expected."

Does therapy help? The broad answer is yes. Though scientific studies haven't been able to demonstrate a big difference in outcome, patients often maintain that therapy was very important to them. In addition, many women who were abused as children have found additional comfort and strength in support groups.

In the final analysis, if you're a victim of abuse it is important to remember that you're not alone, it's not your fault, and you're never too old to heal.

RESOURCES:

Survivors of Incest Anonymous. This 12-step, self-help program has more than 800 groups nationwide. Write P.O. Box 21817 Baltimore, Md. 21222 or call (410) 282-3400.

Voices in Action. This group offers meetings and publications. For information, call (312) 327-1500.

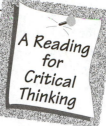

A Reading for Critical Thinking

Why Is Date Rape So Hard To Prove?

By Sheila Weller

With acquaintance rape cases now a TV spectator sport, lots of women I know are having some variation of this black-humored fantasy: You're on the witness stand, watching an expensively suited defense attorney pace around as he spits out accusations: What about those one-night stands six years ago? Your taste for double margaritas? Is it true that you met this man at a nightclub? And weren't you wearing a lace camisole under your blouse? That's the last straw. You stand up, rip the fuzzy blue dot off your face and say, "I give up! Let the bastard walk. It's not worth this trying to convict him."

After the past year's parade of well-publicized rape cases, such fantasy seems all too black and none too humorous. First there was the William Kennedy Smith case, during which the New York Times implied that rape complainant Patricia Bowman's speeding tickets bolstered a schoolmate's claim of her "little wild streak." More recently, when a young Manhattan architect accused three New York Mets of rape, her ex-boyfriend, Mets pitcher David Cone, reportedly told her that no one would believe her and her reputation would be ruined. He turned out to be right on both scores. The *New York Post* trumpeted the headline: "Mets accuser was 'No Vestal Virgin.'" And in early April, the Florida state attorney, pointing to a lack of physical evidence, decided to drop the case. The message to women has been clear: Many of us would not make believable accusers.

Not that a woman who says she's been raped shouldn't be scrutinized. After all, what about the reputation of the accused? There's no getting around the fact that acquaintance rape is a crime in which the victim and the sole eyewitness are often one and the same. Both sides admit they had intercourse. The only issue is consent. When it's her word against his, it's only fair that her credibility and ulterior motives be questioned.

But that doesn't mean the woman is the one who should go on trial. All too often the legitimate question "Did this woman consent to intercourse?" leaps dangerously to "Was she leading him on?" In another recent case, a group of young men from prominent Tampa families admitted to drugging a woman and then raping her. The defense argued that by willingly accompanying the men after a night of drinking, she invited the ensuing events. The men were acquitted.

No wonder so few women actually report being raped. A new study by the National Victim Center estimates that one in eight women in the United States has been raped, in most cases by someone she knew, but that only about 16 percent of the rapes were reported. Of those cases that are reported, the majority are dropped by the prosecutor, according to Gary LaFree, a sociologist at the University of New Mexico and author of *Rape and Criminal Justice*. Only the rare resilient case, roughly one to 5 percent of all rapes, actually reaches the courtroom.

The road into and out of that court room can be so treacherous that even some rape counselors question whether it's worth it. "When I first started working here," says Colleen Leyrer of the Washington, D.C., Rape Crisis Center, "I was uncomfortable not encouraging a woman to prosecute. Now, after seeing victims go through a second trauma as a result of prosecuting, I urge the woman to decide for herself."

It's a tough decision — one that a woman should make with both eyes open. "If it's likely the case will end in acquittal, and if the woman's wavering, then I

From *Health* (July/August 1992), pp. 62-64. Reprinted with permission from *HEALTH*. © 1992.

probably wouldn't recommend prosecution," says Andrea Parrot, a rape expert and psychologist at Cornell University.

But how does a woman know whether her case is likely to end in acquittal? How can she know if it will even make it to the courtroom? The people who deal with acquaintance rape cases daily — prosecutors, judges, defense attorneys — know firsthand why so few of them end in conviction. Here's what they say makes acquaintance rape so hard to prove.

Unless the woman is a girl scout or virgin, the jury will give more weight to her character than to the evidence.

Even the Mike Tyson conviction seemed to confirm this theory: Wasn't Desiree Washington a naive, churchgoing teenager? "A woman who has a good reputation, does not dress suggestively, has a nine-to-five job, and goes home after work will be looked on more favorably by a jury," says Brooks Leach, sex crimes prosecutor in Columbia, Alabama.

In a study of 880 rape cases, sociologist Gary LaFree found that a complainant's "questionable" character was the best predictor of a defendant's acquittal. "We found that juries were most swayed by things like whether she had been drinking or even if she had birth control pills in her pocket," says LaFree. Juries find it more important that a woman frequents bars than that the man had a gun; more important that she had sex outside of marriage than that she was physically injured in the rape; more important that she was a "party girl" than that her clothes were torn that evening.

But you don't have to be a wanton woman for your morality to be suspect. Anyone who's had multiple sexual partners or an abortion is vulnerable. Even though 40 states now have "rape shield" laws making details of an accuser's past sexual life inadmissable in trials, such legislation is hardly foolproof. "There's an insidious way to get around the law," says sociologist Susan Caringella-McDonald. "Defense attorneys question the woman about her past sexual activity; the prosecutor objects; the judge sustains the objection — but the jury's already heard it so the damage is done."

Many well-off defendants hire private investigators to scout for information on accusers that can either be "leaked" at the trial or used to derail a case before it reaches the courtroom. "We'll do a surveillance of a rape complainant to find out: Does she go to parties and bars? Leave with somebody? Come home drunk?" says attorney Marshall Stern of Bangor, Maine. "You can't use these findings on the stand, but it's a bargaining tool with the prosecutor. If

you say, 'See, she smoked dope here . . . ,' he may not think he has the winning case he once had."

Even a woman who's been sexually abused in the past might be considered less credible if that comes out in court, says Nancy Hollander, president of the National Association of Criminal Defense Attorneys: "If she has a history of abuse, we can use it to suggest that it's left her misunderstanding signals and thinking she was raped when she wasn't."

The more romantic contact the woman had with the man, the tougher her case is to win. "You can almost diagram it," says Nancy Diehl, assistant prosecuting attorney for Detroit's Wayne County. "Fair to good is: The woman was in her or his house with him voluntarily, but she didn't have a previous relationship with him, it wasn't late at night, and she didn't kiss him. The more of those conditions that change from negative to positive, the harder it gets to win the case."

Patricia Bowman's case, for instance, was crippled by the lateness and the kissing. "When a woman has been acting in a way that juries see as encouraging a sexual encounter, they tend to say, 'Lady, you can't act like that and then change your mind,'" says Rock Harmon, deputy district attorney in Oakland, California. One of the most outrageous examples of this kind of bias occurred in the Tampa case. A defendant (later acquitted) explained at the trial that the complainant used profanity, smoked cigarettes, and dressed in green stretch pants: "She was not commanding as much respect from the guys as we would normally give other, more ladylike females."

Women jurors can often be hardest on women, perhaps because they want to deny that they too could be victims. Larry Donoghue, head of one of the sex crimes units of the Los Angeles district attorney's office, finds that female jurors are especially biased against assertive, ambitious women. Men are often surprisingly empathetic. "Fathers and grandfathers

Juries don't have much sympathy for a woman who was a willing participant up to the time of the alleged rape.

seem to take a protective attitude toward the victim," says Des Moines–based trial consultant Hale Starr. "But religious home makers are the worst jurors for the victim. Their attitude is, 'I would never have gone to that room with that man . . .' They're unforgiving."

Still, there are some surprising exceptions. In a recent Detroit case, jurors convicted a man for the rape of a topless go-go dancer who had accepted a ride from him, changed into her street clothes in the back of his van, and driven with him in search of cocaine. Nancy Diehl says an eyewitness's testimony and strong physical evidence pushed the jurors past the tendency to believe that the woman "got what she deserved."

Rarely are there broken bones with acquaintance rape, but that doesn't mean there's no physical evidence. Even if a woman is uncertain whether she wants to pursue a complaint, she should go immediately to a doctor's office or the hospital for an examination. Forcible as opposed to consensual sex is often medically verifiable, even in long-sexually-active

Unless there's physical evidence, it's her word against his.

women. "When a woman is having consensual sex with a man, she needs to do what is referred to as a 'pelvic tilt' to accommodate his penis," says D.A. Donoghue. "In forcible sex, the last thing that she wants is to accommodate him. His force can lead to anything from reddening to bruises to lacerations. If it's just reddening, you've got to identify it fast, or it fades. It's not perfect evidence, but it can make the difference between winning and losing."

Immediate report of the assault also makes a rape victim appear more genuine. "Juries look for an immediate outcry. They want to see that she wasted no time telling the authorities," says Barry Levin, a defense attorney in the St. John's College case in which seven men were charged with gang-raping a black woman student. Levin, who plea-bargained his client down from a felony to a misdemeanor, says he got his biggest boost from the complainant, who waited a month before reporting the rape. The same holds true for the woman who accused the three Mets players a year after the rape. The prosecutor said her long delay and the resulting lack of physical evidence meant she didn't have a case.

"If you delay, the defense is going to say, 'See? She made it up to get back at the guy,' and the jury will believe it," says D.A. Nancy Diehl. "My advice always is: Report first, then decide. If you choose not to pursue the complaint, you can always back out of it."

The accuser should be calm but not robotic, testifying with feeling but not appearing overly emotional. Despite the harrowing experience she's endured, a victim who cries may be viewed as unstable. A calm but concerned woman, able to summon up the trauma without relapsing into it — like Desiree Washington — appeals more to juries.

Believability is crippled when the accuser tells a story that contains even a few loose threads, which defense attorneys use to unravel her entire story. Many prosecutors say that this is what most damaged Patricia Bowman's case: Her story was inconsistent and prosecutor Moira Lasch did her no favor by letting those inconsistencies reach the court room. "I did not find Bowman's story credible, and Lasch did not confront this before trial," says Karvn Sinunu, head of the sexual assault division of the Santa Clara County, California, district attorney's office. "I listened to Bowman say that she kissed him 'but it wasn't sexual' and I thought, You can kiss a husband of twenty years good-bye in the morning and it isn't sexual, but you don't kiss someone you've just met and it isn't sexual.' When you try to make your story sound better, the jury ends up seeing through it."

Even when a prosecutor catches all evasions well before the trial, they can come back to haunt the complainant and end up destroying her case. D.A. Donoghue tried a case in which a very credible woman had initially told police she was forced into the rapist's car: "She was too embarrassed to admit she had misjudged the man's moves when he offered her a ride home and had gotten into the car voluntarily." Though she corrected her story by trial time, the original falsification was bandied about by the defense attorney: If she had lied about that, then she could have lied about the whole thing. The defendant walked.

A skilled prosecutor plays devil's advocate early on, gently pushing the woman past her urge to apply face-saving spin control to her memory of the ordeal. "The woman needs to convince me that she was raped," says D.A. Nancy Diehl. "I say, 'Look, I need the whole truth. No matter how bad you think it looks, if you tell me, I'll be able to explain it to the jury.'"

Emotional or conflicting testimony can destroy a woman's credibility.

These days, with Desiree Washington's success as inspiration, prosecutors say more women are deciding to press charges on a crime that has mostly been endured in silence and shame. But individual women can't be expected to live their day-in-and-day-out lives as political symbols, or as statistics in a war against apathy. In the end, the decision to pursue prosecution is deeply personal. "Victims and psychiatrists tell me it's therapeutic to prosecute," says Donoghue. Wanda Jones, who became a victims' service officer in Birmingham, Alabama, after she was raped by seven men, says the experience of seeing her rapists brought to justice was empowering. Says sociologist Andrea Parrot: "Some women, even understanding the likelihood of the man's acquittal, need to go through with prosecution to feel whole and vindicated. In those cases, I'd say go ahead."

Sheila Weller is the author of Marrying the Hangman, *recently published by Random House.*

PART 3

Reproductive Health Issues

Reproductive health is often at the forefront of discussions of women's health. The reasons for this emphasis are obvious: women have monthly cycles and can bear children. But women's health issues also tend to be limited by this association. Sometimes we hear about reproductive issues at the expense of other health concerns.

This section focuses on some of the emerging discussions about fertility and/or infertility. The readings on fertility present a variety of perspectives. The controversial reading on "Conception at Any Cost?" examines the expenses involved in treating infertility, the low success rate of many of the treatments, and the pitfalls of insurance coverage, or lack thereof, for these treatments. Couples spend time, money, and emotional energy on fertility treatments. But have we fully examined the costs of these treatments and the ethical considerations of assisted reproduction?

Another reading deserves special mention as well. The reading on the maternal birthing position (Reading 19) shows how the manner in which women give birth in the United States has evolved and changed over time. The reading illustrates, as with so many other issues in women's health, that standard medical practices may not always be in a woman's best interest. (Please see the **Quick Reference Guide to Topics/Readings/WWW Sites** and **Appendix A: WebLinks: A Directory of Annotated World Wide Web Sites** to select WWW sites that coordinate with the readings in this part.)

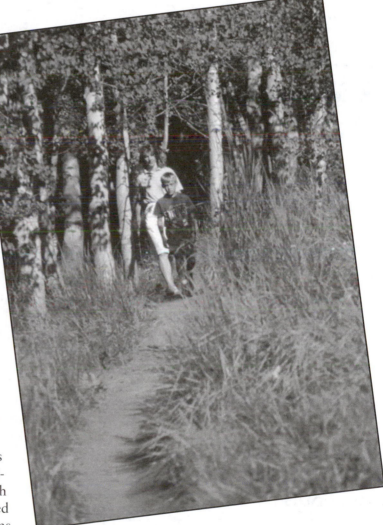

Conception at Any Cost?

One in six couples is infertile, though some of them are already parents.
In the quest to conceive, are they being given false hope?
And are they paying too high a price — in time, money,
and mental and physical well-being — to get pregnant?

A Reading for Critical Thinking

By Rosemary Black

When their daughter, Kaitlyn, turned 2, Karen and John Kilduff, who live in New Jersey, stopped using birth control. Two years, several thousand dollars, three doctors, and six cycles worth of fertility drugs later. Karen, 35, still wasn't pregnant. She decided to stop taking the fertility drugs, and her doctor scheduled a procedure called a laparoscope to see whether she might have a problem he hadn't diagnosed.

But two days before the procedure, Karen took a required pregnancy test — just in case. As it turned out, she was pregnant. "I was ecstatic," says Karen, who is due in August.

So far, Julie Mitchell, 35, hasn't been as lucky. She and her husband, David, 37, who live in upstate New York, began trying to conceive when their daughter, Katie, now 5½, was 1½. At one point, Julie took the drug Clomid for three months. "I was miserable, screaming half the time and crying the other half," she recalls.

Julie says she's been trying to get pregnant for so long that she's not even sure she wants another child.

However, she and David are still being treated by fertility specialists. "I don't want to be sorry in 10 years," she says. "So I'm not leaving any stone unturned."

One in six couples — about 5.3 million — in the U.S. is infertile, but not all of them are childless: The American Society for Reproductive Medicine (ASRM) in Birmingham, Alabama, estimates 1.3 million women suffer from secondary infertility.

Infertility patients can now take advantage of high-tech procedures that were unheard of even a few years ago. But these advancements in infertility treatment come at a price. It's not unusual for an infertile couple's out-of-pocket medical expenses to reach $30,000. Infertility treatment often takes over a couple's life, and it can put a major strain on the marriage. It extracts an emotional toll as well, which even the best-intentioned doctor may not tell you about. Likewise, your physician may not tell you when to call it quits.

And according to a few studies, fertility drugs may increase your chances of getting ovarian cancer. So how can a couple evaluate when to continue and

Conception

The Road to Fertility	Unprotected sex three times a week for a year	Semenalysis	Ovulation test	Cervical mucus test
While fertility treatments vary from couple to couple, depending on the nature of each couple's problems, the following are some of the steps that infertile couples commonly go through.	If no results, see a doctor about underlying physical conditions.	In this procedure, motility, morphology, and quantity of sperm are tested by a urologist.	Using various methods, doctors see if woman is ovulating.	Have sex an hour before going to the gynecologist who will test cervical mucus to check that it's healthy.

when to give up? Here's the latest on the options, the risks, and your odds of bringing home a baby.

INFERTILITY TODAY

Although overall infertility rates have remained fairly constant in the last three decades, The National Center for Health Statistics (NCHS) in Hyattsville, Maryland, reports that the infertility rate has increased for the segment of the population most likely to have trouble getting pregnant: women between the ages of 35 and 44.

Many factors play a role in infertility — exposure to pollutants; use of alcohol, cigarettes, and recreational drugs; the proliferation of sexually transmitted diseases. However, waiting to have kids is a major cause of infertility today, says Zev Rosenwaks, M.D., director of the Center for Reproductive Medicine and Infertility at New York Hospital-Cornell Medical Center in New York City.

According to the ASRM, nearly 40 percent of infertility cases are due to male conditions, such as sperm problems. Another 40 percent of problems may be traced to a female condition. In the remaining 20 percent of cases, either both partners are infertile or doctors can't identify the problem.

But for most couples, the options these days are truly wondrous. Zygote intra-fallopian transfer (ZIFT) is a variation of in-vitro fertilization (IVF) in which the egg is fertilized in the lab and the embryo is placed in the fallopian tube, allowing for natural movement to the uterus. With gamete intra-fallopian transfer (GIFT), another IVF variation, a sperm and egg are placed, unfertilized, in the fallopian tube, where fertilization and, hopefully, implantation occur.

Both ZIFT and GIFT have a slightly higher success rate than IVF. Pamela Madsen, 33, president of RESOLVE New York City, a local chapter of the national advocacy and support group for infertile couples, tried to get pregnant for two years before she had Tyler, now 6, with GIFT. Four years later, with the help of IVF, she gave birth to Spencer. "The procedures

Is Bad Sperm to Blame?

By Rebecca Baumgold

A study of French sperm donors just published in *The New England Journal of Medicine* found semen quality is on the decline.

However, "the studies to date don't prove that sperm count and quality are changing in the general male population," says infertility expert Richard Sherins, M.D. Dr. Sherins's chief faults with this study: It included only sperm donors, not a representative sampling of men. It relied on only one sample per subject, and sperm count can vary from week to week. Finally, it didn't look at whether reduced sperm counts affected subjects' fertility.

involved surgery and anesthesia, but I looked at it like this: Everything we do in life has a risk," she says.

Infertility treatment doesn't come with any guarantees. In fact, "The chances of failure are pretty good," says Arthur Caplan, Ph.D., Philadelphia based author of *Moral Matters: Ethical Issues in Medicine*. "And while I've never seen a group more desperate to have a child than infertility patients, there's also a need for honesty. It's the physician's responsibility to say when it is hopeless to continue."

Fortunately, new federal laws help protect couples from fertility clinics' exaggerated claims. All fertility clinics are now required to report their pregnancy success rates to the Centers for Disease Control and Prevention in Atlanta, which will publish them annually.

Just what are your chances for success? Many experts estimate that 65 percent of those who seek treatment will eventually have a baby. In the process, though, many women endure years of expensive, physically invasive procedures — and the treatment is fraught with risks.

Studies have found a link between fertility drugs and ovarian cancer (see "The Clomid-Cancer Connection"). Leslie Laurence, a New York City-based co-author of *Outrageous Practices: The Alarming Truth*

Laparoscopy
In this surgical procedure, doctors check the fallopian tubes, uterine lining, and ovaries.

Infertility specialist
An infertility specialist may prescribe fertility drugs, like Clomid or Perganol, or try in-vitro techniques.

Artificial insemination
This is a procedure in which sperm is separated out of partner or donor semen and placed directly in the uterus or fallopian tube.

In-vitro fertilization
A fertilized egg, or embryo, is surgically inserted in the fallopian tube.

The Clomid-Cancer Connection

A study at the University of Washington and the Fred Hutchinson Cancer Research Center in Seattle describing a possible link between Clomid and ovarian cancer is just the latest of many studies to implicate certain fertility drugs with this disease.

Ovarian cancer is difficult to diagnose. In its early stages, it produces no symptoms, and three-fourths of all cases are not diagnosed until the cancer has spread beyond the ovary. At that point, fewer than 10 percent of women are cured.

But even doctors involved in fertility drug studies are quick to note that they aren't conclusive. "The data is preliminary," says Alice Whittemore, Ph.D., of Stanford University in Palo Alto, California, who co-authored a study linking ovarian cancer and fertility drugs. "Women who can't get pregnant may be at a higher risk for ovarian cancer because of problems with their ovaries, not because of the drugs."

Follow-up studies are underway. Meanwhile, the medical community is not sounding a big alarm. Physicians say women should be counseled on the possible risks of drugs and shouldn't take them for extended periods. The latest study found no increased risk for women who took Clomid for less than a year.

About How Medicine Mistreats Women, worries that doctors may not know the risks of the treatments because their long-term use hasn't been studied. She points to women's health scandals such as breast implants and the Dalkon Shield IUD. "Some were used for decades before the risks became apparent," she says. Women have a legacy of not knowing the dangers of drugs we're taking."

EMOTIONAL COSTS

And yet the longing for a baby can be overpowering, leaving a woman feeling isolated from friends and relatives with kids. Guilt is common too, especially in women who put off having kids to pursue a career. Alice Domar, Ph.D., director of the Behavioral Medicine Program for Infertility at New England Deaconess Hospital in Boston, compared the psychological distress in those suffering from infertility with those who are HIV positive and who have heart disease, cancer, hypertension, or chronic pain. "The depression and anxiety experienced by infertile women are equivalent to that in women suffering from a terminal illness," she says.

Because infertility is a chronic stressor that has a cyclical effect on a woman's mood (women often mourn each time they get their period), treating the mind as well as the body is crucial, experts say. Counseling and support groups can reduce a sense of isolation and help women regain control.

Having — as well as being — a supportive spouse is also important. "Women say that their husbands never want to talk about the infertility, and husbands say they feel like it's all their wives ever want to talk about," explains Dr. Domar. "We help them learn to respect that the other person feels differently."

Couples dealing with secondary infertility need to stay attuned to their children, too. Even very young kids can pick up on parents' escalating anxiety level and change of routine. "Children know on some level something's wrong," says Harriet Fishman Simons, L.I.C.S.W., Wellesley, Massachusetts-based author of *Wanting Another Child: Coping With Secondary Infertility*. "Sharing information in an age-appropriate manner can be a way to introduce your child to ways

Infertility Causes and Cures

Here's a guide to the most common causes of infertility, plus the procedures and drugs used to treat them. Predicting the rate of success with each treatment is impossible because of various factors, a woman's age being the biggest one.

Problem	Treatment	Success Rate
Male factors (account for 40 percent of problems): low sperm count, poor sperm motility, varicocele	Surgical correction (of the varicocele), fertility drugs, artificial insemination, Intra-Cytoplasmic Sperm Injection (ICSI)	Highly individual; varies from 15 to 40 percent
Failure to ovulate (accounts for 15 percent of conception problems)	Clomid, Pergonal (by injection), HCG (sometimes used with Clomid and Pergonal)	5 to 35 percent; Pergonal's success rate is higher than Clomid's
Tubal damage (35 percent of problems): due to Pelvic Inflammatory Disease, ectopic pregnancy, or endometriosis	Tubal surgery to repair the tubes, IVF, ZIFT, GIFT	Anywhere from 15 to 65 percent
Unexplained infertility (accounts for 10 percent of conception problems)	Fertility drugs, IVF, artificial insemination	Anywhere from 15 to 35 percent

of coping with crises. Reassure your child that you'll be able to take care of her and that though you have a lot of doctor appointments, you're not sick."

THE ADOPTION OPTION

Another path to parenthood is adoption. More than 60,000 children (about half of them healthy, U.S.-born infants) are adopted through private or agency adoptions each year, according to Adoptive Families of America, a Minneapolis-based support group. "Nearly everyone can get a child in two years," says Susan Freivalds, executive director of the organization. "If you want a baby born in this country, the typical wait is one to five years."

For Ann Cohen, 41, of Chicago, adopting a baby helped end the sense of loss she felt at having been unable to conceive a second child. Less than two years after stopping fertility treatments, the Cohens adopted a baby boy. "Every child is special," Ann says. "But when you have had trouble having a baby, then you really look at your children as treasures."

Rosemary Black, an editor at The New York Daily News *lives in Pleasantville, New York, She has six children.*

Baby Love

Fertility treatments are expensive, risky, and often ineffective. Yet banning them would be a setback for women.

By Rickie Solinger

Reports of technological breakthroughs in reproductive technologies have tended to focus on the sensational and the singular: on the putative grotesqueries of post-menopausal pregnancies; and on surrogacy cases, which are invariably transformed into melodrama described as if gender, class and sometimes race exploitation were not at their heart. The media trendsetter, of course, was the "Baby M" case, reported as if it were about one lowdown, unstable and insufficiently maternal female welching on the good-faith deal she made with a proper middle-class couple — lacking only a baby in their quest for perfection.

The media dishes out these tales of perversity with relish: but the big impact of the new technologies is on the lives of ordinary women, hundreds of thousands of them, who have participated in fertility-enhancing programs in recent years. These women, who for one reason or another are apparently unable to conceive in the usual way, undergo treatments ranging from IUI (intra-uterine insemination) to egg harvesting, embryo implantation, embryo and egg freezing, the micro-injection of sperm and the micro-manipulation of ova.

Lately there has been a great deal of controversy among feminists, most often expressed in heated political terms, about the broader implications of such treatments. Such discussion generally proceeds as if it

is possible to embrace or reject any given modality of procreation for straightforwardly political reasons.

But, in this arena as in so many others, the personal is always threatening to trump the political — in ways that might be familiar, say, to progressives who feel compelled to go to extraordinary expense and other inconveniences in order to raise their children in a safe neighborhood with good schools, despite their commitment to improving the lot of all children in society. In a capitalist society, it is the rare individual who forgoes on principle the chance to buy what one values — in this instance motherhood — if one has the resources, even when it takes a special effort to fit an essentially personal choice into a deeply held politics of justice.

And so, to begin with, I'd better identify my own reproductive history: I have two biological children conceived through intercourse. It may also be relevant that I have a close relative deeply enmeshed in the full array of new reproductive technology treatments. I say this because I have the feeling that readers of this kind of article are, like me, always sleuthing the subtext. Is the writer herself a mother? And if so, what kind? A biological mother? An adoptive mother? A technologically assisted mother? Or is she a voluntarily child-free person?

The differences between those supporting and those opposing the new technologies is stark. Those who oppose them insist that the new technologies constitute a new form of violence against women, alienating them from their reproductive processes, reducing them to what critic Janice Raymond, author of *Women as Wombs*, calls "experimental raw material" or "womb environments." Supporters, such as Carol Sternhell, director of women's studies at New York University, argue that the technologies can be potentially liberating for women. "All the new alternative forms of family building are . . . challenges to our culture's dominant ideas about family," Sternhell suggests.

Raymond and the other critics can draw upon a great deal of history to back up their opposition to the new technologies. One need only recall the horrifying examples of thalidomide and the Dalkon Shield to prove that real danger can lurk in the heart of technology's promise to women desperate to manage their fertility. And it is clear that technologically assisted conception has been overhyped. The statistics are terrible, yet desperate women keep coming, a fact

From *In These Times* (September 19, 1994), pp. 17-20. Reprinted with permission from *In These Times*, a bi-weekly newsmagazine published in Chicago.

suggesting that the customers are actually being duped and even coerced into undergoing treatments that are not only physically risky but often futile.

Equally troublingly, the new technologies use up vast social and financial resources that could potentially be better spent solving existing problems such as high infant mortality rates in some parts of the United States and around the globe. (In the United States alone, fertility clinics do $2 billon of business a year.) And the technologies pose tougher issues for the ethicists. They mandate a "normalcy" standard for fetuses: all participants in the programs have the right to demand perfect babies, so fetuses that fail the test will be selectively eliminated.

In addition, the mere existence of the new technologies creates new worldwide inequities. The procedures are terribly expensive: in vitro fertilization, for example, costs $10,000 or more. And so there are multiple new opportunities for exploitation, both of women desperate to be pregnant and of poor women who, out of an extreme lack of resources, can be pressed into service as egg donors or so-called surrogate mothers.

The new technologies, Raymond suggests, are dangerous to women and to feminism because they take power and control over fertility away from desperate women and hand it over to doctors and technicians who manage and profit from the infertility empire. "Women as a class have a stake in reclaiming the female body," Raymond argues, "by refusing to yield control of it to men, to the fetus, to the state, and most recently to those liberals who advocate that women control our bodies by giving up control."

Given this house of horrors (and the sci-fi scenarios any one can conjure up, based on what seems to be possible and acceptable in the realm of reproduction today), the theorists believe that the only effective check on the evils inherent in the new technologies is a curiously "liberal" one — that the State must outlaw the whole business on the grounds that these technologies are necessarily used in ways that are unethical, dangerous for women, costly and out of sync with the common good.

While the feminists who categorically oppose the new technologies are a relatively homogeneous group, those who support them share no common analysis or creed. No single ideology fits the diverse perspectives of researchers, doctors, business types and participants in fertility programs. And, of course, the doctors and technicians who develop and deliver the new technologies and the average women who buys them may or may not identify with feminism in any form.

While Raymond and her colleagues concentrate on the big picture, the supporters of the new technologies focus on the rights of individual women. They may sometimes have the less powerful argument, medically and politically. But I am struck by their references to the sheer number of women moving through infertility programs — women ready to make sacrifices and take risks simply to be able to give birth. In some ways, their desire for control over their own reproductive capacities is not all that different than that of the countless women who sought abortions even when a large measure of social opprobrium was attached to women trying to determine their fate that way.

The woman entering a fertility program simply wants to be a mother, probably in pretty much the same way that most other women, feminist or not, want to be mothers. She wants to be a mother so badly (maybe partly because of the cultural mandate that presses women into motherhood, partly because motherhood seems so genuinely, emotionally grand) that even though she knows something about the lousy stats, the painful procedures, the possible risks, she enrolls in an fertility program anyway, glad to have the *choice* to do so, and glad to have the resources to pay for it. The odds tell her there is a good chance that at the end of the process she will be frustrated, disgusted, depressed and much poorer — though not necessarily sorry she tried everything she could.

This woman may also see herself as a feminist, someone who cares about ethics and justice and issues of equity. She simply wants her life to meet her expectations, and having a baby is a key expectation. And so she justifies her participation in the program on roughly the same principles as her like-minded friends when they explain why they choose to live in safe neighborhoods or send their children to private schools or colleges or why they use so much of their disposable income to pay for summer vacations instead of, let's say, sending all their excess dollars to organizations devoted to ending world hunger.

What's more — and this is the most painful part — she doesn't believe it is her personal responsibility to engage in orphan-saving just because she or her partner is infertile, or lesbian, any more than it is the responsibility of the lawyer couple next door with one conventionally conceived 6-year-old and tons of money. She is concerned about the high infant mortality rate in the United States and abroad, but she doesn't see how her forbearance from participating in a fertility-enhancing program will reduce the rate of infant deaths. She doesn't believe that her infertility or her sexual orientation requires her to redress this particular human problem. She herself would find paying another woman to be a "surrogate mother" repugnant and unacceptable. Like the theorists, she assumes that the state should have a role in this arena, but for her, the much more limited role of regulator is sufficient.

Given the competition between the logic of the opponents of reproductive technology and the strength of the desire of unwillingly childless women to become pregnant, how does one formulate a position regarding the new technologies? Surely we have to find a position that allows us to reject the medico-cultural mandates that rigidly define infertility as a disease requiring a medical "cure" and that leaves it to the infertility establishment alone to define what is and is not a legitimate mode of procreation. And certainly we must insist that the possibility of male infertility be equally scrutinized in each case where appropriate, and treated accordingly.

Just as important, we need to evaluate the controversy between the supporters and the opponents of the new technologies in light of what we know about the politics of parental worthiness in the United States at the end of the 20th century and the enduring race and class biases that continue to shape these politics. Specifically, it would not do to consider the politics of fertility without attention to the fact that the new technologies can contribute, on the one hand, to the enduring anxiety about poor and non-white women who have "too many" children and must have their fertility controlled, while, on the other hand, it drums up sympathetic concern for "deserving" white middle-class women beset by infertility problems who must be given the chance to enhance their child-bearing possibilities.

These issues cut to the heart of gender and class politics in this era. Together with the politics of abortion and welfare of which they are a part, they define the huge, problematic terrain in which many women now live, a terrain substantially unreconstructed after 20 years in which feminist politics has had an impact on many facets of our national life.

And yet, to construct a meaningful position with regard to the new technologies, one must listen carefully to the voices of women who use them. We must ask why women keep on seeking out and undergoing fertility treatments, despite the poor statistics and the political implications.

And it would be best if we could imagine that these legions of women filing into burgeoning infertility programs around the country are just like those of us who conceived in the old-fashioned way. They've sized up the options, and they've sized up their hearts, realizing that the costs (emotional, financial, medical and political) of the new technologies — like the costs of living through one's child's adolescence or paying for a child's college education — are very high. But no one can tell them — or me — that it's not worth it. Nor, in the end, does it seem fair to me to impose a demographic politics of justice on the backs of women who simply want the same thing that I got without even trying.

Rickie Solinger is a visiting scholar at the University of Colorado. She is the author of Wake Up Little Susie: Single Pregnancy and Race Before Roe v. Wade *(Routledge) and* The Abortionist: A Woman Against the Law *(The Free Press).*

REPRODUCTIVE HEALTH

A Father's Role

By Patricia Thomas

There are many reasons to worry about the consequences of environmental destruction and proliferating toxins. One emerging cause for concern, according to some scientists, is the adverse influence that parental exposure to various drugs, chemicals, or pollutants may have on the health of a developing fetus.

Clearly not every life has a good beginning. Over l0% of pregnancies end in miscarriages or stillbirths about 3–5% of children enter the world with a recognizable birth defect, and over 10% of babies in the United States are born too small to catch up easily. Some youngsters seem fine at first but later show developmental or behavior abnormalities.

In a perfect union, male and female contribute equal amounts of healthy genetic material to their offspring. But when something goes wrong, scientists have traditionally examined the egg to find out why. The assumption has been that eggs are fragile and susceptible to the damaging effects of radiation, poisons, and the hazards of everyday living. It is not surprising, then, that researchers have focused on the roles that maternal age, nutrition, and use of recreational drugs play in conditions such as Down's syndrome, neural tube defects, and developmental problems.

SUSCEPTIBLE SPERMATOZOA

Fathers were completely absent from this picture. Their role didn't attract much attention because many reproductive biologists assumed that the sperm, a tight little capsule of DNA with a tail, is largely impervious to environmental factors. During the past decade, however, geneticists have learned how to unbundle the sperm and scrutinize its contents. These examinations have revealed that some 8–10% of sperm from apparently healthy men with no history of heritable disease are abnormal: some carry the wrong number of chromosomes; others have bits and pieces of genetic material out of place.

Laboratory scientists aren't entirely sure how these abnormalities might translate into problems for any children conceived by such sperm. Both basic scientists and epidemiologists who track paternal exposure to drugs, alcohol, radiation, and workplace toxins say that these factors may be implicated in miscarriages, stillbirths, congenital defects, low birth weight, behavioral or learning difficulties, and even some types of cancer.

REDISCOVERING OLD WISDOM

The idea that both parents' personal habits or occupational exposures may influence a child's well-being is not entirely new. Because a child conceived by intoxicated parents was thought likely to be unhealthy, the ancient cities of Carthage and Sparta had laws prohibiting the use of alcohol by newlyweds. During England's "Gin Epidemic" of 1720–1760, long before the scientific method had been brought to bear on the reproductive hazards of alcohol, physicians worried that drunken fathers — as well as debauched mothers — would breed "feeble or distempered" offspring.

More than a century passed before researchers published the first reports linking a specific occupational exposure with a pattern of reproductive problems. In one of those investigations, which was published in 1860, a French scientist noted that the wives of lead workers were less likely than other women to become pregnant, and if they did they were more prone to miscarrying. Since then, many other studies have detected a similar pattern. In some cases such observations caused government authorities to ban women —

From *Harvard Health Letter* (October 1992), pp. 5-7. Reprinted by permission of *Harvard Health Letter*. © 1992, President and Fellows of Harvard College.

but not men — from workplaces where lead was handled. Today the response is apt to be much the same when reproductive hazards are suspected.

UNEQUAL PROTECTION

The current surge of concern about environmental exposures that may damage a man's offspring has been bolstered not only by a growing body of provocative research but also by a Supreme Court decision. In February 1991, the American Association for the Advancement of Science sponsored its first symposium on the topic. One month later the United States Supreme Court handed down its ruling in *International Union, UAW v. Johnson Controls*. In this case, a manufacturing company located in Wisconsin removed fertile women (who could have borne children if they wanted to) from jobs where they were exposed to lead while assembling batteries. Fertile men were not steered away from the assembly line, which paid better than other jobs in the factory. The Supreme Court ruled that the company, even though it claimed to be acting in the best interests of female workers, could not single out women in this manner. Some observers believe that this case heralds a new era for both men and women where occupational exposures are concerned.

HAZARDOUS WORK?

Proving that the sins or circumstances of the father will be visited upon the child is extremely difficult. It would be unethical for researchers to expose anyone to poisonous chemicals, or to feed them copious quantities of alcohol or illicit drugs, in order to see if anything out of the ordinary occurs when they produce children.

Because such experiments cannot be done, epidemiologists have focused on workplace exposures of fathers whose offspring have diseases such as brain cancer or leukemia. Several studies suggest that men who work in the aircraft industry or handle paints or chemical solvents may be at higher risk for producing children with brain tumors. Paternal exposure to paints has also been linked with childhood leukemias. And investigators have observed elevated rates of leukemia and non-Hodgkin's lymphoma among children of men who were exposed to low-level radiation while working at a nuclear power facility in England. There are also preliminary indications that firemen, subjected to a potpourri of potential toxins in smoke, may produce an unusually high number of abnormal sperm and be less fertile than other males.

At least one investigation indicates that malignancies are more likely to occur among children whose fathers smoke tobacco, even if their mothers do not.

The results of some studies contradict these observations. In a few instances, geneticists have scrutinized sperm from small groups of male cancer patients treated with chemotherapy or radiation. Although their chromosomes were broken or rearranged in abnormal ways, and these changes persisted for years after treatment was stopped, there was no apparent harm to the offspring of these cancer patients. When the wives of these men became pregnant, they were no more likely to miscarry, or to bear children with cancer or birth defects, than were women in any other group.

Human studies are difficult to interpret, simply because there are so many variables involved. Fire fighters and industrial workers are exposed to so many potential toxins that a specific causative agent cannot be identified. And even if the offender is known, determining whether an individual has gotten a dose big enough to affect his reproductive capacity may be difficult. Finally, it may be impossible to tell if a man has been harmed by something at work or during leisure activity.

OF MICE AND MEN

Animal experiments may shed more light on the connection between paternal exposures and reproduction — in part because rodents don't complicate matters by stopping for a drink on the way home. In a typical experiment, a large number of male mice or rats are exposed to a potentially harmful food, drug, or airborne chemical. Researchers then look for physiological abnormalities such as smaller testes and decreased spermatogenesis (sperm formation). Some of these animals are bred to females that have not been subjected to the substance in question, and their offspring are compared with those of unexposed parents. Investigators note any health problems, delays in development, and premature deaths in the second-generation rodents.

Scientists have used such studies to evaluate the paternal effects of many drugs and workplace toxins including alcohol, the anticancer drug cyclophosphamide, and both opiate and nonopiate narcotics. Male mice dosed with cyclophosphamide — the most extensively studied of these agents — remain fertile but act and look different from unexposed ones. They undergo permanent genetic changes that are inherited by successive generations of their offspring.

At least one study indicates that chronic alcohol use has a more pronounced effect on sexually immature rats than on older ones. When given alcohol every day, young rodents were slow to achieve normal testis size and testosterone levels and fathered smaller litters than did the more mature animals. Offspring of the hard drinking youngsters appeared normal at first

Good News for Older Dads

Jack Nicholson and Warren Beatty are just the tip of the iceberg. Plenty of men who've never graced the cover of a magazine are fathering children over age 50, and an obvious question for them — and their partners — is whether their age increases the chance of having a child with physical or mental disabilities.

Definite answers are in short supply because scientists have only been able to explore this possibility for about a decade. So far, most geneticists agree that the incidence of some single-gene mutations rises with paternal age. The majority of the conditions produced by these changes are so rare — occurring approximately once in every 25,000–100,000 births — that the likelihood of producing an afflicted child remains quite low even for older fathers, according to geneticist Renee H. Martin, a professor of pediatrics at the University of Calgary.

Dr. Martin is one of a handful of scientists who have analyzed chromosomal aberrations in sperm from healthy men of various ages. "My research shows that abnormalities in the number of chromosomes, such as Down's syndrome, actually decrease with paternal age. But abnormalities in the structure of chromosomes — caused by breaks — increase," she said. Other researchers have made the same observation.

In a structural abnormality, a bit of chromosome breaks off and is lost or exchanged with another piece of genetic material. Such alterations cause several mental retardation syndromes including Prader-Willi (which involves obesity) and cri du chat (characterized by a plaintive, catlike cry). Instead of leading to the birth of a disabled child, however, the odds are that fertilization with a structurally abnormal sperm will lead to an early spontaneous abortion that goes unnoticed, Dr. Martin said.

Although it may take longer for a woman married to an older man to become pregnant, no high-tech genetic tests are indicated and there's no reason to lie awake at night worrying about broken chromosomes, she said.

but later turned out to have endocrine abnormalities that slowed their sexual development.

A survey of animal data indicates that paternal exposure to environmental toxins — ranging from recreational drugs to industrial chemicals — apparently contributes to problems ranging from fetal loss and stillbirth to diminished aptitude for learning to perform tasks such as running a maze.

PROMOTING HEALTHY PATERNITY

Where does this leave prospective parents? The first step is being aware that either parent's exposure to a variety of agents — in a factory or at home — may pose a risk to the future children. And, given a choice between just saying no and ingesting or inhaling a drug, people must weigh the benefits against the potential risks. Prudence dictates that during their peak reproductive years, both men and women should be judicious about the use of alcohol, tobacco, or other recreational drugs. When a medicine is needed to treat a specific health problem, potential parents should discuss any possible reproductive effects with their physician.

Now that sperm are recognized as being susceptible to environmental dangers, some researchers are seeking strategies to protect them against harm. One recently published study found that free radicals ravaged sperm of men on a diet that limited vitamin C intake to 5 mg a day. When the same men increased their vitamin C to 60 or 250 mg daily, however, such damage to their sperm was minimal. Although there is not enough evidence to justify recommending that prospective fathers head for the vitamin counter, there is certainly no harm in eating a few more servings of fresh fruits and vegetables every day.

Public Health Then and Now

The Evolution of Maternal Birthing Position

By Lauren Dundes, MHS

INTRODUCTION

The birth of a child is one of the most significant events in a woman's life. Practices associated with the birthing process are, therefore, important to the woman's health and well-being as well as the successful outcome of her pregnancy. Included among these practices is the horizontal birthing position which has been the subject of a great deal of controversy.[1-4] This position has been widely used in Western cultures only for the last 200 years. Prior to this time, the recorded history of birthing indicates upright birth postures were used extensively.

Both the dorsal position, where the parturient is flat on her back, and the lithotomy position, where she lies on her back with her legs up in stirrups, have been challenged in the last 100 years.[1-5] Since the decline in the use of scopolamine and morphine "Twilight Sleep", there has been a trend encouraging parturients to utilize lateral, dorsal, and reclining positions to give birth. but such practices are far from universal.[5]

This paper will explore the historical roots of the dorsal and lithotomy birthing positions now practiced in most hospitals in the United States. Although various explanations for the change in position have been proposed, including facilitation of forceps usage, promotion of men's power over women (both midwives and parturients), and requirements with the use of anesthesia, none adequately explains the confluence of events which led to the shift away from the upright to the horizontal maternal birth position. Conflict between midwives and surgeons and interaction of the disciplines of obstetric surgery and lithotomy surgery which emerged 300 years ago appear to have contributed to this change. The transition was greatly influenced by the French who were at that time considered the leaders in obstetrical practice.

WORLDWIDE PRACTICES

Most cultures throughout the world either use, or have used, such birthing positions as kneeling, squatting, sitting, and standing for labor and delivery (Figures 1–4).[15-18] Earliest records of maternal birth positions show the parturient in an upright posture, usually squatting or kneeling. A bas-relief (see Figure 1) at the Temple of Esneh in Egypt depicts Cleopatra (69?–30 BC) in a kneeling position, surrounded by five women attendants, one of whom delivers the child.[15] The birthing chair (Figure 2) dates back to the Babylonian culture, 2000 BC. It then spread to many parts of the world.[19] In some parts of the world, various traditional birthing chairs are still used, while a modern version is now available in some Western hospitals.[20]

In a 1961 survey of 76 traditional cultures, Naroll, et al., found that in only 14 (18 per cent) did the women assume either a prone or dorsal birthing position.[17] The findings and conclusions of this cross-cultural survey are in accord with extensive work done earlier by Engelmann (1882), and Jarcho (1934).[7, 15] Currently in many developing countries, traditional birth attendants (usually women) attend parturients. The birth position they use differs from

Address reprint requests to Lauren Dundes, MHS, doctoral student, Department of Maternal and Child Health, School of Hygiene and Public Health, Johns Hopkins University, 615 N. Wolfe Street, Baltimore, MD 21205. This paper was accepted for publication on November 3, 1986 by Barbara G. Rosenkrantz, PhD, Editor of the Public Health Then and Now section of the Journal.

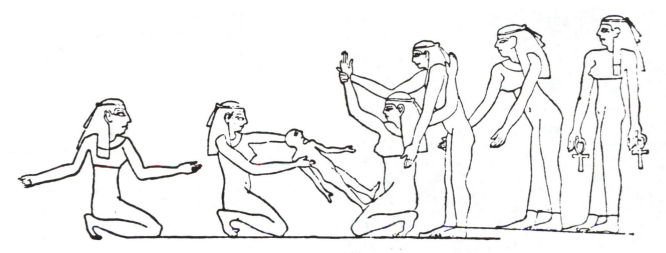

FIGURE 1—The accouchement of Cleopatra. Bas-relief from the temple of Esneh, a town on the Nile in Upper Egypt.

that suggested by physicians and by trained midwives who have been taught the Western practice of horizontal labor and delivery positions. [21, 22]

INTERPROFESSIONAL RIVALRY

In Europe until about 1550, midwives were the only attendants at births[23] (see Figure 3). When Paré, the famous surgeon-obstetrician, practiced medicine (1517?–1590), barber-surgeons began to compete with midwives for obstetric cases.[24] Initially, these surgeons were poorly trained; their social rank remained on a par with that of carpenters, shoemakers, and other members of guilds, known collectively as the "arts and trades" until the 18th century.[25] As time progressed, they sought recognition for the obstetric

skills they had acquired in delivering women whose lives were threatened as a result of obstetric complications. Achieving recognition for their skills was made difficult, due to their status and because exposure of women's bodies to men was considered indecent. Physicians, granted special privileges and accorded higher status than surgeons, were not eager for this advancing profession to encroach on any of their territory. Neither did midwives, many of whom had received formal training, welcome the surgeons' intrusion as it represented a threat to their livelihood and recognized area of expertise.

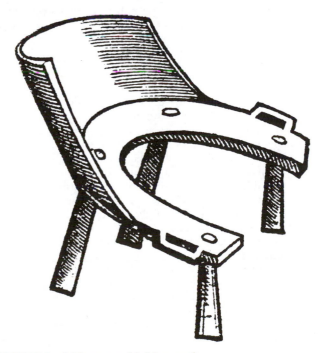

FIGURE 2—14th century birthing stool.

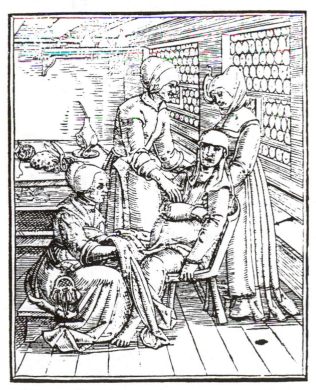

FIGURE 3—Midwives attending woman in labor on birth chair, 16th century.

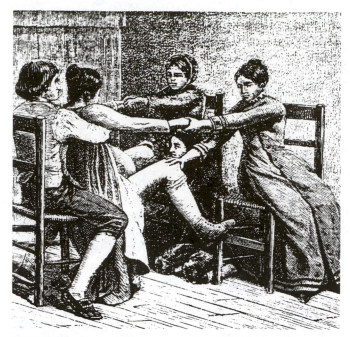

FIGURE 4—Pioneer birth scene after Engelmann's illustration showing woman, husband, midwife, and two attendants.

Mauriceau (1637-1709), a prominent French physician at this time, recorded the climate of the times and the co-existence of the intense interprofessional rivalry:

> "There are many Midwives, who are so afraid that the Chirurgeons should take away their practice, or to appear ignorant before them that they chuse rather to put all to adventure, then to send for them in necessity: others believe themselves as capable as the Chirurgeons to undertake all . . . and some do maliciously put such a terror and apprehension of the Chirurgeons in the poor women (for the most part undeservedly), comparing them to Butchers and Hangmen, that they chuse rather to die in Travail with the Child in their Womb, than to put themselves into their hands."[26]

Although midwives continued to retain their long-standing position as the primary birth attendants (see Figure 4), barber-surgeons were increasingly called in cases likely to result in fetal and/or maternal morbidity or mortality: often they practiced manual extraction of the fetus from the mother in order to save her life.[23] The practice of obstetrics offered surgeons a plausible entry into the medical field. Their attendance at traumatic cases helped them develop a disease orientation to childbirth, and they held a competitive advantage over midwives due to their skills or practice in dealing with complications. Derogated by the physicians and forced to compete with midwives, they had to make themselves marketable. If most women viewed pregnancy as a normal, natural event, then the surgeons' services would not be required. If, however, pregnancy was seen as an illness,

then their presence might appear more appropriate. Midwives did at times promote their own services by proclaiming the need for intervention, although intervention within a disease orientation benefited the male accoucheurs.

Guillemeau (the pupil and son-in-law of Paré) had advocated reclining bed birthing in 1598, supposedly for women's comfort and to facilitate labor[27]: the techniques used by surgeons to handle difficult births 50 years later could also be best performed in a reclining position. This led to using the bed as the place to perform childbirth, and the reclining position developed into the one practiced for normal as well as complicated deliveries. Women at the Paris Hotel Dieu (a large hospital with a maternity section) delivered in a special bed; by the end of the 17th century, bed delivery had become a common practice in France except among rural women.[28]

Although convenience is continuously pointed to in the literature as the primary reason for changing to the supine birth position, the experience varied by country. By the 11th century, when births began to occur in bed, many women, especially in England, lay on their sides, which differed from the reclining position used in France that accommodated the birth attendant.[28]

INFLUENCE OF MAURICEAU

Despite Guillemeau's earlier advocacy of the reclining position and the influence of the barber-surgeons, the person generally credited with greatly influencing the change in birth position is François Mauriceau.[8,30] He claimed that the reclining position would be both more comfortable for the parturient women as well as more convenient for the accoucheur. In his 1668 book, *The Diseases of Women with Child and in Child-Bed*, he recommended the change of position and offered the following recommended rationale for doing so:

> ". . . all women are not accustomed to be delivered in the same posture: some will be on their Knees, as many in Country Villages; others standing upright leaning with the Elbows on a Pillow upon a Table, or on the side of a Bed . . . but the best and surest is to be delivered in their bed, to shun the inconvenience and trouble of being carried thither afterwards;
>
> The bed must be so made, that the Woman being ready to be delivered, should lie on her Back upon it, having her Body in a convenient Figure, that is, her Head and Breast a little raised so that she be neither lying nor sitting; for in this manner she breaths best, and will have more strength to help her Pains than if she were otherwise, or sunk down in her Bed . . . and have her feet stayed against some firm thing . . ."[26]

Mauriceau also was affected by prevailing views of pregnancy as an illness. His 1668 work on midwifery in which he claimed that pregnancy, properly

PART 3 – REPRODUCTIVE HEALTH ISSUES

construed, was a "tumor of the Belly" caused by an infant was among the first of many early references to medical problems during pregnancy and childbirth[31] that defined all births as inherently pathologic and abnormal, leaving no room for the midwife.[32] Change in position was a natural accompaniment of the shift in concept.

ROLE OF KING LOUIS XIV

Some scholars claim that the change in birthing position was a perverted caprice of King Louis XIV (1638–1715), a contemporary of Mauriceau (1637–1709).[30,33] Since Louis XIV reportedly enjoyed watching women giving birth, he became frustrated by the obscured view of birth when it occurred on a birthing stool, and promoted the new reclining position. He also insisted on male accoucheurs attending births. The influence of the King's policy is unknown, although the behavior of royalty must have affected the populace to some degree. Louis XIV's purported demand for change did coincide with the changing of the position and may well have been a contributing influence.

King Louis XIV not only promoted the use of the male accoucheur, but also granted favors to a well-known lithotomist Frère Jacques (born Jacques Beaulieu in 1651).[34] For unknown reasons, the procedures of obstetrics and lithotomy were preoccupations of this head of state. The lithotomy surgery of the urinary bladder for removal of a stone had been performed since at least 200 BC,[35] and was used extensively in France in the 17th century. Paré (1517-1590), who has been called the father of modern obstetrics,[23] was also involved in lithotomy surgery. The interaction of the evolving sciences of lithotomy and obstetrics is not surprising since techniques used in Obstetric surgery (e.g., cesarean section) had features in common with those used in lithotomy. The lithotomist, Frère Jacques, a name made famous by the French folksongs,[34] was taught anatomy by Fagon, who served as a surgeon to Louis XIV. At one point, Frère Jacques so impressed Louis XIV that the King gave instructions for him to be lodged with the Royal Valet and to be given the King's License to do lithotomy operations.[34,35] Frère Jacques performed the lithotomy operations at the same Hôtel Dieu during the time period in which the new birth position was instituted. Although a precise relation between the reclining birth position — the forerunner of the lithotomy position — and the lithotomy operation is difficult to establish, the adoption of the lithotomy position for birthing and extensive practice of the lithotomy operation occurred at the same time and place in France in the 17th century.

FORCEPS AND ANESTHESIA

It has also been argued that the change in birthing position was instituted because it provided improved access to the perineum when forceps were used.[8,9] Forceps had been known in obstetrics since the third century[36] and were also used in lithotomy procedures by Paré in the mid-1500s.[35] Obstetric forceps fell into disuse, however, until 1588 when they were rediscovered by Chamberlen. To guard their secret, the Chamberlen family, French Huguenots who fled to England for safety, carried the forceps in a locked case, and used them under a sheet with the patient blindfolded.[37,35] Mauriceau, because of his prominence, was offered the secret of the forceps by a descendant of Chamberlen in 1670. He declined to buy the instrument (which he never actually saw)[24] because he had witnessed their unsuccessful use in the delivery of one of his patients.[6]

It is reported that forceps were not used by others outside of the Chamberlen family until 1700,[24,31,37] and that the secret of forceps construction emerged around 1720 at which time their utilization increased dramatically.[39] Forceps could not initially have played a major role in affecting the birth position, since the birthing position had been changed many years before forceps came into wide usage, although they have been an important factor in the retention of the reclining and lithotomy positions.

A number of scholars believe that the advent of general anesthesia eliminated women's ability to participate at all in labor and delivery, requiring them to lie down to be delivered.[40] However, a relationship between general anesthesia and the change in birth position is unlikely, since anesthesia was not used until almost 200 years after the reign of Louis XIV. In Europe, Sir James Simpson of Edinburgh introduced the use of chloroform in 1847, and the use of general anesthesia in obstetrics increased after chloroform was administered to Queen Victoria in 1853.[39]

FLAT MATERNAL BIRTH POSITION IN US

Neither the lithotomy position nor the flat horizontal position was recommended by Mauriceau in the mid-1600s. He advocated the reclining posture which may be more favorable physiologically and more comfortable for the woman. The controversial flat position[41] (in contrast to reclining) first began to be used in the United States.[42,43] This position differed from that used in European countries. In Cazeaux's 1884 obstetrics book, it is reported that women in the United States lie flat on their backs, French women lie back on an inclined plane, English women lie on their left side, and German women use the birthing chair.[42]

Since European practices greatly influenced those of the United States, it is understandable that American accoucheurs could have emulated the European practice of birthing in bed. Exactly why the United States deviated from the European reclining posture is not clear, however.

The employment of the flat dorsal birth position (circa 1834) is attributed to William Potts Dewees, the third chairman of obstetrics at the University of Pennsylvania.[8,44] Dewees advocated the dorsal birth posture, although he recommended side-lying for labor. The site of implementing his recommendation is uncertain, since Dewees does not define the term "sick room."[43] His writings support the contentions that the United States had deviated from European practice, and that convenience of the accoucheur was crucial.

> "The British practitioner almost invariably directs the patient to be placed upon her side . . . while the Continental accoucheur has her placed on her back . . . the woman should be placed so as to give the least possible hindrance to the operations of the accoucheur — this is agreed upon by all; but there exist a diversity of opinion, what that position is. Some recommended the side: others the knees, and others the back. I coincide with the latter . . . Therefore, when practicable, I would recommend she should be placed upon her back, both for convenience and safety."[43]

Since he "coincides" with an established position, evidently he was reflecting an existing opinion and the flat position had been advocated by others preceding him.

LINKS BETWEEN LITHOTOMY AND OBSTETRICS IN US

William Shippen, Jr., the first chairman of Obstetrics and Anatomy at the University of Pennsylvania, was an influential leader and teacher in obstetrics until his death in 1808. Writing of Shippen, one scholar stated: "Among colonial physicians specializing in midwifery, no one deserves a more prominent place."[45] Shippen established a lying-in hospital in Philadelphia in 1765.[46] Yet when Shippen is discussed in midwifery literature, his career as an esteemed lithotomist is not explored. In fact, according to the lithotomy literature Shippen is considered one of the most influential bladder stone lithotomists although only a few of his writings are extant.[47] Another connection between the two specialties involves Hugh Hodge, who followed Dewees as the Chairman of Obstetrics at the University of Pennsylvania Medical School. Like Shippen, Hodge was a student of lithotomy. His mentor (Caspar Wistar) was a bladder stone lithotomist and a pupil of Shippen's. Thus we have an additional link between obstetrics and lithotomy in the United States during the late 18th century.[44]

From the mid-18th to the 20th centuries, obstetric practices were not standardized, and various forms of horizontal positioning prevailed. Moreover, there was almost no control of or examination for medical licensing, and medical schools enforced only minimal requirements.[48] Such circumstances would delay the spread of Shippen's influence on birth position, which was also undoubtedly greatly affected by accoucheur advantage of horizontal positioning.

CONCLUSIONS

The pros and cons of childbirth in the dorsal and lithotomy positions have been discussed at least since Engelmann's time (1882)[7]; however, little has been done until recently to encourage alternative birthing positions that may be better accepted by and more beneficial to the parturient woman, her child, and the birth attendant (see Figure 5). The adoption and use

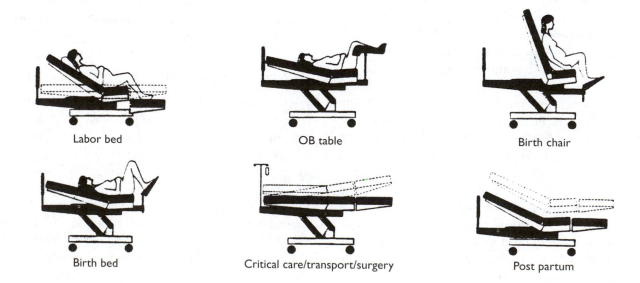

Labor bed

OB table

Birth chair

Birth bed

Critical care/transport/surgery

Post partum

FIGURE 5—The modern multipurpose birthing bed has many uses in today's labor-delivery-recovery (LDR) room.

of the lithotomy position was not based on sound scientific research. By exploring the circumstances that existed when the maternal birth position changed, we see that the position was altered as a result of interprofessional struggles of surgeons and midwives and by the development of obstetrics as affected by the practice of lithotomy. A position was implemented without verifying its appropriateness. Today, with more women and their families exercising their rights to actively participate in the birth experience and to make it a more personal and more physiologically and psychologically advantageous experience, the time is ripe for further scientific investigation of the lithotomy position. Unlike our historical precedent, where an important change seems to have been influenced by the reputation of prominent persons and the prevailing circumstances of the times, it is currently possible to design and plan studies that evaluate the different birthing positions — options that have an important bearing on the health and safety of the parturients and the newborns.

ACKNOWLEDGMENTS

I would like to thank Donald A. Cornely, MD, MPH, Professor and Chairman of the Department of Maternal and Child Health, Johns Hopkins University School of Hygiene and Public Health, for his careful reading of this paper; I am also greatly indebted to Woodrow S. Dellinger, MS, MPH, Research Associate, Department of Maternal and Child Health, Johns Hopkins University School of Hygiene and Public Health, for his many valuable suggestions.

REFERENCES

1. Dunn P: Obstetric delivery today — for better or for worse. Lancet 1976; 1:7963, 790–793.
2. Kitzinger S: Experiences of obstetric practices in differing countries. In: Zander L (ed): Pregnancy Care for the 1980s. London: Royal Society of Medicine, and Macmillan Press, 1984.
3. Shaw NS: Forced Labor: Maternity Care in the United States. New York Pergamon Press. 1974.
4. Leifer M: Psychological Effects of Motherhood: A Study of First Pregnancy. New York: Praeger Special Studies. 1980.
5. Carlson JM, Diehl JA, Sachtleben-Murray M, et al: Maternal position during parturition in normal labor. Obstet Gynecol 1986: 68:443–447.
6. Wertz RW, Wertz DC: Lying-In, A History of Childbirth in America. New York: Free Press, 1977.
7. Engelmann GJ: Labor among Primitive Peoples. St. Louis: J.H. Chambers, 1882.
8. Caldeyro-Barcia R: The Influence of maternal position on time of spontaneous rupture of membranes, progress of labor and fetal head compression. Birth Fam J 1979; 6:7–16.
9. Carr KC: Obstetric practices which protect against neonatal morbidity: focus on maternal position in labor and birth. Birth Fam J 1980: 7:249–254.
10. Haire D: The Cultural Warping of Childbirth. Milwaukee: International Childbirth Education Association (ICEA), 1972.
11. Fenwick L: Birthing. Perinatology/Neonatology 1984: 8: 51–62.
12. Roberts J. Mendez-Bauer C, Wodell DA: The effects of maternal position on uterine contractility and efficiency. Birth 1983: 10:243–249.
13. Stewart P. Hillan E, Calder AA: A randomized trial to evaluate the use of a birthing chair for delivery. Lancet 1983; 1:1296–1298.
14. Roberts J: Alternative positions for childbirth — Part I: first stage of labor. J. Nurse-Midwifery 1980; 25:11–18.
15. Jarcho J: Posture and Practices during Labor among Primitive Peoples. New York: Paul B. Hoeber. 1934.
16. Russell JG: The rationale of primitive delivery positions. Br J Obstet Gynecol 1982: 89:712–715.
17. Naroll F. Naroll R. Howard FH: Position of women in childbirth. Am J Obstet Gynecol 1961: 82:943–954.
18. Jordan B: Birth in Four Cultures. Montreal: Eden Press, 1983.
19. Lagercrantz VS: Zur verbreitung des geburtsstuhles in Afrika. Mitteilungen der Anthropologischen Gesellschaft. Vienna, 1939: 69:261–272.
20. Johnson TRB, Repke JR, Paine LL: Choosing a birthing bed to meet everyone's needs. Contemp Ob/Gyn 1987: 29:70–73.
21. Cosminsky S: Traditional midwifery and contraception. In: Traditional Medicine and Health Care Coverage. Geneva: World Health Organization. 1983.
22. Cosminsky S: Knowledge and body concept of Guatemalan midwives. In: Artschwager M (ed): Anthropology of Human Birth. Philadelphia: F.A. Davis. 1982.
23. Townsend L: Obstetrics through the ages. Med J Aust 1952: 1:558–565.
24. Ackerknecht EH: A Short History of Medicine. Baltimore: Johns Hopkins Press, 1982.
25. Gelfand T: From the guild to profession: the surgeons of France in the 18th century. Texas Rep Biol Med 1974: 32:121–132.
26. Mauriceau F: The Disease of Women with Child and in Child-Bed. London: John Darby. 1683. (Translated by Hugh Chamberlen from the original work published in French in 1668).
27. Guillemeau J: Child-Birth or the Happy Delivery of Women. London: A. Hatfield. 1612.
28. Eccles A: Obstetrics and Gynecology in Tudor and Stuart England. Kent: Kent State University Press. 1982.
29. Shorter E: A History of Women's Bodies. New York: Basic Books. 1982.
30. Arms S: Immaculate Deception. Boston: Houghton Mifflin. 1975.
31. Wilbanks E: Historical Review of Obstetrical Practice. In: Aladjem S (ed): Obstetric Practice. St. Louis: C.V. Mosby. 1980.
32. Rothman BK: Anatomy of a Compromise: Nurse- Midwifery and the Rise of the Birth Center. J Nurse- Midwifery 1983: 28:3–7.
33. Mendelsohn RS: Male Malpractice: How Doctors Manipulate Women. Chicago: Contemporary Books, 1982.
34. Ellis H: A History of Bladder Stone. Oxford: Blackwell Scientific Publications. 1969.
35. Riches E: The history of lithotomy and lithotrity. Ann R Coll Surg Engl 1968: 43:185–199.
36. Speert H: Iconographia Gyniatrica: A Pictorial History of Gynecology and Obstetrics. Philadelphia: F.A. Davis. 1973.
37. Corea G: The Hidden Malpractice: How American Medicine Treats Women as Patients and Professionals. New York: William Morrow. 1977.

38. Chaney JA: Birthing in early America. J Nurse-Midwifery, 1980: 25:5–13.
39. Edwards M. Waldorf M: Reclaiming Birth-History and Heroines of American Childbirth Reform. Trumansburg: Crossing Press. 1984.
40. Walton VE: Have it Your Way. Toronto: Bantam Books. 1976.
41. McKay S: Maternal position during labor and birth: a reassessment, 1980: 9:5. 288–291
42. Tarner S: Cazeaux's Theory and Practice of Obstetrics. Philadelphia: Blakiston, Son and Co., 1884.
43. Dewees WP: A Compendious System of Midwifery. Philadelphia: Crey, Lea, and Carey, 1828.
44. Baas JH: Baas' History of Medicine (translated by H.E. Handerson), New York: J.H. Vail, 1889.
45. Donnegan JB: Midwifery in America. 1760–1860: A Study in Medicine and Morality. (Dissertation for History Department. Syracuse University, 1973).
46. Hiestand WC: Midwife to Nurse-Midwife: A History: The Development of Nurse-Midwifery Education in the Continental United States to 1965. (Dissertation for Education in Teachers College, Columbia University, 1976).
47. Bush RB: Lithotomy, Its practice and Practitioners in Philadelphia during the Colonial and Early Republican Period: An Essay in the Transit of Culture. (Dissertation in the Department of History, New York University, 1976).
48. Rosenberg C: The Practice of Medicine in New York a Century Ago. Bull Hist Med 1967: 41:233–252.

Photo Acknowledgments

The Journal is grateful to the National Library of Medicine,. History of Medicine Division, for providing the photographs for Figures 1, 2, 3, and 4, from the following sources: FIGURE 1, Speert H: Iconographia Gyniatrica: A Pictorial History of Gynecology and Obstetrics, Philadelphia: F.A. Davis, 1973. This publication contains a wealth of historical photographs on the history of OB/GYN. The accouchement of Cleopatra also appeared in Witkowski GH: Historie des accouchements chex tous les peuples. Paris, 1887, p 344. fig. 218. FIGURE 2, Roeslin E: Der swangern Frauwenund Hebammen Rosegarten. Strassburg, 1513, fol, Dii verso, woodcut. FIGURE 3. Ruff, 1554, from a wood engraving. FIGURE 4. Witkowski GJ: Histoire des accouchements chez tous les peuples. Paris: Steinheil, 1887. p 418. FIGURE 5, A multipurpose birthing bed. Borning Corporation, Spokane, WA 99204.

The Truth About . . . . . . PMS

What Causes Premenstrual Syndrome?
Is PMS an Illness?
What Can You Do About It?

By Nancy Wartik

It's part of the universal language of women. Snap at a coworker, burst into tears or go on a chocolate-eating spree, and any fellow sufferer will sympathize once you utter three letters of the alphabet: PMS.

Premenstrual syndrome is an array of physical and psychological symptoms triggered by ovulation (the midcycle release of an egg from the ovary) and ending with menstruation. First identified in the 1930s, PMS has gained wide recognition — even notoriety — only in the past two decades, due in part to two British murder cases in the early 1980s in which the defendants invoked PMS as an extenuating circumstance.

Despite hundreds of PMS studies, the condition remains perplexing and controversial. It's estimated that 5% to 10% of all menstruating women are seriously affected, while at least that many more have symptoms that could benefit from treatment. Though it's undoubtedly linked to monthly hormonal fluctuations, there's little agreement on exactly what causes PMS or at what point ordinary premenstrual discomfort turns into a medical disorder. Some doctors question its very existence, while others feel that the severe depression, anxiety or violence it can trigger in its extreme form makes PMS a psychological illness.

Then there are those in the middle, who acknowledge the symptoms but question their classification as a medical disorder. "We're making a disease out of normal changes in mood and body," asserts Dr. Jerilynn Prior, an endocrinologist at the University of British Columbia in Vancouver. "The symptoms are real, but we shouldn't be labeling them as an illness. It's one of the many ways by which we've medicalized women's experience."

The debate continues, but in the meantime, women who seek help may find themselves facing questionable remedies, unethical practitioners, or treatments that aren't always appropriate, such as hysterectomy. Their best defense is to get the facts.

Dozens of symptoms have been attributed to PMS, including moodiness, fatigue, insomnia, broken concentration, food cravings, backaches and breast pain. (Menstrual cramps, however, are not considered part of PMS.) Women who have asthma, migraine headaches or other chronic illnesses often find that these conditions worsen as their period approaches.

But for many women it's the emotional turmoil that's hardest to take. "Women may have sore breasts, bloating or food cravings, but that's not what they come in and complain about," says Dr. Ellen Freeman, codirector of the University of Pennsylvania Medical Center PMS program. "They talk about feeling like a different person in the premenstrual phase. They're afraid they'll hurt their children, they're angry and they're upset. Some get extremely depressed; they withdraw, want to sleep, don't want to leave the house."

"I've had people tell me PMS is just an excuse for being crabby," says Mary Brooks, 35, a St. Louis administrative assistant. "But if you're not in my shoes, it's hard to understand what it feels like. Each

From *American Health* (April 1995), pp. 64-67, 87. Reprinted with permission of *American Health* © 1995 by Nancy Wartik.

month like clockwork, 10 days before my period, I have a total personality change. I want to cry at the drop of a hat; I pick fights. It affects my work, because I'm tired as soon as I wake up. I don't have any energy. I have headaches, bloating. I walk into a room and can't remember what I wanted there."

No matter how many doctors insist that women only imagine such distress, new studies suggest that specific physiological changes, including variations in sleep patterns and body temperature, take place prior to menstruation in women who have PMS. What's more, the syndrome isn't limited to American women. When researchers at the State University of New York at Buffalo and other institutions compared women from the U.S., Italy and Bahrain (a Middle Eastern nation), they found that although many of the foreign women had never heard of PMS, they nevertheless reported many of its typical symptoms. "This supports the idea that PMS isn't simply a media-created phenomenon, as some have suggested," says Dr. Lisa Monagle, a certified nurse midwife, who headed the study.

Women who have had a major episode of depression or whose mothers or sisters have PMS may be more prone to develop the condition. Age also seems to play a role, though researchers don't know why. A 1992 study from the University of Calgary in Alberta, for instance, found that women in their late 20s to mid 30s are likeliest to experience mood problems.

Getting the Facts

For more information, consult the following resources:

- The National Women's Health Resource Center, 2440 M St. NW, No. 325, Washington, DC 20037; 202-293-6045. Send $15 for an information packet on PMS.

- National Women's Health Network, 514 10th St., NW, Washington, DC 20004; 202-628-7814. Send $7.50 for an information packet on PMS and referrals to local clinics.

- American College of Obstetricians and Gynecologists, Resource Center, 409 12th St. SW, Washington, DC 20024. Send a business-sized SASE for a free copy of "Premenstrual Syndrome."

- *A Woman Doctor's Guide to PMS: Essential Facts and Up-to-the-Minute Information on Premenstrual Syndrome* by Dr. Andrea J. Rapkin with Diana Tonnessen (Hyperion).

- PMS Access, 800-222-4767. Call for a free packet of information, but keep in mind that although the packet discusses many treatment approaches for the syndrome, the company itself markets a vitamin and mineral supplement for PMS.

There's little doubt that PMS is linked to hormonal changes during the menstrual cycle. Estrogen levels rise gradually during the first two weeks of the cycle. After ovulation, estrogen production decreases, while the other female hormone progesterone dominates the last two weeks. A decade ago, it was thought that PMS resulted from a progesterone deficiency. But scientists have so far failed to find evidence that women with PMS have different levels of progesterone — or of any other reproductive hormone — than unaffected women. It's now believed that some women may simply be extra sensitive to the effect of normal hormonal fluctuations and that the syndrome has multiple causes. These include:

Serotonin imbalance. Changing hormone levels may affect neurotransmitters (chemical messengers) in the brain. Serotonin imbalances, for example, have been linked to depression, violent behavior, and appetite and sleep disturbances. PMS sufferers seem to have abnormally low levels of this chemical in the 10 days before menstruation.

Endorphins. The monthly hormonal tides may also affect endorphins, opiate-like compounds that act as natural pain relievers. It's possible that symptoms are triggered by an endorphin decline around the time of ovulation, mimicking what addicts experience during withdrawal from a drug: depression, anxiety, increased appetite and insomnia.

Body chemistry. Other possible PMS triggers include deficiencies or imbalances of nutrients, such as zinc or magnesium, or abnormal levels of prostaglandins, hormone-like substances with wide-ranging effects on body function.

Stress. Many experts believe psychological factors and life stresses contribute strongly to premenstrual woes. "If two individuals have the same degree of biochemical imbalance," say Dr. James Chuong, director of the PMS program at Baylor University College of Medicine in Houston, "but one woman has marriage or job problems, her symptoms will be more severe. It's not that PMS is only a psychological problem, but the way a woman experiences it has to do with a combination of biological and situational factors."

Dr. Joseph Mortola, a reproductive endocrinologist and psychiatrist at Harvard Medical School, disagrees. "Stress doesn't cause PMS," he says. "PMS causes stress. In the high-progesterone state preceding menstruation, a woman may be more reactive to the same event and experience it with more intensity. We've studied women over three consecutive cycles, and when we add up all the stress someone has in a given month, it's no prediction of how bad PMS will be that month. Your most stressful month is just as likely to be your mildest PMS month."

What should you do if you think you have PMS? First, since there are no specific tests for it, your best chance to identify it is by carefully charting your daily physical and emotional symptoms for two months. If you don't have at least a week's reprieve following the cessation of menstruation, PMS isn't your problem, In fact, more than 50% of women who see a doctor for suspected PMS discover they have a different ailment. "A lot of women think they have it, because they've seen so much about PMS in the media." says UCLA gynecologist Andrea Rapkin, author of *A Woman Doctor's Guide to PMS.* "About half turn out to have clinical depression or anxiety." Other conditions that may produce PMS-like symptoms include diabetes, thyroid disorders and anemia.

If you do have PMS, you may have to do some experimenting to find a treatment that's right for you. In some cases, simply identifying what's going on may help. That was true for a 30-year-old woman whose premenstrual moodiness was straining her marriage until her husband pointed out that their worst fights always happened before her period.

"Now when I get upset," she says, "I think, Does this have to do with the time of the month? I try to stay away from stressful situations, because I know if I start an argument when I have PMS, I can't control myself."

If you can't deal with the problem alone, talk with your gynecologist or look for a PMS program at a local medical school. A team approach — including doctors, psychologists and registered dietitians — may be helpful. But be wary of those freestanding PMS clinics that are more interested in your wallet than in helping you. "If they give you an immediate diagnosis or try to sell you a treatment program or special PMS products right away, go elsewhere," warns Dr. John Renner, a board member at the National Council Against Health Fraud. Unless the problems is severe, experts advise taking a conservative approach to treatment, say, changing diet or exercise habits or trying stress reduction techniques.

Diet. Try cutting back on sugar, caffeine and alcohol during the premenstrual period, though it's unclear whether these substances exacerbate PMS or whether women use them as self-medication. Caffeine, however, is thought to aggravate breast tenderness. If bloating is a problem, decrease premenstrual salt intake. Snacking on several small meals during the day may help allay food cravings and have a beneficial effect on energy and mood.

Ilene Fox, 40, executive director of a New York City nonprofit organization, saw her PMS symptoms decrease dramatically after she altered her diet. "It used to be that just before my period I couldn't sleep at all." Fox recalls. "My brain was racing. I was anxious, angry, bloated. My breasts were sore. When I got my period, I'd just crash; I was exhausted. When I went to my gynecologist, he didn't take it all that seriously."

But after Fox read a book describing dietary treatments for PMS, she cut way back on caffeine, and a week before her period curtailed salt and started eating smaller, more frequent meals. "Since then, I haven't had a single sleepless night," she assets. "I don't get the mood swings, breast tenderness or bloating. It's a real success story."

Some women may also benefit from carbohydrate loading. Several studies have linked carbohydrate consumption to an increase in sertonin in the brain, and some scientists now think that premenstrual cravings for sweet, starchy foods are the body's attempt to combat moodiness and irritability by increasing serotonin levels. But if you carbo load, opt for lowfat, low-salt foods such as whole-grain bread and pasta or baked or sweet potatoes, and eat them over the course of the day, rather than bingeing on sweets and fattening fare.

Supplements and Nonprescription Drugs. Like other poorly understood disorders. PMS is a magnet for purveyors of unproven remedies and treatments. "Most are based on a lot of hype and very little science," says Renner. For instance, evening primrose oil, available in health food stores, has long been promoted as a PMS cure. But most studies have failed to support the claim, and the FDA took action against it when it was promoted as a treatment for serious diseases, It's still available in some stores, however. Those who want to try standard vitamin or mineral supplements should be aware, says UCLA's Dr. Rapkin, that there's little evidence to support the efficacy against PMS. And above all, avoid megadosing.

Among supplements, a current favorite is vitamin B6, used by the body to make several neurotransmitters, including serotonin. But studies of B6's effect on PMS have yielded conflicting results, and an overdose — more than 200 milligrams (mg) a day — can cause neurological problems.

A 1992 U.S. Department of Agriculture study found that women who consumed 1,300 mg of calcium a day had fewer mood swings and concentration problems and less bloating than when they took only 600 mg daily. An ongoing study at the National Institute of Mental Health suggests that IV magnesium may alleviate PMS mood symptoms over the short term. If you'd like to try these minerals, Rapkin recommends consuming 1,500 mg of calcium a day and about half that amount of magnesium, in food (say, beans and greens) or in supplements. Zinc deficiency may also be linked to premenstrual symptoms, according to

Baylor's Chuong, who has found decreased zinc levels in the blood of PMS patients. Nevertheless, experts warn against popping zinc pills, because the mineral is toxic in high doses.

Over-the-counter PMS medications such as Diurex may relieve minor aches and pains, says Rapkin, but won't do much for mood problems. Typically these drugs contain the analgesic acetaminophen, the mild sedative pyrilamine maleate and a diuretic to combat bloating. Some also contain caffeine which should be limited.

Exercise. Vigorous activity may be one of the best PMS antidotes. A 1993 Duke University study compared a group of women who did aerobic exercise for one hour three times a week with a group who did strength training. PMS symptoms improved to some degree for all the women, but the aerobic group reaped especially significant benefits, particularly for depression.

Stress reduction. While the experts debate the role of stress in PMS, there's evidence that stress reduction techniques — say, meditation or deep breathing — can alleviate symptoms. A 1990 Harvard Medical School study found that women with severe PMS who practiced meditation twice daily for 15 to 20 minutes experienced a 57% improvement in physical and psychological symptoms.

Light therapy. Light therapy was initially used to treat seasonal affective disorder (SAD), a depressive illness that strikes as the days shorten in winter. Now researchers at the University of California at San Diego have found that exposing PMS patients to bright light every day in the week before menstruation significantly decreases depression. The link between SAD and PMS isn't understood, but it's possible that abnormalities in melatonin, a light sensitive hormone that helps set the body's internal clock, is a factor in both.

Hormonal treatments. If conservative measures fail, medication may be the next step. Since the mid 1980s, progesterone (via vaginal suppository) has been the drug prescribed most often for PMS. In a 1990 study, however, Penn's Freeman found progesterone suppositories no better than a placebo. Many doctors now prescribe progesterone in oral form, because they believe it's more effective taken this way. But Freeman, who has just completed a study of oral progesterone, says the results are unconvincing.

Doctors may also advise PMS patients to try birth control pills, which disrupt the normal hormonal cycle and thus block ovulation. For about a third of women, the Pill does seem to help, but for the majority, it either has no effect or makes symptoms worse.

Drugs. Certain drugs target specific premenstrual symptoms, but some may create more problems than

Is It an Illness?

Is severe premenstrual syndrome (PMS) a medical disorder that makes women "crazy" and incapable of functioning normally? Or does it merely fall at the far end of the spectrum of normal behavior — a natural, if uncomfortable, aspect of being a woman, like morning sickness in pregnancy or hot flashes at menopause?

Such questions lie at the heart of an ongoing controversy fueled by a diagnosis in the *Diagnostic and Statistical Manual of Mental Disorders*, fourth edition (*DSM-IV*), published by the American Psychiatric Association. When the latest edition of the venerable guide to psychiatric disorders was released last spring, it included a listing for premenstrual dysphoric disorder. PMDD, as it's called, is defined as bouts of marked premenstrual depressed mood, anxiety, sadness or anger that, together with one or more physical symptoms such as breast tenderness or bloating, impair a woman's ability to "function socially or occupationally in the week prior to menses." The APA estimates that 3% to 5% of all women who say they have PMS suffer from PMDD.

But labeling even a small group of women as mentally unbalanced on the basis of monthly hormonal changes bothers some experts. One consultant on the *DSM-IV* task force, University of Toronto psychologist Paula Captan, severed her connection with the *DSM-IV*. "In many cases, they're taking a normal woman's behavior and saying it's sick," she says. "I'm not saying women don't get PMS, but that does not mean they're mentally ill. There's also concern that the PMDD diagnosis will lend support to a long-standing myth that women become incompetent once a month."

On the other side of the debate are those who argue that classifying severe PMS as a disorder allows women's premenstrual discomfort to finally be taken seriously. "This way, we encourage the psychiatric community to look at it and develop standards for how PMS should be researched," says psychiatrist Sally Severion of the White Plains, N.Y., division of New York Hospital-Cornell Medical Center. She served on the APA's task force and felt PMDD should appear in the *DSM-IV* appendix.

"Although feminists disavow the idea of any cyclic dysfunction in women," adds Dr. Judith Gold, the Halifax, Nova Scotia, psychiatrist who chaired the PMDD work group of the task force," individual women continue to report symptoms and request treatment. Just because only women have this disorder doesn't mean we should deny it in a well-meaning attempt to avoid stigmatizing them."

Some experts think a partial solution might be to classify severe PMS as a physical disorder, rather than a mental one. For now, the criteria for PMDD remain confined to the *DSM-IV* appendix, meaning further research and debate are required before PMDD is classified as a mental disorder.

they solve. Bromocriptine (Parlodel) suppresses a hormone called prolactin, which may cause premenstrual breast tenderness, but the drug is linked to a risk of seizures and strokes in a small percentage of patients. Alprazolam (Xanax) is often prescribed for premenstrual anxiety, but studies of its effectiveness are conflicting, and it can be habit-forming.

For severe PMS, doctors are increasingly turning to medications that correct serotonin imbalances, including antidepressants such as Prozac and Zoloft. These may help physical, as well as mood-related, symptoms. A 1992 study by researchers at the University of California at San Diego found that Prozac reduced the emotional symptoms of PMS 75% and physical symptoms such as breast tenderness 40%. More recently, Harvard's Mortola has shown that women may benefit even if they take the drug only in the second half of the cycle.

For women disabled by PMS, a possible, though drastic, tactic is to induce artificial menopause by prescribing synthetic forms of gonadotropin releasing hormone agonists — Lupron or Synarel, for example — which eventually suppress estrogen and progesterone production. Women taking these drugs, which are otherwise used to treat fibroid tumors and endometriosis, often take small amounts of estrogen and progesterone as well to counteract menopause-related osteoporosis and heart disease. In a 1991 study, Mortola found that GnRH drugs and hormonal "add back" therapy decreased premenstrual distress 60%. But the treatment is relatively expensive, and its long-term effects have not been fully studied. "When we give a patient GnRH agonists," says Chuong. "we need good documentation that her symptoms are really affecting her life and that no other medications have helped."

If GnRH drug therapy helps, some doctors may advise a patient to consider having a hysterectomy, but only as the very last resort. "I treat one of the severest populations in the country, and I've never done one," says Mortola. "I think you'd have to reach a point where a woman was housebound for a week each month, or unable to control her rage, or suicidal."

If you are seeking help for PMS, be willing to experiment, and keep in mind that it may take a while to find relief. "We can help everyone who comes to see us," says Rapkin. "But it may take time. You have to be willing to try different approaches and, if possible, try them for at least two cycles. PMS isn't something you can just give a pill for and make go away."

Nancy Wartik is a Contributing Editor at American Health.

PART 4

Reproductive Choices

This section looks at the choices that women (and men) have regarding reproductive control. The general theme that emerges from all the readings in Part 4 is this: there are ongoing safety concerns with the birth control options that women have, and the choices women can make regarding their own fertility remain limited. Although several new methods of birth control have appeared on the market in the last couple of years, these methods have their complications.

Newer methods of birth control, for example Norplant, provide a reasonable standard of protection against contraception, but they do not prevent the transmission of sexually transmitted diseases, and may also have complicating side effects. Many students ask what about birth control for men? That is an issue that provides a good basis for classroom discussion! (Please see the **Quick Reference Guide to Topics/Readings/WWW Sites** and **Appendix A: WebLinks: A Directory of Annotated World Wide Web Sites** to select WWW sites that coordinate with the readings in this part.)

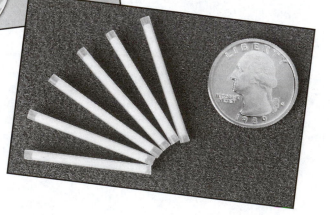

Still Fumbling in the Dark

Contraception: With all the condoms, pills and foams, why are so many women getting sterilized?

By Michele Ingrassia, Karen Springen, Debra Rosenberg

Jennifer Wohlenberg is just 22, but she can already tick off a lifetime's worth of contraceptive disappointments. She tried the pill, but couldn't stand the weight gain, the nausea, the yeast infection that lasted a year and a half. She and her husband, Brad, hated condoms — lubricated condoms, non-lubricated condoms, condoms with spermicide, condoms without spermicide, they all irritated her. After that, the alternatives dwindled rapidly. Diaphragm? Wohlenberg finds even tampons painful. Norplant? She considered the implant sticks, "but then I read these stories about how you have to dig them out." Her mother had an IUD scare, and two of her sisters got pregnant on the progestin-only minipill. So for now, she reluctantly uses the only method she feels is left: nothing. (Well, they do watch the calendar.) "It kind of puts a damper on your sex life," says the South Pasadena, Calif., marketing coordinator. "It's like being a teenager again, being scared of what will happen."

When it comes to birth control, Americans are still fumbling in the dark. Thirty years after the pill promised a contraception revolution, the effort to find a cheap, easy-to-use, safe and effective method has proven a bitter failure. Men and women feel cheated. And not even researchers talk in terms of magic pills anymore. Instead, at a time when more than half of all pregnancies are unplanned and sexually transmitted diseases are growing at the rate of 12 million to 13 million new cases a year, the options are shrinking. The manufacturers of the Today Sponge pulled it off the market in January; the IUD has all but disappeared, and the diaphragm is literally as unpopular as abstinence.

PERMANENT OPTIONS

Our frustration is playing out not just in the bedroom but in the operating room. A stunning new National Center for Health Statistics survey reports that, for the first time, more women are opting for sterilization than any other form of birth control — a trend that used to be associated with Third World countries, not leading industrialized nations. But while few were paying attention, voluntary sterilizations have risen sharply in the last decade. Of all American women using contraception in 1990, the last year for which figures are available, 29.5 percent had tubal ligations, surpassing even the once dominant pill. Add in vasectomies and the number of women relying on some type of sterilization tops 42 percent.

Worldwide, Americans rank near the top of the list of women relying on sterilization. In 1988, the last year for which comparable data exist, more than 36 percent of married American women used sterilization. That puts the United States up there with China (35 percent) and India (31 percent) and well ahead of Westernized countries like Britain (23 percent) and the Netherlands (15 percent). Not surprisingly, most Americans getting sterilized are in their 30s and 40s, a sign that baby boomers are nearing the end of their child-bearing years. But the steady increase in couples of all ages opting for permanent methods underscores how fed up they are with the choices.

Yomari Ortiz is planning to get her tubes tied next month — and she's only 21. After two children in two years, Ortiz has mapped out her life — a high-school-equivalency diploma, college, a job as a radiology technologist and marriage — and more children are not in the equation. Neither is hassling with birth control. The young Chicagoan says she was using condoms when she conceived her son, who is now 3, and was on the pill when she got pregnant with her daughter, who's 2. And though her doctor's assistant tried to talk her out of sterilization, her boyfriend supports her. Ortiz is adamant. "I might as well just cut my tubes now and throw them away," Ortiz says with a chilling matter-of-factness.

Is this where the Sexual Revolution was supposed to lead us? Symbolism aside, the pill was designed to let women control when and if they got pregnant. Of course, it also freed them to go to work and allowed them — and their partners — to view sex as recreation. But that was before sexual freedom gave way to increasing numbers of out-of-wedlock births. In the years since, policymakers have grown frustrated trying to stem the tide — to the point where a new, unabashedly conservative Congress threatens to take welfare benefits from single mothers who bear more children. Abortion isn't a solution. With anti-abortion protests becoming more violent, the number of counties with doctors willing to perform abortions has shrunk to 16 percent.

Politics, coupled with the high cost of developing new contraceptives, has taken a mighty toll. "The pharmaceutical industry has washed its hands of birth control," says the father of the pill, Stanford University chemist Carl Djerassi. In the space-race '60s —

when women demanded, "If we can put a man on the moon, why can't we come up with decent birth control?" — nine major American companies were doing contraceptive research; now only one is still committed. Djerassi blames U.S. regulators for being hypercautious. It took Depo-Provera, a progestin that's injected every three months, 25 years to win Food and Drug Administration approval, in 1992. Even benign methods aren't immune. The sponge wasn't the most effective option on the market; tales are legion of teenage girls who read the "wet before inserting" instructions and thought they could use spit or Coca-Cola. It *was* cheap and readily available. Yet Today Sponge manufacturer Whitehall-Robins Healthcare pulled it off the shelves, saying it would cost too much to upgrade its plant to meet new FDA safety rules.

ABORTION PILL

Nowhere are the battles more fierce than with RU-486, the so-called French abortion pill. It isn't close to getting on the market here. U.S. firms refused to touch it, frightened by controversy and threatened boycotts by abortion opponents. And the French manufacturer, Roussel Uclaf, handed over U.S. rights to the drug — a potential $50 million market — to the non-profit Population Council, which is conducting clinical trials. It's not just RU-486. Companies have fled the entire contraceptive market because the risk of lawsuits outweighed any possible jackpot. "We live in a very litigious society,' says Polly Harrison of the National Academy of Science's Institute of Medicine.

With all the talk of high-tech solutions, it's no small irony that the only contraceptive to get excited about these days is the old low tech condom. The first polyurethane condom, Avanti, is slated to go on sale nationwide this fall. Its British manufacturer, London International Group, says it's thinner and more sensitive than the standard latex condom — but thinner and more sensitive isn't likely to alter the sort of biases that most men pick up long before they've had their first date. As Sam, a 28-year-old carpenter from Worcester, Mass., puts it: "Nobody likes making love to a balloon." Even if it's a woman wearing it. In the nearly two years since Reality, the female condom, was introduced, it's been applauded for giving women control over STD prevention and criticized for esthetics: it looks like an oversize male condom, feels like Crisco and squeaks. It takes getting used to. "I had never used a diaphragm, so it's an awkward feeling," says Rita Wanser, 35, of Middletown, N.Y.

But even if people don't *like* condoms, a decade's worth of public-service campaigns against AIDS and STDs have forced a growing number to agree they're essential. Condom World, on the funky end of

Options, But No Solutions

In 1990, nearly 60 percent of women age 15–44 used contraception. Surgical sterilization was the most-used method; in 1982, it was the pill.

FEMALE	%
Sterilization	29.5
Pill	28.5
Condom	17.7
Male sterilization	12.6
Diaphragm	2.8
Periodic abstinence	2.7
IUD	1.4
Other methods	4.8

Source: National Center for Health Statistics

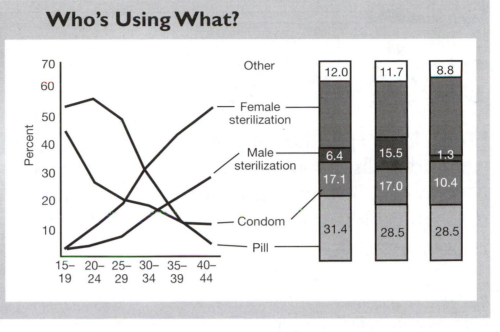

Who's Using What?

Younger women are more likely to use condoms and other reversible birth control, according to 1990 data, while older women opt more for sterilization. Black women rely the most on tubal ligation, followed by Hispanics and then whites. The pill is most popular among Hispanics.

*Other includes IUD, Diaphragm, periodic abstinence and other. Source: National Center for Health Statistics

Boston's Newbury Street, sports more condoms than a frat house — more than 150 varieties in all. The atmosphere here is far different from a corner drugstore, where condoms are still dauntingly hidden away. Indeed, on a sunny Saturday, customers browse the way they do at neighboring Tower Records. "It's just a fact of life these days." says Zeb Robbins, 25, an engineer from Newton who wandered into the shop with two female friends. The young blond allows how condoms have helped his sex life; women, he says, like that he's willing to use them.

WHO'LL USE

The more pressing question is, how willing are teenagers to use condoms — or anything else? Susie Carrillo and her boyfriend, Sam Vongkorad, tried to use condoms, but she concedes that "sometimes they weren't at hand." Two months ago Susie, an Aurora, Ill., 17-year-old, gave birth to a girl. Even a few years ago doctors rarely debated that the first choice for a teenager was the pill. Now they're not so sure. By the age of 21, according to the Centers for Disease Control, one in four young people is already infected with an STD. But the chances of getting kids to "double Dutch" — as teens in the Netherlands call the pill-and-condom combo — are small. So health experts find themselves in the troubling position of having to decide between putting teens at risk for pregnancy or AIDS.

The solution, of course, is a method that does it all — which puts us back on the magic-pill hunt. Researchers are already trying to develop microbicides, "detergent" suppositories or foams that kill off anything from sperm to disease. Next best, they say, would be a "menses inducer," a pill that women could take if they've had unprotected sex. Actually, morning-after methods already exist — a doctor can prescribe large doses of birth-control pills to a woman or insert an IUD — but no company is willing to market a morning-after label.

All the confusion leaves women like Jennifer Wohlenberg still searching. After running through the entire contraceptive medicine cabinet, she's more frustrated than ever. "I wish there was a pill for men," she sighs. But the promise of a male contraceptive by the millenniun is unlikely. Instead, Djerassi suggests, men could freeze their sperm and then get vasectomies. But that won't protect against AIDS and STDs. And it won't affect men who refuse to get involved. Which makes even that futuristic option no option at all.

Michelle Ingrassia with Karen Springen in Chicago and Debra Rosenberg in Boston

Blood and Tears

Medicine: How do the new 'abortion pills' really work? *Newsweek* followed two women through clinical trials of the controversial drug RU-486.

*By Debra Rosenberg,
Michele Ingrassia, Sharon Begley*

When the name RU-486 washed up on this side of the Atlantic 12 years ago, it accomplished the seemingly impossible: it gave pro-life and pro-choice advocates something in common. Both thought that if the "French abortion pill" ever became available, it would change the landscape of abortion in America. Pro-choicers believe that a nonsurgical method of terminating a pregnancy would remove abortion from the public arena, taking it away from easily targeted clinics and into the privacy of a physician's office. They hope that it would be made available to the millions of women who live days away from a willing doctor. Abortion foes also foresee a revolution, one so repugnant that they have successfully fought for years to keep RU-486 from being made or marketed in the United States. They fear that medical abortion — in which a physician gives a woman a few tablets that, within days, cause her to expel her fetus — would make the procedure as easy to get as the local newspaper.

Now America may be about to find out whether either side is right. This summer *Newsweek* was granted extraordinary access to the clinical trials of RU-486. Named after its French manufacturer, Roussel Uclaf, it is called mifepristone in the United States. For the last year the New York-based Population Council (a private research and advocacy group) has run tests of the safety and efficacy of mifepristone among 2,100 women at 17 clinics. The experiences of the women at two of these clinics — Aurora Medical Services in Seattle and Planned Parenthood of Westchester and Rockland in White Plains, N.Y. — show that medical abortion is neither the panacea that pro-choicers believe nor the nightmare that pro-lifers dread. Their experiences also show that abortion by any means will never be just another trip to the doctor. This is the story of two women who volunteered to test mifepristone.

Becky, 30, is a full-time geology student and a married mother of three daughters. Her youngest, 4, has spina bifida, a congenital defect that exposes part of the spinal cord; the little girl needs a ventilator at night and requires near round-the-clock nursing. Becky and her husband, Richard (who asked that their last name not be used), did not want to risk bringing another crippled child into the world. Becky, a cherubic Hispanic woman whose brown bob is pulled off her face with a white cloth headband, has chosen Aurora because she had two surgical abortions as a teenager. She still remembers the slurping noise of the suction machine, the loneliness, the doctor's coldness. "It's surgery," she says. "You get all afraid you're going to die. When they close the door on that tiny little room and that suction machine goes on, it's terrifying."

Sarah (not her real name) is a waitress and single. Her diaphragm failed one morning when she made love with her boyfriend, Neal, a bicycle messenger. In addition to not feeling ready to be a mother, Sarah, 25, had done a fair amount of drinking and smoking before she realized she was pregnant, and worried about the health of the fetus. She had resigned herself to another suction abortion — she had had one when she was 18 — until she heard from a friend about the abortion pill.

Becky is eight weeks pregnant when she arrives at Aurora one Wednesday morning in July. The nurse-midwife, Beth (who didn't want her last name revealed for security reasons), explains how mifepristone blocks the effect of the hormone progesterone, without which the uterine lining sloughs off as during a menstrual period and a pregnancy cannot continue. The drug misoprostol, taken two days later, induces uterine contractions that expel the fetus. Beth gives Becky a pelvic exam, a blood test and a sonogram to be sure she is not more than nine weeks pregnant, the cutoff for a medical abortion. Becky decides to go ahead with it. She swallows three yellowish oval tablets of mifepristone and goes home.

Nothing much happens at first. On Thursday evening Becky feels some back pain and bleeds a little while she fries chicken for dinner. Sarah, who took the mifepristone the same morning as Becky, has it worse. At 2 a.m. she is vomiting and reeling from a headache. "I lay there for a while, trying to figure out if there was actually anything going on," she recalls.

'PMS PILLS'

On Friday morning, both Becky and Sarah return to Aurora, which is tucked discreetly into a corner of a professional building, for their three white misoprostol pills. Sarah, a tall, muscular brunette with a golden tan, gets fidgety waiting for something to happen. She goes to the bathroom down the hall and then looks over the rack of videos in the waiting room. "I'm a little nervous. I'm a little weenie when it comes to pain," she admits. She can't lean back in the upright chair in the waiting room. "They need some La-Z Boys," she says. After 45 minutes, Sarah gets cramps and decides to lie down in patient room 3. She tries to get comfortable between the stirrups on the exam table (Aurora has no special beds for the medical-abortion patients). Neal sits next to the table. Sarah curls up under a blanket and tries to read her Isabel Allende novel. The bleeding starts around 10:35. At 11:15, she dispatches Neal for what she calls "PMS pills," big sugary doughnuts. While he's gone Nancy, the counselor, checks Sarah's blood pressure. "I just passed something incredibly huge." Sarah tells her. "I'm wondering if that was it." 'Was it white?" Nancy asks. Sarah doesn't think so. Then it probably wasn't the sac containing the fetus, Nancy says. Sarah closes her eyes, but doesn't sleep. When Neal returns with a dozen doughnuts, she wolfs down a sugar doughnut and half a maple bar. Neal wanders through the waiting room to offer a doughnut to Becky. "The cramps are getting a little worse," Sarah says at 12:15. She tells Nancy that she passed another large clot, but that it sank into the toilet before she could get a good look at it. "A lot of times people just know [that they've expelled the fetus]," Nancy assures her. "They just know." But Sarah isn't sure at all. She is surprised by the size and number of the blood clots — many as big as a half dollar. She is mildly nauseated. Another ultrasound reveals that the sac containing the fetus is no longer viable but not whether it is still clinging to the uterine wall.

Becky fares better. Half an hour after she swallows the misoprostol, her usual chatter slows. She can't get comfortable in the waiting-room chair. "Leave me alone," she snaps at Richard when he tries to rub her back. She curls up in a blanket on the floor near the TV. "Oh, it hurts," she wails as waves of cramps wash over her. "It just feels like your uterus is trying to s--t out a watermelon." Becky takes some Tylenol with codeine, paces the hallway, eats the doughnut Neal gives her, goes into the bathroom and throws up. She says she's "gushing" blood. She returns to her chair, rocks gently, hugs a hot-water bottle to her abdomen, tries to vary her breathing. "How long will the cramps last?" she pleads. Richard corners a nurse. She assures him his wife's pain is normal. Becky's face is ashen. Her limbs feel shaky. Then, suddenly, something seems to shift inside her. The pain stops abruptly and Becky relaxes, her face glistening with sweat. She exhales and leans her head back against the wall. Minutes later, around 1:20, she goes into the bathroom and yells: "Richard! Come here — look at this!" There is a fist-size glob of red and white at the bottom of the toilet. Becky can see the curled-up fetus, the size and color of a cocktail shrimp. "Look at that, honey," Becky says to Richard. Its hands are curled into tiny fists. "It's sad. It's sad," Becky murmurs, turning away.

DOWN THE DRAIN

Unlike Becky, Sarah has not expelled the fetus within 24 hours of taking the misoprostol. She is among the 10 percent of women whose mifepristone abortion takes more than a day. Sent home in the late afternoon, Sarah bleeds heavily for the next few days but manages to go in to work. The following Sunday — nine days after the misoprostol — she is taking a shower when she suddenly expels the pregnancy sac. It doesn't go down the drain. She scoops it up, wraps it carefully in toilet paper and flushes it away. "It really emotionally hit me," she says later.

Despite the nine days of bleeding and cramps, and despite seeing the fetus swirling around the shower drain, Sarah preferred the medical abortion to the surgical one she had as a teenager. "It just seemed a little healthier," she says. "It seemed a little less traumatic." Claudia, a 23-year-old computer programmer from Connecticut who lives with her boyfriend, had an experience starkly different from Sarah's: the night after taking the drug at the Planned Parenthood clinic she passed the fetus, without even taking the contraction-inducing misoprostol. She had never had an abortion before. "At first I cried," she says. "It's a mourning process. It's respect for life. But it wasn't guilt . . . Maybe I would have had more guilt with a surgical abortion because I wasn't connected with it." Becky preferred the medical abortion to her surgical ones, even though it was more emotionally draining. She wanted to experience the pain, both emotional and physical, she says. She felt she should suffer for terminating her pregnancy, since for her, as for many women who have an abortion, the certainty that she did not want to carry the fetus to term did not make the decision any less morally or emotionally ambiguous. "There was a little bit of regret about seeing [the fetus], because it had little hands," Becky says. "I remember little fists. I felt more responsible this time."

The clinical trial of mifepristone ended last week, and for now the drug is unavailable. Now the Population Council will spend several months collecting and analyzing the data; it hopes to submit a request for FDA approval by the year-end. Approval could come as soon as next year. Studies in Europe, as well as preliminary results in this country, suggest that the drug regimen is safe and effective. And late last month a New York gynecologist announced the results of another abortion-drug trial: he found that two common prescription drugs, used to fight cancer and ulcers, can also be used successfully to end an early pregnancy (*Newsweek*, Sept. 11). This regimen could win FDA approval by 1997.

But it is unclear whether medical abortion would bring about the changes that pro-choice forces envision. Although the activists hope that abortion-by-prescription will be more widely available, especially in rural areas, there is no guarantee that physicians will have any more enthusiasm for it than they do for surgical abortion. There are, however, some hints. In a study scheduled for release later this month, the private Kaiser Family Foundation, a health-policy research group, finds that one third of obstetricians/gynecologists who do not now offer abortions say they would prescribe mifepristone. No matter how many doctors offer it, pro-life activists say they will have little trouble finding them. "We will be able to find out where they're doing [medical] abortions," vows Ann Scheidler of the Pro-Life Action League.

Whether the political landscape of abortion would change with the availability of a pregnancy-ending pill depends, of course, on how many women opt for it over surgery. A Population Council survey finds that 60 to 70 percent of women who had a medical abortion preferred it to the surgical option: But the population at large might not be so enthusiastic. In fact, medical abortions will almost certainly cost just as much as surgical abortions. They could have a higher failure rate, since surgery is almost foolproof but drugs act differently in different women. Medical abortions are also less convenient. The expulsion of the fetus could happen anywhere, any time, after the first pills are swallowed. It is not clear how many women really want to see, or dispose of, their fetus. "I think medical abortion is being portrayed as easier than it is," says Vicki Saporta executive director of the pro-choice National Abortion Federation. "This is not like taking an aspirin and your headache goes away."

But these are just practical concerns. The turmoil that comes with the decision to abort will be no less if a woman knows she will double over with cramps rather than brace herself for the cold steel of the stirrups and the suction hose. Abortion-by-prescription may indeed make the procedure a private matter between a woman and her doctor once again. And that would undoubtedly make women's ordeals easier. But never easy.

Just ask Becky or Sarah.

Debra Rosenberg in Seattle, Michelle Ingrassia in White Plains and Sharon Begley

Means to an End: Three Abortion Techniques

Though their results are the same — the termination of a pregnancy — medical and early-stage surgical abortion work in different ways. The benefits and disadvantages of three methods:

PROCEDURE	SIDE EFFECTS, RISKS	COST, TIMING, STATUS
RU 486 Mifepristone (RU 486) pills block hormone sustaining pregnancy; misoprostol pills two days later induce contractions.	Intense cramping and bleeding can last more than a week. Four percent failure rate.	About $300. Effective until the 9th week of pregnancy. FDA may approve it next year.
Methotrexate and Misoprostol A shot stops fetal cells from dividing. A vaginal suppository 5 to 7 days later induces contractions.	Nausea and diarrhea in rare cases. Four percent failure rate.	Drugs are $10, M.D. visits bring tab to $300. Effective up to 9th week. Could be approved in 1997.
Surgery Usually vacuum aspiration of the fetus through the vagina. Performed under a local anesthetic.	Slight chance of perforation of the uterus or injury to the cervix.	About $300. Used from 6th to (in rare cases) 24th week. Legal, but 85% of U.S. counties have no practitioners.

DIMINISHED CHOICE

Why it's harder than ever to get an abortion

By Monika Bauerlein

At age 79, Dr. Jane Hodgson still regularly makes the 150 mile trip from St. Paul to the Duluth Women's Center, a reproductive health clinic in northern Minnesota that she helped found. The veteran abortion-rights crusader does it in part because she "can't let go" and in part because — more than two decades after the Supreme Court legalized the procedure — the clinic can't find a local doctor to terminate pregnancies.

Abortion rights have gone through a lot of ups and downs since Hodgson first got active after seeing too many women bleeding to death from back-alley attempts. The issue has faded from the headlines a bit since the Supreme Court narrowly reaffirmed the right in 1992; even conservative groups have been holding their fire, focusing on things like budgets and taxes instead. But away from the limelight, the abortion landscape has been shifting in ways that could affect women's options more dramatically than any amount of political debate. Some observers warn that between a growing doctor shortage, financial obstacles, and a variety of other quiet de facto restrictions, women may keep the right to choose but find it harder and harder to actually exercise that right.

The issue hasn't attracted a lot of headlines; one of the few media to take note has been the *Journal of the American Medical Women's Association* (*JAMWA*), which considered the topic hot enough to devote its entire September/October 1994 edition to it. The journal's first warning is directed at the fact that, as Hodgson's generation of frontline abortion doctors retires, fewer and fewer young physicians are learning the procedure. In 1976, reports Dr. Carolyn Westhoff, almost one out of four ob-gyn programs required students to learn how to terminate a first-trimester pregnancy. Another two-thirds offered the training as an option. But in 1994, fully one-third of programs didn't offer abortion training at all, and most of the rest made it voluntary — an option. Westhoff warns, that busy med students won't necessarily choose when they know that "harassment, poor pay, low prestige, and tedium" are among the rewards awaiting abortion doctors.

Ironically, Westhoff and others note, the problem is exacerbated by the fact that in the years since *Roe*, independent clinics have picked up an ever greater share of women's reproductive health care. Doctors get their basic training as residents in hospitals, where only 7 percent of abortions were performed in 1992; as a result, many ob-gyn residents end up doing tubal ligations more often than abortions. Clinics are also much more likely to be targets of protests, further discouraging doctors from practicing there. And though clinics are usually more accessible than hospitals, they often can't or won't perform some of the more complicated abortion services: 43 percent don't terminate pregnancies past the first trimester, and one third won't serve HIV-positive women.

The first to notice the effect of doctor shortages are women in rural areas. Already, according to the Alan Guttmacher Institute in New York, which studies the economics of reproductive health issues, nine out of ten abortion providers are located in metropolitan counties; 27 percent of women seeking an abortion have to travel more than 50 miles. And while that kind of trip may not faze a financially secure adult woman who has a car, it can be a daunting obstacle for poor women and teenagers.

From the *UTNE Reader* (September/October 1995), pp. 18, 20. Reprinted by permission of Monika Bauerlein, Managing Editor of *City Pages*, the alternative weekly in Minneapolis/St. Paul.

The same groups, not surprisingly, have the most trouble with the other big practical obstacle to abortion: money. Thirty-seven million Americans, including nine million women of childbearing age, had no health coverage as of 1993, according to census figures, and one-fifth of those who do must show some kind of medical problem to get an abortion paid for. Medicaid, the federal/state health care program for the very poor, hasn't been required to cover abortions since Congress passed the Hyde amendment in 1976; only six states currently choose to cover the procedure, while nine more do so by court order.

According to the Guttmacher Institute, first-trimester abortions currently cost $300 on average. And raising that money out of pocket is more than an inconvenience: Frequently, delays due to financial problems result in a more complicated second trimester abortion or none at all. Kathryn Kolbert and Andrea Miller, writing in *JAMWA*, cite one stunning statistic: "Between 18 and 23 percent of Medicaid-eligible women living in those states that do not provide coverage for abortion carried unwanted pregnancies to term because they could not afford to pay for the procedure." Those figures may rise as more states enact the kind of restrictions the Supreme Court found constitutional in the 1992 Casey decision: 24-hour waiting periods, statescripted lectures from physicians on the risks of abortion, parental consent for minors, and so on. Those restrictions can be financially tough on clinics — when, for example, they require doctors rather than nurses or social workers to do the mandatory counseling. That burden, plus violent protests and the doctor shortage, could drive some clinics out of business.

There are some signs that the problems are starting to register in the medical profession. In an article for the Women's Feature Service, Leslie George notes that after the 1993 killing of Dr. John Britton outside a Pensacola, Florida, abortion clinic, young doctors-to-be formed Medical Students for Choice with the goal of pushing for increased abortion training; some of their older counterparts hold workshops to train family practitioners and other doctors in the procedure. *JAMWA*'s Westhoff reports that a medical committee charged with setting standards for ob-gyn training is considering language under which "experience with induced abortion and management of its complications must be part of residency training, except for residents with moral or religious objections to the former"; some hospitals are working out rotation arrangements with abortion clinics for their residents. And there are efforts to encourage other medical professionals, like physician assistants, to do abortions in areas where the doctor is many miles away.

Lest all this sound too encouraging to pro-choicers, the bad news comes in one final *JAMWA* article: If access to abortion is becoming a problem in the United States, Deborah Maine, Katrina Karkasis, and Nancy Bolan report, the issue is one of life and death for women in much of the rest of the world. They note that about one in 21 women in Africa will die as a result of complications from pregnancy or childbirth, compared to one in 6,366 in North America. Complications of induced abortions — fully or partially outlawed in countries containing more than half the world's population, but widely performed nevertheless — account for an estimated 14 percent of maternal deaths, totaling between 70,000 and 200,000 worldwide annually; in other words, every day 200 to 550 women die trying to terminate a pregnancy. In Latin America, botched abortions are the leading cause of death among women aged 15 to 39. For most of the world's women, the authors conclude, "the bad old days are still here."

Monika Bauerlein is managing editor of City Pages, *the Minneapolis/St. Paul alternative weekly.*

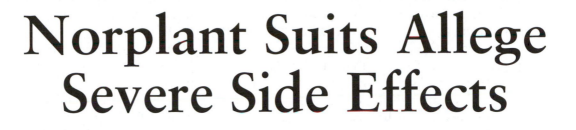

A Reading for Critical Thinking

Norplant Suits Allege Severe Side Effects

By Jamie Talan

Deciding that her family was complete, Rose Ann Friedman says she was enticed by the ease of an implanted contraceptive device that could end her worries for at least five years.

No more skipped pills. No more diaphragms. No more bother.

But soon after the six hormone-filled capsules were surgically placed in her arm, the New York City woman found herself suffering from mood swings, adolescent type acne on her face and scalp, clumps of dark chin hair, almost constant headaches and a 2 pound weight gain.

"I was a wreck," the 34 year-old mother of two said recently. "I kept attributing my problems to everything else in my life."

But eventually, she began to think it might be the Norplant. "Finally, after 10 months, I came in and begged my father (a gynecologist/obstetrician) to remove it."

THICK SCAR TISSUE

But even that was no easy matter, she said. When Friedman's father — Dr. Anthony Sgarlato of New York City — cut a tiny incision in his daughter's arm to remove the matchstick-sized implants, he said he was horrified at what he found. The first two came out easily, but the remaining four were covered by thick scar tissue, requiring a second, larger surgical cut to remove them.

Sgarlato said he had been against Norplant from the beginning and had not received training in removing it, but as a surgeon he believed removal would be routine. Sgarlato said the procedure took four hours — much longer than the 20 minutes described in pamphlets produced by Wyeth-Ayerst Laboratories of Wayne, Pa., the company that sells the implant.

"Don't even mention Norplant," Sgarlato said recently. "I've delivered thousands of babies, performed hysterectomies, removed ovarian cysts . . . but I've never seen anything like this. The capsules migrated . . . they were stuck in scar tissue. My daughter was crying."

Friedman is not alone.

During the past several months, the contraceptive has been the target of class-action lawsuits in Chicago, Dallas and Florida, alleging that the removal of Norplant is much more difficult, and potentially more dangerous, than advertised. Also, attorneys involved in the Chicago suit broadened their case two weeks ago to include a second charge: that Wyeth-Ayerst has failed to adequately warn women about the potential severity of the contraceptive's side effects.

COMPANY'S DENIAL

Spokesmen for Wyeth-Ayerst deny the charges. Dr. Marc Deitch, vice president of medical affairs for the company, describes the removal procedure as being "affected by a number of variables" including

Side Effects of Norplant

Side effects and other problems associated with the contraceptive implant Norplant:

- Headaches
- Nervousness
- Dizziness
- Acne
- Weight Gain
- Removal of the implants is much more difficult than the makers acknowledge, according to class-action lawsuits.

"how the capsules were originally inserted, the procedure used for removal and the circumstances that are unique to a given patient." Because of this, the company contends, a class action is inappropriate.

But attorneys at Holstein, Mack and Klein of Chicago disagree, arguing that the problems are too widespread to be considered individually. They say that since their suit was filed as a class action in June, they have received more than 1,000 calls from women with stories similar to Friedman's.

Corey Berman, a lawyer with Holstein, Mack and Klein, said the firm is seeking damages and an injunction ordering Wyeth-Ayerst to train all doctors who dispense the implants and to strengthen its warnings on potential removal problems and possible side effects. The company's existing labeling, fails "to disclose what can happen to these women," Berman said.

A MILLION U.S. WOMEN

Since its introduction in the United States in February 1991, Norplant has been used as a contraceptive by nearly a million U.S. women. The insertion takes 15 to 20 minutes, and doctors charge $450 to $750, including removal.

The six capsules — which are implanted by a doctor in the arm, just above the elbow — work by releasing controlled bursts of the hormone progestin.

However, about 20 percent of Norplant users drop the method in the first year, either because of side effects or because they want to become pregnant, according to the nonprofit Center for Reproductive Law and Policy in New York City. And that, the attorneys have charged, is when problems can really arise.

In addition to problems like those reported by Sgarlato, some doctors said some of the capsules had ruptured, sending an overload of steroid hormone into the blood stream and causing pronounced side effects.

Wyeth-Ayerst, meanwhile, says it has trained 28,000 doctors to implant and remove Norplant, although the training is not a condition for dispensing the contraceptive.

The problems with Norplant are no surprise to federal regulators and company officials. According to Dr. Lisa Rarick, an FDA medical officer who worked on Norplant throughout the approval process, 13 percent of the removals in experimental trials were considered difficult.

"There are benefits and risks to most procedures," Rarick said. "Patients should be made aware of the risks, but it doesn't mean we are going to pull Norplant from the market."

As for the side effects, the company says patients are being properly warned. Patients, it said, should receive from their doctors a recently updated brochure that includes warnings about headaches, nervousness, dizziness, acne and weight gain, as well as rare reports of birth defects when women got pregnant while using Norplant.

WARNINGS TO PATIENTS

The brochure also warns that some women have complained of mood swings, arm pain, strokes and heart attacks, though company officials say "association with the Norplant system has been neither confirmed nor refuted."

It is unclear whether news coverage of the court cases has hurt sales of Norplant. But Dr. Jerry Wider, an obstetrician gynecologist with a large group practice on Long Island, said recently that he thinks there is a "low patient acceptability" for the contraceptive right now.

Lisa Kaeser, a policy analyst at the Alan Guttmacher Institute of New York, a nonprofit agency specializing in population issues, also points out that — unlike some other contraceptive methods — "a woman can't just wake up in the morning and say 'I don't want it.'"

The Pill: What It's Done For Us … and to Us

By Anne Glusker

Few things in our world go by no brand name, need no descriptive adjective. Just an article and the generic name of the thing. There's the moon, the sun, and . . . the Pill. There is certainly a universe of other tablets and capsules at the pharmacist's disposal, there may be plenty in our own personal medicine chests, but only one is "the" Pill. This year marked the 35th anniversary of the introduction of the birth control pill in the U.S. The Pill has become such a part of common parlance that it's easy to forget how powerfully liberating this new method of contraception seemed at first (and how disturbing and disappointing were the later revelations of its severe health risks. While the Pill was more effective in preventing pregnancy than its predecessors — with a failure rate of only 3 to 6 percent — its truly radical nature was the way in which it separated the actual sexual moment from the act of contraception.

Not long after the Food and Drug Administration (FDA) approved it in 1960, however, the Pill was implicated as a cause of blood clots and pulmonary embolisms, heart attacks, and strokes. Spurred by Barbara Seaman's book, *The Doctors' Case Against the Pill*, and the then-nascent women's health movement, the Senate held hearings on the Pill in 1970, and the super-strength version (containing as much as 150 micrograms of estrogen) was eventually replaced by lower dosages of 35–50 micrograms.

In recent years, in its less-powerful form (now as low as 20–30 micrograms), the Pill has experienced something of a renaissance — with some doctors even asserting its health *benefits*. Although women's health activists dismiss such claims, the Pill's place as a

Perhaps pleasure isn't best attained by ignoring one part of our physical selves in favor of another.

vortex of controversy, debate, and feminist critique has been supplanted by Norplant and Depo-Provera. But, far from any headline or spotlight, women are still using the Pill — at least 65 million women around the world currently take it, and according to the most recent statistics from the Centers for Disease Control, almost 10 million women in the U.S. were using the Pill for birth control in 1990.

There's a simple reason the Pill is up there with the moon and the sun in name; recognition — it did nothing less than revolutionize the way our culture sees sex. With a condom or a diaphragm, somebody had to blearily reach over to the nightstand, walk to the dresser, or stumble down the hall to the bathroom. There might be awkwardness, there might be annoyance, certainly there was interruption. In the heady days of the sixties and seventies — that era that we now set off in quotes and call the "sexual revolution" with more than a bit of irony — the Pill helped broker a disconnection between women and our reproductive capacity that was seen by many of us as immensely freeing, as aiding us in the quest for pleasure. But we've learned a thing or two since those days. Not that pleasure isn't one of the most important things in life. Not that we shouldn't proceed, full-force, in search of it. But perhaps Dionysian delight isn't best attained ignoring one part of our physical selves in favor of another. One thing we've learned for sure is that the actions we take to prevent pregnancy have ramifications. So, as long as we choose to have intercourse, and long as we can conceive, we have to confront this reality. Words like "ramifications" and "consequences" have an ominous ring these days —

they sound like punitive imprecations from the Christian right or Chairman Newt. Nevertheless, we must think about long-term effects: the risks to our overall physical well-being — and to our future fertility, should we desire to have children — of any drug or device we ingest or insert into our bodies. If we don't, we run the risk of compartmentalizing ourselves into (a) human beings who are sexual and (b) human beings who worry about health and reproduction. It's ironic that the very thing that seemed so liberating in the Pill's early days — the separation of birth control and sex — now seems archaic in its illusion of isolating one part of being a woman from another.

In the imperfect world we live in, there is no obvious winner in the contraceptive contest. While we lobby and pray for the contraceptive of our dreams — one that is safe, affordable, and easy to use — we also have to make our selection from what's available. Any current contraceptive choice involves some sort of trade off: greater or lesser risk of pregnancy; more or less protection from AIDS and other sexually transmitted diseases (STDs); more or less convenience (i.e., interruption of sex); greater or lesser possibility of breast cancer and heart attack.

The women who select the Pill as their method of birth control today certainly face far fewer health risks than did the first users of the Pill, back in the sixties. Although conflicting opinions exist in the medical community, the major health threat still associated with the Pill seems to be breast cancer — a risk that appears to increase when use begins at an early age and continues for a prolonged period of time. According to Cindy Pearson of the National Women's Health Network, there is evidence of an increased chance of breast cancer in women who start using the Pill before they are 20 and who stay on it for about five years. "Minor" side effects include depression, weight gain, and irritability. Women who smoke (especially smokers over 35) and women who have high blood pressure, diabetes, or a history of blood clots are advised to stay away from the Pill; their risk of heart attack or stroke may increase if they take it. Through decreasing hormone dosages, the major risks of the old, high-estrogen Pill — chief among them blood clots and pulmonary embolisms — have "been almost solved, almost licked," according to Barbara Seaman, one of the staunchest enemies of the Pill. But even today, Seaman bluntly says, "any woman over 35 who smokes and takes the Pill is asking for a heart attack." Although in 1990 the FDA lifted its warning that nonsmoking women over 35 refrain from using the Pill, this is still the advice of many in the women's

health community. Women who have had liver disease, breast cancer, or cancer of the reproductive organs are also urged to avoid the Pill. In addition, since the Pill is not a barrier method, it does nothing to battle pelvic inflammatory disease (PID), usually caused by untreated STDs. A woman can have PID for years without knowing it, and the ensuing complications can result in infertility. A great deal is still unknown about the Pill. Questions of negative interactions with some commonly used drugs — such as penicillin — haven't been sufficiently investigated or publicized. Furthermore, much of what we do know is based on studies of the old, high-dosage Pill. As Barbara Seaman observes, "We don't know that the low-dose pills have the same risks or benefits as high-dose pills."

We became used to a no-conversation-necessary approach to sex in the post-Pill era.

The fact that the Pill is not a barrier method has become a crucial disadvantage in the age of AIDS. While condoms and spermicides may bring back the grope for the nightstand that we thought we'd left behind, they do offer protection against HIV. As Dr. Adriane Fugh-Berman, a scientist and board member of the National Women's Health Network, says: "In the sixties we were only worried about being pregnant — now we worry about dying." The ideal method of birth control provides a highly effective barrier against both pregnancy and HIV; Fugh-Berman makes the point that "good family planners tell their patients to use condoms with the Pill." In practice, however, few women who are on the Pill are likely to ask their partners to use condoms. We became used to a no-conversation-necessary approach to sex in the post-Pill era. In the age of AIDS, it is all-important that sex partners have the very kinds of conversations that we abandoned.

Even with the threat of AIDS and other STDs, "women will put up with almost anything in order not to be pregnant," says Julia Scott of the National Black Women's Health Project — which can mean making pregnancy prevention a higher priority than disease protection. This is particularly true of young women. who have a higher risk of infection with HIV and other STDs, but who often use the Pill by itself because it's convenient. The problem is compounded by health care providers who recommend methods like Norplant or the Pill to girls. They are focusing on girls' reproductive lives without "thinking of the health of the whole girl," says Luz Alvarez Martinez of the National Latina Health Organization.

Apart from convenience, some women may opt for the Pill for its supposed health advantages: much has been made recently of its role in helping to prevent certain types of cancer. Earlier this year, the American College of Obstetrics and Gynecology, in marking the 35th anniversary of the FDA's approval of the Pill, announced that it was embarking on a campaign to promote both the safety of the lower-dosage Pill and its "benefits." What the organization was not so eager to publicize was the fact that one of the major manufacturers of the Pill, Ortho Pharmaceuticals, was a funder of this publicity effort. Although women who take the Pill do seem to run a lower risk of getting both endometrial and ovarian cancers, most women's health advocates agree that such benefits are hardly the basis on which to select a method of birth control. As Cindy Pearson says, any discussion of the Pill's health advantages is "kind of dancing away from the real issues."

Clearly the age of zipless contraception is over — if indeed it was ever truly with us. Not only do we need to think through our decisions, but we must also get up the nerve (if such is required) to talk to our partners about birth control. Scott observes: "Women say they prefer methods not associated with the act of sex. They don't want to break up 'the moment.'" But perhaps the separation of sex and birth control only created a fetishized image of sex, a Hollywood script of seamlessness, wherein all goes off without a hitch, no one has a pimple, there's no interruption, and no conversations need ever take place.

As long as we are living in the age of AIDS, barrier methods will continue to be the contraceptive choice of health care providers. But other methods lurk on the research horizon. Some — like the one-size-fits-all diaphragm — are improvements on what we now have and know to be safe. Other potential

The Vital Statistics

Amost 80% of women in the U.S. try the Pill by the time they're 35. Nearly 30% of all contraceptive-using women ages 15 to 44 choose it as their method of birth control; the number drops off sharply — to 4.7% — for women ages 35 to 44. And 20% of single women use it, compared to 14.5% of married women. White women and women of color use the Pill at about the same rates.

methods — such as a contraceptive vaccine or a male birth control pill — hold the same promise of convenience that the Pill once did. But because they are systemic, hormonal methods, they may pose some of the same health dangers as the Pill.

Women will probably never again welcome any method of contraception with the open arms with which we greeted the Pill. But by the same token, we will never again see sex in quite the same way. The Pill may well have been a necessary phase in the evolution of thinking about sex: it has become a given that women have the right to pursue sexual pleasure with as much vivacity and purpose as men. We can never lose the freedoms the Pill bequeathed to us, the sense of entitlement to pleasure. For in spite of the present need to use condoms and the risks of the currently available methods, now that contraception and sex have been unbundled, they can never be bound together so tightly again.

Anne Glusker is a senior editor at The Washington Post Magazine.

PART 5

Consumer Awareness and Health

We each have choices to make regarding our health and behavior. What we eat, drink, smoke, as well as how we take care of ourselves in general, impacts our health. Most researchers think that if we took better care of ourselves, we would reduce the incidence of cancer, heart disease, and other diseases that have been linked to our modern lifestyle. Of course, education about what constitutes good health is the foundation for making healthy choices. There are, however, factors over which we have limited or no control, such as environmental toxins and the genes we've inherited. Although we may be able to mediate the effects of these factors through our behavior, we cannot control the circumstances of our birth, or what we are exposed to in our environment. In this part, there are readings that discuss topics related to health and our genetic inheritance and the environment in which we live.

Then there is the issue of the lengths to which some women will go in pursuit of changing their looks, even at the expense of their health. The readings on breast implants and fingernail treatments discuss the possible risks women face with these procedures.

A controversial reading in this section is the one on the confusing issue of genetic testing for the breast cancer gene. How should these tests be used, and by whom, and for what purposes?

Reading 31 on female circumcision examines an issue that has emerged at the intersection of international policy and women's health. As women from other countries where female circumcision is performed move to the United States and Canada, should western societies permit this practice to continue? This is a cultural issue and a public policy issue, not only a health issue for individual women. (Please see the **Quick Reference Guide to Topics/Readings/WWW Sites** and **Appendix A: WebLinks: A Directory of Annotated World Wide Web Sites** to select WWW sites that coordinate with the readings in this part.)

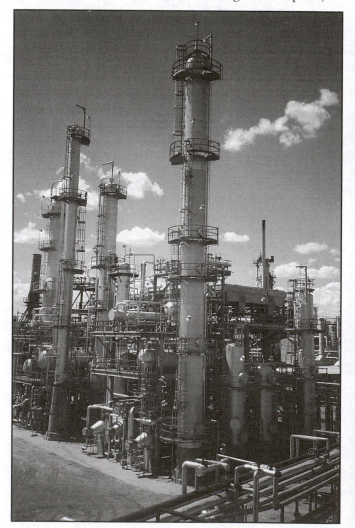

A Reading for Critical Thinking

In 1994 researchers found mutations in a gene — now known as BRCA1 — that dramatically increase a woman's risk of breast cancer. Currently the National Institutes of Health is testing women who have a family history of breast cancer as part of a series of studies designed to gain a better understanding of the gene. In the meantime, private genetic laboratories have begun offering tests of their own.

Pro Con

Should the breast cancer gene test be available to any woman who wants it?

By John Hastings

YES

It's arrogant to say no to a woman who wants this test. Women who have breast cancer can use the information when deciding on treatment, since a mutation in the BRCA1 gene greatly increases the likelihood that the cancer will return. And BRCA1-positive relatives of women who have cancer can take preventive measures to reduce their risk.

Doctors will begin to treat women differently knowing that someone with a BRCA1 gene mutation has an 85 percent lifetime risk of breast cancer and a 50 percent risk of having breast cancer by the age of 50. The simplest step is early and frequent mammograms. Usually doctors don't recommend mammograms to young women because the odds of seeing a tumor in a general screening are low. But if you take a group — women with a mutation — for which the odds of seeing a tumor are quite high, then the measure is worth taking.

Another reason to get tested is that early childbearing helps prevent breast cancer. If a woman learns at a young age that she has the mutation, she may choose to order her life differently.

Understanding of the gene will increase rapidly when the test goes into use and we can identify large groups of women with the mutation. Researchers will be able to learn whether preventive measures work.

Many people argue that there is no guaranteed prevention. What you can do — the best you can do — is try to alter your risk based on knowledge.

Walter Gilbert teaches molecular biology at Harvard and serves on the board of directors at Myriad, a company now developing its own BRCA1 test.

NO

Not everybody who has a BRCA1 mutation is going to get breast cancer. A number of mutations are possible in this gene, and we don't know what they all mean yet. The estimates of cancer risk are based on what we know about a small number of families with specific mutations. We don't yet know how to estimate an individual's risk.

Even if we knew all there is to know about the gene, the question is, What can women do about it? Those who come from high-risk families are already encouraged to get regular mammograms and do regular self-exams — they're already scared about getting breast cancer.

On top of that, there are questions about whether preventive measures work. We hope they do, but we have no studies to support them. Mammograms are very tough to read in young women. Some doctors want to use the drug tamoxifen for prevention, but that drug is still being studied; it's extremely controversial because it may raise a woman's risk of other cancers.

I'm also concerned that a woman who's found not to have a mutation may assume her risk has dropped to normal. Yet she could have a mutation that the test could not detect, and her risk would still be high.

I don't believe we should hold back for a hundred years, until we make every unknown known, but we need to understand more about what the test means before we offer it to the public. Otherwise, we may do more harm than good.

Barbara Biesecker is codirector of the Genetic Counseling Research and Training Program at the National Center for Human Genome Research at NIH.

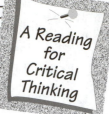

A Reading for Critical Thinking

IS THE MODERN WORLD GIVING US CANCER?

Maverick Scientist Devra Lee Davis is Afraid She Knows the Answer

By Amanda Spake

Is that her? Is that the doctor?" A small, round woman is inching toward the stage. "Oh, she looks like I thought she would," the woman says. "Tall . . . dark hair."

There's a snowstorm outside, but the auditorium in Long Island's Adelphi University is full for tonight's forum on breast cancer. The star attraction, researcher and scientific gadfly Devra Lee Davis, is adjusting the microphone when she sees the woman at the edge of the stage. "I'm Margaret Riva," the woman introduces herself.

Davis walks over, leans down, and clasps her hand warmly. "Margaret!" Davis says, as though greeting an old friend.

But the two have never met. Several months ago, Riva called Davis's office with questions about the health effects of environmental pollution and was shocked when the scientist herself picked up the phone to talk to her. Starstruck now, Riva hangs on Davis's words, smiling and nodding like a shy girl.

Next week, Margaret Riva will learn she has breast cancer — one more victim of what some see as an epidemic of breast cancer sweeping Long Island. Rates of the disease in communities in this suburban area have drawn national attention in the past few years: They jumped during the 1980s and are now as much as 6 percent higher than in the rest of the country. Some scientists believe that the increase, while distressing, is probably due to nothing more than better

detection or an unusually dense concentration of women who happen to be at high risk of breast cancer. But many Long Island women, and their doctors, fear the rates are due to a very specific local threat — the indiscriminate use in years gone by of DDT and other pesticides on the island's once vast potato fields.

That's where Davis comes in. For more than 15 years, she's argued that environmental pollutants are causing an increase in some cancers, particularly in people over age 55. "These cancers may be preventable," she says. "We just need to be smart enough to figure it out." This is an appealing message for a public terrified of cancer, especially since cancer will soon top heart disease as our number-one killer. Davis is an unlikely cult figure — an epidemiologist, she's a policy adviser in the Department of Health and Human Services. But she draws fan letters from cancer survivors and fistfuls of speaking invitations from the doctors who treat them. (This month, she moves to the World Resources Institute, a research center in Washington, D.C.)

Her lecture tonight focuses on chemicals she has dubbed xenoestrogens, coining the word two years ago from *xeno*, meaning strange or foreign, and estrogen, the female sex hormone. Davis believes that a vast number of man-made chemicals — in some pesticides used on crops and lawns, and in some cosmetics and plastic bottles, among other things — can behave

From *Health* (October 1995), pp. 52-56. Reprinted by permission of Amanda Spake, author.

in the body like hormones, mimicking estrogen or blocking testosterone.

For decades, animal biologists have been drawing similar conclusions, documenting the fact that pollutants can destroy animals' ability to reproduce and can reduce their immunity to disease. Once considered outlandish, that evidence is no longer debated.

But Davis goes further. She believes xenoestrogens affect humans, too. Pesticide residues leach into groundwater; DDT and PCBs are found in fish caught in many lakes around the country; dioxin is stored in the fat of beef cattle and other animals consumed by humans. Davis believes exposure to such chemicals may be partially responsible for an increase in infertility as well as in hormone-related breast, testicular, and prostate cancers.

The auditorium darkens. A videotape begins. We see a clip of Diane Sawyer on "Prime Time Live" talking with Davis. Then we see Long Island women who

California, Berkeley, and inventor of the test commonly used to determine whether a chemical can cause cancer. He argues that plant estrogens and natural pesticides — toxic compounds that plants produce to protect themselves from predators — present a greater risk than the tiny amounts of synthetic chemicals most people encounter. "Our food is filled with compounds that have estrogenic activity," says Ames. "Some of them turn out to be billions of times more potent than a little bit of DDT.

Ames believes that synthetic chemicals cause relatively little cancer. Despite widespread public suspicion to the contrary, many scientists agree with Ames. The view was underscored recently by the National Cancer Institute, which reported that man-made hazards don't seem to be having much effect on cancer rates.

"We've been eating natural pesticides throughout history," Davis answers her questioner, "and have

"We used to believe only a woman's natural estrogen could turn the key that causes breast cancer," Davis says. "It's now clear chemicals in pesticides can turn the key as well."

have breast cancer. "As you know," Davis says, raising her voice over the din of the audience, "some of the women in that video tape are dead."

Silence. Click. A slide comes up on the overhead projector as Davis explains that a woman's lifetime exposure to estrogen affects her risk of breast cancer. Scientists believe that one of the forms of estrogen women make naturally — estradiol — activates estrogen receptors, stimulating breast cell growth and, sometimes, damaging cell DNA. If a woman begins menstruating early, enters menopause late, never gets pregnant, never breast-feeds, or is obese, she'll be exposed to more estradiol, increasing her risk of breast cancer.

"We used to believe that only a woman's natural estrogen could turn the key on these receptors and cause breast cancer," Davis says. Click. We see a long list that includes chemicals in pesticides, detergents, cosmetics, plastics . . . "It is now clear that many chemicals in plastics and pesticides can turn the key as well."

A man stands up to ask Davis a question. "Dr. Bruce Ames has talked about natural pesticides being far more potent than anything man-made," he says. "I suppose you disagree?"

This is the Bruce Ames question, one Davis is often asked. Ames, one of Davis's most ardent critics, is professor of biochemistry at the University of

probably built up resistances. Synthetics have increased astronomically since the fifties and we also have increasing rates of cancer."

This is a more tactful response than the one Ames gives when asked about Davis's work on xenoestrogens. "It makes absolutely no sense," says Ames. "I used to think Devra Davis was always wrong. Then I decided she wasn't that reliable."

Davis has an impressive résumé — in her position at the National Academy of Sciences, she was responsible for the ban on smoking aboard domestic plane flights — but she has alienated many leading epidemiologists with her theories about cancer. Even her friends in the field say she sometimes gets overzealous, drawing conclusions that go beyond the research. Most scientists meticulously develop one area of expertise; Davis goes off in many directions. But her supporters think there are advantages to her whirling dervish approach. "Devra synthesizes information and finds new ways of looking at the data," says Aaron Blair, an epidemiologist at the National Cancer Institute. "We need people who can do that."

Take the data on xenoestrogens and breast cancer. Scientists have known for 25 years that DDT and similar chemicals are stored in human fat, where they accumulate. Suggestions that there might be a link with breast cancer date back to the late seventies. But the idea wasn't taken seriously by cancer researchers, in part because no one could explain *how* these chemicals might influence cancer.

Four years ago, Davis began bugging endocrinologist H. Leon Bradlow, who researches estrogen metabolism at Strang–Cornell Cancer Research Laboratory in New York — calling repeatedly to suggest that some pollutants might alter the way the human body breaks down estrogen.

"I was convinced she was totally wrong," says the scientist. Bradlow had shown that estrogen can take two forms in the body. One he called a "good" estrogen, since, in test-tube studies, it has no effect on tumor cells. The "bad" estrogen fuels tumor growth and can prompt normal breast cells to turn cancerous.

Some pesticides, Davis suspected, boost formation of "bad" estrogen. The idea could be easily tested: Just add pesticide to breast cancer cells in a lab dish and measure the various estrogens.

"And I finally said to her, 'Look, you've bothered me enough about this,'" Bradlow remembers. "'I'll do the experiment and prove to you that you are wrong.'

"And the only problem was," he says, "she was right."

Davis has a nickname, earned after a day and night of meetings at the National Academy of Sciences. Dinner had concluded, but conversation was continuing in the clubby atmosphere of the NAS library. One board member wanted to talk about a project. Cigar and cognac in hand, the man leaned forward. "Listen, honey . . ." "Uh," Davis said, "it's Dr. Honey."

Impressions of "Dr. Honey" are seldom tepid. "She makes people uncomfortable because she raises issues," says NAS colleague and epidemiologist Marvin Schneiderman. "She steps on people's toes, and she may step on their whole foot."

She jumped on some very illustrious feet in 1990 with a scientific article on what she saw as ominous trends in cancer. New treatments were drastically cutting the death rate in young patients. But, she said, cancer was on the rise among older people because of an increase in lymphoma, multiple myeloma (a bone marrow cancer), and cancers of the breast, brain, and kidney, among others.

Her claim raised the ire of the grand masters of cancer epidemiology — Sir Richard Doll, the Oxford University researcher who established the link between smoking and lung cancer, and Doll's colleague, Richard Peto. Not only do Doll and Peto, like Ames, say there's no evidence that synthetic chemicals are of much importance in the total cancer picture, they dispute Davis's contention that cancer, in general, is rising.

"I think it's a really serious and misleading misjudgment to believe that there is a generalized increase in cancer," Peto says. Look at the number of people dying from the disease, he says: If you subtract the cancers caused by tobacco, mortality is actually falling slightly.

How can the number of cancer cases be in dispute? Isn't it a simple matter of addition? Unfortunately, the math problem isn't so easy. Take breast cancer: Between 1973 and 1991, the number of cases jumped by nearly 24 percent. But it's clear that much of this increase reflects better cancer detection. With more women getting mammograms, more breast cancers are being found at earlier stages. For that matter, doctors worried about malpractice suits have become more likely to diagnose and treat growths that are borderline — abnormal but not clearly malignant. So cancer statistics now include cases that 20 years ago might not have been reported.

Even if there is a genuine increase in breast cancer, it may be the result of changes in lifestyle, not an environmental villain. Women are postponing childbirth or having no children at all, girls are menstruating earlier — all known to increase breast cancer risk.

There is ample room for disagreement about other kinds of cancer, too. Is brain cancer on the rise? Davis says cases have doubled in 25 years. Doll and Peto argue it's likely that, before the CAT scan came along, many deaths due to brain cancer were probably attributed to stroke or other diseases.

These are difficult arguments, and loaded ones. If cancer is not on the rise, then it seems unlikely that there are unknown dangers lurking in the environment. So why spend research dollars looking for them? But if Davis is right, then danger is all around us.

"What's the downside here?" she says. "Are we so sure all the increases are due to better detection that we want to run the risk of missing some avoidable factor — something we could change?"

One of the first clues that pollutants might affect the hormonal lives of animals came almost by chance. In 1977, a researcher studying sea gulls on Santa Barbara Island off the Los Angeles coast, noticed something bizarre: Female gulls were pairing up and sharing nests. In one area, there were 19 females for every male. What had happened to the males?

Bird toxicologist Michael Fry knew that for over 20 years, beginning around 1950, 4 million pounds of DDT had been pumped into the ocean from a nearby chemical plant. While the pesticide had left California pelicans and other birds producing eggs too fragile to survive, gulls had seemed immune. In his lab, Fry injected DDT into uncontaminated gull eggs collected at a lake. Female hatchlings were more or less normal. But the male hatchlings were hermaphroditic, with both testes and ovaries.

When Fry published his research in 1981, his conclusions were met with disbelief. But over the next decade, wildlife experts worldwide reported declining births, hermaphroditic offspring, and lowered sperm counts or testicular deformities in fish, panthers, alligators, and other animals in polluted habitats.

"If you look at people," says Timothy Gross, a wildlife endocrinologist at the University of Florida, in Gainesville, "the same pollutants are in our bodies. What is a safe level? We don't know. But I'd be a pretty naive scientist to conclude there couldn't be the same effects in humans."

People don't dine exclusively on fish from polluted lakes, as wild creatures might, or drink as often from contaminated rivers. And our larger bodies may be more resistant to doses that can harm many animals. But there are suggestions — though they are anything but conclusive — that something is messing with human hormones. For instance, endometriosis seems to be on the rise. A 1992 German study reported that women with this painful disorder of the uterine lining were more likely than other women to

cancer, some without. This was the first big study to try to isolate the effect of xenoestrogens by taking into account other cancer risk factors, such as family history or having children late in life. Wolff found that the women whose blood showed the highest levels of DDE — a breakdown product of DDT — were four times more likely to have breast cancer than women with the lowest levels in their blood.

In another large study, epidemiologist Nancy Krieger measured DDE levels in the blood of 300 women, half of them diagnosed with breast cancer. She found that women with high levels of the chemical in their blood were no more likely than the other women to have breast cancer. Still, Krieger, at the Harvard School of Public Health, doesn't dismiss the possibility that xenoestrogens play a role.

Davis and Bradlow write that they know that xenoestrogens cannot be the single factor responsible for increases in breast cancer. But, they say, "If reducing avoidable exposures to xenoestrogens allowed us to avert only 20 percent of all breast cancers each year, we would spare more than 36,000 women and

Critics say Davis tends to hype the risk, but no woman who suspects that pollutants caused her breast cancer is likely to object.

have elevated levels of PCBs in their blood. And monkeys exposed to dioxin developed endometriosis in proportion to the dose they received.

At the same time, sperm counts appear to be declining. According to a 1992 Danish study, sperm counts in men around the world are only about half what they were before World War II. Some researchers call decades-old statistics on sperm counts unreliable and say it's not clear that the drop is real. But if it is, xenoestrogens could be partly to blame: When pregnant rats were injected with tiny amounts of dioxin, their male offspring had abnormal testicles.

What about cancer? "In the United States and Britain, testicular cancer has doubled in the last three decades," says Davis. The rate of prostate cancer has doubled in the last decade, as well. Part of the increase may well be a matter of better detection. But Davis believes that at least part is due to the soup of hormone disrupting pollutants in the environment. As is true, she believes, for breast cancer.

In their papers, Davis and Bradlow discuss ten studies that have looked for links between breast cancer and exposure to xenoestrogens. In one of the largest, Mary Wolff, a specialist in environmental medicine at the Mount Sinai School of Medicine, looked at 229 New York women, some with breast

their families from this difficult disease."

Twenty percent may well reflect Davis's tendency toward hyperbole; it isn't based on data. But no woman who suspects her breast cancer was caused by pollutants is likely to object to a little exaggeration. Certainly not if Davis's forcefulness convinces politicians to fund more research on xenoestrogens and breast cancer.

"In 1990, we spent over $30 billion on cancer treatment alone in this country," she says. "We can't continue to treat all the cancer. We've got to figure out how to prevent it. That's my message."

If Davis is right about xenoestrogens, prevention won't come easy or cheap. Ridding the environment of xenoestrogens would require sweeping changes in agriculture and industry — that is, if we knew where to start.

"Most chemicals haven't been tested to see if they're endocrine-disrupters," Davis says, "and we don't want to abandon one xenoestrogen for an alternative that may be worse."

Clearly, what's needed first is more research, and that's just what scientists around the world called for recently. Last April, an international panel convened by the Danish Environmental Protection Agency released a report pointing to a dramatic decline in sperm counts and increases in the number of European men with testicular cancer and reproductive abnormalities. These signs of declining male reproductive ability, the report said, warrant an international research effort. And scientists at a U.S. conference last year on estrogens in the environment, sponsored by the National Institute of Environmental Health Sciences, also recommended stepped-up research.

But in the current political climate, money for studies may not be forthcoming. "We're relying on Superfund money for research," says endocrinologist Gross. "And who knows what will happen to that? Congress now has a vendetta against lots of this environmental research.

"In my view, the two most important research tracks are, first, what chemicals might we produce that are better? And second, how do we clean up these sites? We have no idea. The technology doesn't exist." Besides, says Gross, even a thorough cleanup is not the whole answer: "DDT is still produced here, then shipped out of this country, let's say to Mexico. DDT that is sprayed in Mexico reaches us in two to seven days."

Davis is more optimistic about the possibility of bringing xenoestrogens under control. She points to the Long Island Breast Cancer Study Project, which focuses on the role played by environmental pollutants in the area's high breast cancer rates. The project got under way in 1994.

A thorough understanding of the hormonal effects of xenoestrogens will take years. "In the meantime, I advise prudent avoidance," Davis says. She doesn't use plastic in the microwave except for the briefest rewarming, for instance, since chemicals may leach from plastic at high temperatures.

To her audience in the Long Island auditorium, she echoed most breast cancer researchers, advocating a diet heavy on fruits and vegetables and low in animal fat, since pesticides and other xenoestrogens are stored in fat. Moderate exercise may help prevent breast cancer and other ills, she said. It's probably a bad idea to drink large amounts of alcohol; it's a good idea for women over age 50 to get regular mammograms.

"I know that people who can pray, who find a spiritual peace, do better," she said. "People who are connected do better."

Perhaps the reason Davis has attracted so many fans is her ability to speak this language of emotion, rare in a scientist who can talk "metabolites" and "oncogenes" among doctors. She cries over old letters from cancer patients who have died, and she joined a group of breast cancer survivors last summer for a money and awareness-raising climb up Mount Rainier in Washington state. To train for the trek, she spent many hot summer days running up and down the Capitol steps with 40 pounds of watermelon strapped to her back.

The climb reminded Davis why she took on her fight. "Before I began working with these women," she says, "I never thought there was a constituency for prevention. I was wrong. Cancer statistics are just human beings with the tears removed."

Amanda Spake lives in Churchton, Maryland.

A Status Report on

Breast Implant Safety

By Marian Segal

Signing a consent form is now part of the procedure for all women undergoing breast implant surgery. They also must be given information about the devices' known and possible risks.

Recently published studies have shown that women with silicone gel-filled breast implants do not have a greatly increased risk of some well-defined autoimmune diseases, which were among the serious health concerns surrounding the devices. These include potentially fatal connective tissue diseases such as scleroderma and lupus erythematosus.

Widespread reports of adverse reactions to silicone gel-filled implants and a lack of evidence supporting their safety led the Food and Drug Administration to order the devices off the market in April 1992. They remained available only to women in clinical studies, mostly women seeking breast reconstruction after breast cancer surgery. (See "Silicone Breast Implants: Available Under Tight Controls" in the June 1992 *FDA Consumer*) Saline-filled implants were allowed to remain on the market for all uses.

The new studies do not, however, rule out the possibility that a subset of women with implants may have a small increased risk of these conditions, or that some women might develop other immune-related symptoms that don't conform to "classic" disease descriptions.

Nor did the studies address other important safety questions, including implant rupture rates and the incidence of capsular contracture (shrinking of scar tissue around the implant, which can cause painful hardening of the breast or distort its appearance). Answers to these and other questions await the results of new or ongoing studies.

REASONS FOR NEW STUDIES

Breast implants had been marketed since the early 1960s — several years before the first medical device law was enacted in 1976, charging FDA with regulation of medical devices. Every year, thousands of American women had had implant surgery for augmentation (to enlarge or reshape their breasts) or for reconstruction following mastectomy (removal of the breast) to treat breast cancer. Most of the implants consisted of a rubber silicone envelope filled with silicone gel; about 10 percent were filled with saline (salt water).

Under the 1976 law, implants and many other devices already in use were allowed to remain on the market, with the understanding that the agency would at some time ask manufacturers to submit scientific data showing these "grandfathered" products were safe and effective.

FDA requested this information for silicone gel-filled implants in April 1991 in response to a growing number of adverse reaction reports that raised safety concerns about the devices. The data submitted did not prove the devices safe, as required by law, so the agency restricted their use to clinical trials designed to resolve the safety questions.

Between Jan. 1, 1985, and March 16, 1995, FDA received 91,322 adverse reaction reports associated with silicone breast implants and 19,296 reports involving the saline implants. These reports included risks clearly associated with the devices, as well as adverse effects attributed to the implants, but not proved to be linked to them.

From *FDA Consumer* (November 1995), pp. 11-16. Reprinted by permission of *FDA Consumer*.

SILICONE IMPLANT STUDIES

Some recent studies comparing the rates of immune-related diseases in women with implants versus those without implants have provided reassurance that women with implants are not at a greatly increased risk of these disorders.

The largest of these retrospective, or "look-back," studies is the Harvard Nurses' Health Study. The study used data from 87,501 nurses followed for other research purposes from 1976 through May 31, 1990, before there was widespread media coverage of the possible association between breast implants and connective tissue disease. None of the women had connective tissue disease at the start of the study.

Between Jan. 1, 1985, and March 16, 1995, FDA received 91,322 adverse reaction reports associated with silicone breast implants and 19,296 reports involving the saline implants.

In an article published in the June 22, 1995, *New England Journal of Medicine*, the researchers reported that 516 of the nurses had developed definite connective tissue diseases. Women with breast implants numbered 1,183. The types of implants included 876 silicone gel-filled, 170 saline-filled, 67 double lumen (silicone gel-filled implants with a saline-filled outer envelope), 14 polyurethane-coated, and 56 of unknown type. Only three of the 516 women with definite connective tissue disease had implants (one silicone-gel filled, one saline, and one double lumen).

The authors reported they "did not find an association between silicone breast implants and connective tissue disease, defined according to a variety of standardized criteria, or signs and symptoms of these diseases."

Similarly, a 1994 study conducted at the Mayo Clinic found no increased risk of connective tissue diseases among implant recipients. The investigators based their conclusion on comparison of the medical histories of 749 women with breast implants in Olmsted County, Minn., with a similar group of women who did not have implants.

"Because of the limitations in the size and type of the studies, however, the true risk of these diseases is not known," says S. Lori Brown, Ph.D., a research scientist officer in the epidemiology branch of the agency's Center for Devices and Radiological Health. "Although the criteria others may be using to assess those studies show that some concerns are eliminated," Brown says, "unfortunately, they don't rule out a small, but significant, increased risk."

An immunology and epidemiology expert, Brown explains that an inherent problem in the studies is that some connective tissue diseases are extremely rare. "If you have a disease that has an incidence of 1 in 100,000 in the general population, for example, and you do a study of 750 women with implants, like the Mayo Clinic Study, then you wouldn't really expect to see even a single case of that disease," she says, "unless there's an exceedingly high — more than a hundredfold — increase in risk."

Small studies like these can rule out huge risks, but not smaller, yet significant risk increases that would only show up in studies that include several thousand women with implants, Brown says. Nor do the studies fully examine or answer whether the implants might in some women lead to symptoms not typical of classical disease manifestations.

OTHER CONCERNS

Brown also stresses that connective tissue diseases are not the only issue of concern, especially since they may affect a much smaller proportion of women with implants. The larger issue, she says, is the local complications that are clearly related to breast implants, such as rupture and migration of the silicone gel, capsular contracture, and infection.

"Of the two groups of women who consider getting implants — for breast reconstruction or for augmentation," Brown says, "the larger group wants them for cosmetic purposes. These are healthy women who may go out and get implants without a clear picture of what the possible risks are. They may end up

---

POLYURETHANE-COATED IMPLANTS

About 110,000 women have silicone gel-filled implants with a polyurethane coating, intended to reduce the risk of capsular contracture. In April 1991, an FDA analysis showed that polyurethane foam could break down under human body conditions to form a chemical called TDA, which can cause cancer in animals. As a result, the manufacturer immediately stopped selling the product.

Recently, however, a study to measure TDA in women with polyurethane implants found that a woman's risk of cancer from exposure to TDA released by the implant is negligible — about one in a million over a lifetime. FDA considers it unlikely that even one woman would develop cancer from these implants. The study supports the agency's original recommendation that women who are not having problems should not have the implants removed solely because of concern about cancer from TDA exposure.

— M. S.

going back in for surgery time and again and never be happy with the cosmetic effect."

In testimony before a congressional subcommittee in August 1995, FDA Commissioner David A. Kessler, M.D., stated that "Published studies to date suggest a rupture rate between 5 and 51 percent — an enormous range — and unfortunately, we do not know with any confidence where within that range the real rupture rate lies." He also cited two studies that indicate the risk of rupture increases as the implants age.

Another concern — increased risk of breast cancer — has not been borne out by studies. "Several

studies have indicated there is no increased risk of breast cancer in women with implants," Brown says. However, she adds, these women are not yet in the age group that is more prone to breast cancer, and it remains to be seen whether they will eventually have a higher incidence of breast cancer than women without implants. Long term studies to look at this are under way.

MANUFACTURERS' STUDIES

The events that led to removal of silicone implants from the market made it clear that prospective, or forward-looking, studies were also needed to answer important safety questions. Implant manufacturers agreed to conduct human trials in three phases: urgent need, adjunct, and core studies.

"The purpose of the first phase [urgent need] actually was simply to quickly provide implants to women who were already in the process of getting them for breast reconstruction or for another medical reason, and to bridge the time until the adjunct studies were begun," says Sahar M. Dawisha, M.D., a rheumatologist and medical officer who joined FDA's division of general and restorative devices in April 1993.

The women did, however, have to sign an informed consent form that summarized the risks and benefits of the implants. This form had not previously been required.

"The second phase, or adjunct, studies were intended to follow reconstruction patients for five years to assess short term safety data, including rates of capsular contracture, rupture, and complications such as infection and hematoma [collection of blood that may cause swelling, pain and bruising]," Dawisha says. "These studies are open to all women wanting breast reconstruction with implants because of mastectomy, traumatic injury to the breast, or a disease or congenital disorder causing a severe breast abnormality. They do not include augmentation patients."

Mentor Corporation of Santa Barbara, Calif., began adjunct studies in 1992. According to Pamela Powell of the company's Clinical Programs Department, as of July 5, 1995, 12,125 patients were enrolled in the studies.

The third phase, or core studies, Dawisha says, were intended to determine the full safety and effectiveness profile of the device, including rupture rates, quality-of-life benefits, extent of interference with mammography, and many more safety concerns — including rheumatologic assessments — that would need a large number of women. They were also to include augmentation patients. The sponsors, however, have not initiated these studies.

Some recent retrospective studies comparing the rates of immune-related diseases in women with implants versus those without implants have provided reassurance that women with implants are not at a greatly increased risk of these disorders.

SALINE IMPLANTS

Although many of the local complications of gel-filled implants are also associated with saline implants, the latter were permitted to remain on the market unrestricted for both reconstruction and augmentation. FDA considers saline-filled implants less risky, because although they have the same silicone rubber envelope as gel-filled implants, leakage or rupture would release only salt water, not silicone gel, into the body.

Nevertheless, FDA is requiring manufacturers to collect data on the saline implants as well, because the incidence of known risks (for example, deflation and capsular contracture) is not well defined. When the Medical Device Amendments were passed, it was determined that these devices would also eventually require premarket approval. In January 1993, FDA notified saline implant manufacturers that they would have to submit safety and effectiveness data for their products. In December 1994, the agency told them what type of safety and effectiveness data were needed, and delineated objectives and time frames for the trials.

Saline implants will stay on the market while the studies are conducted, but the companies must report the laboratory, animal and clinical data in stages, and must provide written information on the known and possible risks of their products.

"Women considering saline implants should ask their doctor for a copy of the manufacturer's information sheet, a copy of the product insert sheet for the specific implant to be used, and a copy of the hospital informed consent form," says Barbara Stellar, FDA's breast implant information and outreach coordinator.

KNOWN RISKS OF BREAST IMPLANTS SURGICAL RISKS

- possible complications of general anesthesia, as well as nausea, vomiting and fever
- infection
- hematoma (collection of blood that may cause swelling, pain and bruising, perhaps requiring surgical draining)
- hemorrhage (abnormal bleeding)
- thrombosis (abnormal clotting)
- skin necrosis — skin tissue death resulting from insufficient blood flow to the skin. The chance of skin necrosis may be increased by radiation treatments, cortisone-like drugs, an implant too large for the available space, or smoking.

Implant Risks

- capsular contracture (hardening of the breast due to scar tissue)
- leak or rupture — silicone implants may leak or rupture slowly, releasing silicone gel into surrounding tissue; saline implants may rupture suddenly and deflate, usually requiring immediate removal or replacement
- temporary or permanent change or loss of sensation in the nipple or breast tissue
- formation of calcium deposits in surrounding tissue, possibly causing pain and hardening
- shifting from the original placement, giving the breast an unnatural look

- interference with mammography readings, possibly delaying breast cancer detection by "hiding" a suspicious lesion.

Also, it may be difficult to distinguish calcium deposits formed in the scar tissue from a tumor when interpreting the mammogram. *When making an appointment for a mammogram, the woman should tell the scheduler she has implants to make sure qualified personnel are on-site. At the time of the mammogram she should also remind the technician she has implants before the procedure is done, so the technician can use special techniques to obtain the best mammogram and to avoid rupturing the implant.*

— M. S.

Women considering saline implants should ask their doctor for a copy of the manufacturer's information sheet, a copy of the product insert sheet for the specific implant to be used, and a copy of the hospital informed consent form."

— Barbara Stellar, FDA Breast Implant
and Outreach Coordinator

Stellar recommends women be given these documents at least a month before surgery is planned, if possible, so they can thoroughly discuss benefits and possible risks with surgeons, radiologists, and other women. These women should also ask their physicians about participating in the saline breast implant trials.

Brown hopes that further studies will more clearly define risks associated with all types of implants.

"We need to be able to tell women considering breast implants — whether for augmentation or reconstruction — the specific risks on which they can base their decision," she says. "It should be made clear that implants do not last forever, that they may break, and in what time period it is thought they might break. Most women have no idea implants break and there's very little information about rupture rates.

"The same is true for other complications, some of which may require further surgery or may cause the woman to be displeased with the cosmetic effect, which, of course, is the reason she got them," Brown says. "For a product that a person is putting in her body presumably for 20 years or more, we should have this information."

Marian Segal is a member of FDA's public affairs staff.

INFORMATION PACKET

To obtain a comprehensive packet of information on breast implant issues, request FDA's publication, "Breast Implants, An Information Update," by calling the agency's breast implant information line at (1-800) 532-4440.

Fingernails
Looking Good While Playing Safe

By Paula Kurtzweil

With the ease that comes from years of practice, Julie Le, of Nails R Us in Alexandria, VA, sets out to remake customer Natalie Harris' nails. She buffs, files, snips, clips, smooths, and then, with a nod from Harris, paints on ruby red polish.

It's a process repeated every day throughout the country as thousands of women like Harris — and men, too — strive for beautiful nails. They seek the services of nail and beauty salons or manicure their nails themselves with a host of nail products available on the market.

The reason, said Kim Siridavong, owner of Nails R Us, is simple: "Everybody wants to look good."

But achieving that look is not without potential hazard. Infections and allergic reactions can occur with some nail services and products. Some chemicals in nail products, if ingested, are poisonous. Many are flammable.

Relying on nail and beauty salons is not risk free, either. They use the same products, and they may present a greater risk for disease transmission.

Federal and state regulations help reduce the risks, but consumers also need to take care that their pursuit of beautiful nails ensures healthy nails.

GROWTH OF AN INDUSTRY

With the increased use of nail services and products in recent years has come growing concern about safety. According to *Nails 1995 Fact Book*, U.S. consumers will spend an estimated $5.2 billion on nail services in 1995, half a billion more than in 1994. They can choose from 34,852 freestanding nail salons across the country — nearly 2,000 more than a year ago — or hundreds of thousands of beauty salons that offer nail services.

The most requested service, according to the *Fact Book*, is artificial nails. Manicures are No. 2. Other popular services include nail jewelry and nail art.

Because of the variety of nail services, the preferred term for a person who provides nail services is "nail technician" rather than manicurist, said Suzette Hill, managing editor for *Nails*, a magazine for professionals and students.

"Twenty years ago, they mainly did manicures," she said. "Now, they're doing so much more."

They use a range of products, including polishes, paints, artificial nails, glues, and laminates, many of which are available for home use, too.

NAIL PRODUCTS AS COSMETICS

Nail products for both home and salon use are regulated by the Food and Drug Administration. Under the Federal Food, Drug, and Cosmetic Act, these products are considered cosmetics because they are "articles other than soap which are applied to the human body for cleansing, beautifying, promoting attractiveness, or altering the appearance."

By law, nail products sold as cosmetics in the United States must be free of poisonous or deleterious substances that might injure users under the usual or customary conditions of use intended by the manufacturer. These uses are printed on the package or on a package insert. Many nail products contain poisonous substances, such as acetonitrile in glue removers, but are allowed on the market because they are not

From *FDA Consumer* (December 1995), pp. 20-24. Reprinted by permission of *FDA Consumer*.

1993-1995 Market Projections for Salons' Top Nail Services

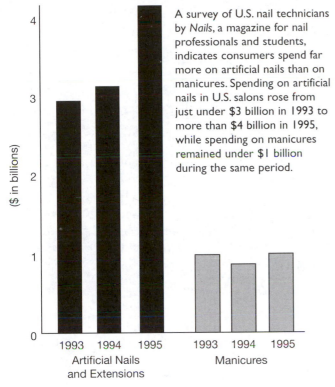

A survey of U.S. nail technicians by *Nails*, a magazine for nail professionals and students, indicates consumers spend far more on artificial nails than on manicures. Spending on artificial nails in U.S. salons rose from just under $3 billion in 1993 to more than $4 billion in 1995, while spending on manicures remained under $1 billion during the same period.

Sources: *Nails 1994 Fact Book* and *Nails 1995 Fact Book)*

harmful when used as directed. They're poisonous only when ingested, which is not their intended use.

Products sold for home use also must he labeled properly, with the names of the ingredients listed in descending order of predominance.

FDA does not review or approve nail products and other cosmetics before they go on the market. However, the agency inspects cosmetic manufacturers and samples and analyzes cosmetics as needed. If a safety problem arises, the agency can take legal action against the product.

FDA also tracks safety problems through its Cosmetic Voluntary Registration Program, in which cosmetic manufacturers voluntarily report to FDA the types of adverse reactions their customers have reported to them. FDA uses this information to determine a baseline reaction rate for specific product categories, such as cuticle softeners, nail extenders (artificial nail ends), and nail polishes. The agency gives this information to participating companies so they can compare their adverse reaction rates to FDA's determined baseline.

FDA also learns about potentially harmful products from manufacturers' competitors, consumers, doctors, and nail technicians, who report adverse reactions directly to the agency.

SALON SAFETY

The salons and their technicians are regulated by the states, usually their cosmetology boards. Lois Wiskur, past president of the National Interstate Council of State Cosmetology Boards, said that as far as she knows, every state has some type of licensing requirements for nail salons, nail technicians, or both.

Under these requirements, salons providing nail services usually must meet certain requirements, such as:

- Employing nail technicians who have had a minimum number of hours of classroom and practical training.
- Properly sterilizing manicure implements. The preferred methods are autoclaving (heat sterilization) or chemical sterilization.
- Undergoing a state inspection periodically.
- Maintaining sufficient equipment, such as at least one manicure table and one sink that runs hot and cold water.
- Making sure that employees wash their hands before beginning work on a customer.

To prevent blood-borne infections, such as HIV and hepatitis, the national Centers for Disease Control and Prevention recommended similar sanitary practices for salon employees in guidelines issued in 1985. The guidelines targeted, among others, personal-service workers, such as manicurists and pedicurists. To date, there have been no reports of transmission of blood-borne diseases to or from a personal service worker, according to CDC.

NAIL INFECTIONS

More common nail problems, dermatologists report, are infections from bacteria, such as *Staphylococcus*; fungi, such as *Candida* (also known as yeast); and skin viruses, such as warts.

Bacterial and fungal infections frequently result from artificial nails, whether applied at home or in a salon. A bump or knock to a long artificial nail may cause it to lift from the natural nail at the base, leaving an opening for dirt to get in. If the nail is reglued without proper cleaning (with rubbing alcohol, for example), bacteria or fungi may grow between the nails and spread into the natural nail.

Also, as the natural nail grows, an opening develops between the natural nail and artificial nail. If this space is not filled in regularly, it can increase the chances for infection.

A fungal infection can take hold when an acrylic nail is left in place too long — such as three months or more — and moisture accumulates under the nail.

PRECAUTIONS FOR ARTIFICIAL NAILS

- If there is any question about sensitivity to the materials in artificial nails, have one nail done as a test and wait a few days to see if a reaction develops.

- Never apply an artificial nail if the natural nail or skin around it is infected or irritated. Let the infection heal first.

- Read the directions for do-it-yourself nails before applying them, and follow the directions carefully. Save the ingredient list for your doctor in case you have an allergic reaction or other injury.

- Treat your artificial nails with care. They may be stronger than your own, but they still can break and separate. Try not to bump or knock them. Find new ways to do ordinary tasks, like using a pencil to dial or depress the numbers on the phone.

- If an artificial nail separates, dip the fingertip into rubbing alcohol to clean the space between the natural and artificial nails before reattaching the artificial nail. This will help prevent infection.

- Never use household glues for nail repairs. Use only products intended for nail use, and follow directions.

- Don't wear artificial nails for longer than three months at a time. Remove them for one month to give nails a rest.

- Keep nail glues and other poisonous substances out of the reach of children.

— P. K.

Reporting Adverse Nail Product Reactions

Doctors, nail technicians, and consumers should report adverse reactions from nail products to the nearest FDA office, listed in the blue section of the telephone book. Or, write to:

Food and Drug Administration
Center for Food Safety and Applied Nutrition
Office of Cosmetics and Colors (HFS-100)
200 C St., S.W.
Washington, DC 20204

Bacterial, fungal and viral infections also can occur from using insanitary nail implements, especially in a salon, where the same implements are used on many people.

Unclean implements are especially dangerous if the skin around the nail is broken. This can occur with overzealous manicuring — if, for example, too much of the cuticle is cut or pushed back too far. If the cuticle is cut or separated from the fingernail, infectious agents can get into the exposed area. This is why dermatologists recommend leaving cuticles intact.

Symptoms of an infection include pain, redness, itching, and pus in or around the nail area. Yellow-green, green, and green-black nail discolorations are signs of a *Pseudomonas* bacterial infection. A blue-green discoloration signals a fungal infection.

If an infection appears while wearing artificial nails, they should be removed and the area cleaned thoroughly with soap and water. If symptoms persist, the person should consult a doctor, who may prescribe a topical or oral anti-infective medicine.

There are no approved nonprescription products to treat fungal nail infections, and over-the-counter products to treat other types of fungal infections should not be used for nail infections. In a review of OTC antifungal products, FDA found that fungal infections of the nails respond poorly to topical therapy, partly because of the nail's thickness. So, in 1993, the agency ruled that any OTC product labeled, represented or promoted as a topical antifungal to treat fungal infections of the nail is a new drug and must be approved by FDA before marketing. This rule, which went into effect in 1994, does not include prescription antifungal products.

Despite the rule, some companies continue to sell unapproved OTC nail products, such as nail glues, with antifungal claims. FDA has warned these companies it might take legal action if they don't stop selling the products.

ALLERGIES AND OTHER HAZARDS

Other common problems associated with nail products are allergic reactions, such as contact dermatitis, a skin rash characterized by redness and itching and sometimes tiny blisters that ooze.

Certain nail ingredients are known for their tendency to cause allergic reactions. Residual traces of the basic building blocks of acrylic resins ("acrylics") used in artificial nails, for example, can cause redness, swelling and pain in the nail bed. In some cases, the reaction is so severe that the natural nail separates from the nail bed, and although a new nail usually grows in, it may be imperfect if the nail root has been damaged.

Nail strengtheners that contain "free formaldehyde" may cause an irritation or reaction, as can certain other chemicals in nail glues and polishes.

In the late 1970s, use of methyl methacrylate, then a common ingredient in artificial nail products, resulted in FDA receiving a number of reports of injuries and allergic reactions, including damage and deformity of fingernails and contact dermatitis. The ingredient now is rarely used because of legal action against a former manufacturer of methyl methacrylate-containing products and numerous seizures and recalls of such products. Methyl methacrylate has since been replaced with other chemicals, such as ethyl methacrylate. However, according to John Bailey, Ph.D., acting director of FDA's office of cosmetics and colors, the replacement chemicals have never been fully studied for safety, and they may be as harmful as methyl methacrylate.

SELECTING A SAFE NAIL SALON

To help you decide if a salon provides sanitary nail services, nail and public health experts suggest considering the following:

● Is the salon licensed? Licenses often are posted. If you don't see one, ask.

● Are the nail technicians licensed? These licenses also are usually posted. Ask if you don't see one for your technician.

● How are nail implements sanitized? Autoclaving (heat sterilization) is best, says Ralph Daniel, M.D., a dermatologist in Jackson, Miss. But most states allow chemical sterilizing as long as the implements are immersed in the solution for at least 10 minutes between customers. Ask the technician what the salon's practices are. If they're using a chemical solution, check the product's label for words like "germicidal" to indicate that it is strong enough to kill bacteria. If in doubt, bring your own implements, Daniel suggests.

● Is there a pre-service scrub? Both the nail technician and the client should wash their hands with an anti-microbial soap before nail work begins.

● Is each customer given a fresh bowl of soapy water to soak their nails in and is a new nail file used for each customer? Both practices should be followed.

● Is the facility neat and clean? Paul Kechijian, M.D., a clinical associate professor of dermatology and chief of the nail section at New York University, compares selecting a salon to selecting a restaurant. "Ask yourself when you walk in: Would you want to eat there?" he says.

● Is there a strong smell of fumes? If there is, it's a sign that the facility is poorly ventilated, says John Bailey, Ph.D., acting director of FDA's office of cosmetics and colors. Inhaling the fumes from nail products can make you sick.

If you have a complaint about a salon providing nail services, contact your state board of cosmetology.

— P. K.

"Our current guidance is that products containing ethyl methacrylate should be used only by trained nail technicians under conditions that minimize exposure and skin contact because of their potential to cause allergies," he said.

Whatever the cause, allergic reactions usually take place where the product has been applied or where it has inadvertently come in contact with other skin surfaces, such as the face, eyelids and neck.

When the offending agent is no longer used, reactions clear up. Sometimes, the user can identify the chemical causing the allergic reaction and avoid it.

Though rare, some nail products can cause illness and even death, particularly if ingested by children. In 1987, a 16-month-old toddler died of cyanide poisoning after swallowing a mouthful of solvent used to remove sculptured artificial fingernails. At least one other youngster was rushed to the emergency room for intensive care after swallowing a similar product. These products contained acetonitrile, a chemical that breaks down into cyanide when swallowed. Since 1990, the Consumer Product Safety Commission has required household glue removers containing more than 500 milligrams of acetonitrile in a single container to carry child resistant packaging. This includes glue removers for artificial nails.

Nail products also can be dangerous if they get in the eyes. And they can easily catch on fire if exposed to the free flame of the pilot light of a stove, a lit cigarette, or even the heating element of a curling iron.

Consumers should read labels of nail products carefully and heed any warnings.

HEALTHY NAILS

From current consumer habits, one might surmise that the main function of nails is to look good. But nails serve several physiological purposes: They enhance fine touch and fine motor skills and protect the fingers and toes. Doctors also may examine them for indications of serious underlying diseases; for example, clubbed nails (a condition in which fingers or toes thicken and the nails wrap around them) is a classic sign of chronic lung and heart disorders. For those reasons, it's important to keep nails healthy.

With proper care and precautions, nails can be both healthy and attractive.

Paula Kurtzweil is a member of FDA's public affairs staff.

Is DNA Destiny?

Genetic Discoveries Raise Women's Expectations — and Tough Questions

Is DNA destiny? It certainly seems so: Discoveries about the genetic underpinnings of human diseases are coming at a breath-taking pace. In September alone, scientists announced that they had found a distinctive mutation of the breast cancer gene *BRCA1* in Jewish women and reported that multiple sclerosis, a disease thought to be triggered by a virus, appears to have a genetic connection as well.

As each new discovery hits the headlines, you may hear predictions that a simple genetic test is on the way. But as it turns out, most of these predictions will be overly optimistic.

Though tests for many common diseases are available, most are still used only in research settings. Nonetheless, genetic testing is, as an industry, about to explode. Before too long, tests will be available and physicians will use them routinely. The question is, are we ready?

WHO'S TESTED NOW?

Dozens of genetic tests have been available for years. The most common are those used before and after birth. Tests are also available for Huntington's disease and for several rare disorders like Wilms' tumor, which affects the kidneys.

Helix, a directory kept at Children's Hospital and Medical Center in Seattle, lists more than 200 labs that now test for genes associated with 275 different disorders. Approximately 25% of these tests are available on a commercial basis to the public through their doctors, says Bonnie Pagon, M.D., the University of Washington pediatrics professor who founded the directory.

The remainder are available only through research studies. However, some studies require that participants have a family history of disease. Moreover some studies require that the DNA from several affected relatives be available, which usually means they must still be alive.

Thus, not everyone can participate in research studies. Even so, there aren't enough studies to accommodate all potential patients, and many of those in progress are closed to new participants.

Nonetheless, there's no need to be discouraged by the shortage of research studies, as more tests are about to make their public debut. A test for the breast and ovarian cancer gene *BRCA1* may be introduced within six months. Other tests likely to follow *BRCA1*'s lead include those for hereditary nonpolyposis colon cancer. Alzheimers disease, thyroid cancer, and melanoma.

NO SIMPLE MATTER

Once these tests become widely available, who should be tested? If you suspect that your family history places you at risk, you might want to be tested. However, before you go ahead, you need to consider the following questions:

● **What do the results really mean?** Genetic test results *can* tell you whether you carry the gene in question. But in most cases, they *can't* tell you whether you'll eventually be diagnosed with the disease, says Patricia Kelly, Ph.D., director of medical genetics and cancer risk screening for Salick Health Care in Los Angeles.

If your results are positive, that doesn't necessarily mean that you're bound to get the disease. For instance, in the case of cancer, as Dr. Pagon points out, "Other events — including environmental ones —

From *Women's Health Advocate* (November 1995), pp. 1, 7-8. Reprinted with permission from *Women's Health Advocate Newsletter*. For subscriptions call 1-800-829-5876 and ask for the introductory price of $16 per year, a 33% discount.

Where's the Breast Cancer Test?

The whole point of genetic testing is to get the jump on preventing or treating a particular disease. But that strategy isn't as simple as we wish it were, and that's why many genetic tests are being detained on the launch pad.

Many of the complications can be illustrated by the test for *BRCA1*, a gene that increases the risk of breast and ovarian cancer.

As with most other genetic tests the *BRCA1* test has been studied in high-risk populations — that is, in women who have three or more closely related family members with the disease. Among these women, those who have certain *BRCA1* mutations face an 80% to 90% chance of getting breast cancer and a 40% to 70% chance of getting ovarian cancer. (In the most recent report, scientists announced that one mutation is eight times more common among Jewish women of Eastern European origin.)

But researchers don't know whether those statistics will hold true for women in the general population. "The risk might be much lower," says Barbara Biesecker M.S. co-director of the National Institutes of Health's genetic counseling research and training program.

One problem is that there are many possible mutations of the gene, and researchers haven't identified all the mutations or the risk of cancer associated with each. "There may be some mutations that don't confer any increased risk," Biesecker notes. "Others may increase the risk by 20%."

Then again, a finding of no *BRCA1* mutations doesn't completely rule out breast cancer. There are other breast cancer genes, including *BRCA2*. And defects in a recently discovered gene called *ATM* (for ataxia telangiectasia, mutated) may be twice as common as *BRCA1* mutations. Researchers speculate that *ATM* defects may be linked to about 8% of all breast cancer cases. *BRCA1* to about 5%. (*ATM* defects raise the risk of getting other diseases as well.)

And even if doctors know that a woman carries *BRCA1* or *ATM*, they don't know what the next step should be. Some doctors say that women with *BRCA1* mutations should go ahead and have their still-healthy breasts and ovaries removed. But even that preemptive strike can't guarantee that breast cancer won't develop, as it's difficult to surgically remove all breast tissue.

What about stepping up screening? Though that move seems logical, there may be difficulties here as well. Because the *ATM* gene predisposes carriers to an extreme sensitivity to x-rays, some researchers fear that even the small doses of radiation from mammograms might be enough to increase an *ATM* carrier's chance of getting cancer. Even though that risk is only hypothetical, it's cause for concern.

When you add other concerns to the mix, such as the possibility of losing health insurance, it's clear that this brave new world of genetic testing is a profoundly complex and challenging one.

---

may have to happen for cancer to occur; in some people, that second event will never take place."

And even if your test results come up negative, that doesn't mean that you won't get the disease for other reasons. In truth, most cases of many diseases can't be attributed to heredity.

- **Is any treatment available?** At the moment, doctors and geneticists can't always advise you what to do if you carry a defective gene. "Medically, we have no idea what surveillance or prevention measures to take for people who test positive for cancer genes," says Barbara Biesecker, M.S., who's co-director of the National Institutes of Health's genetic counseling research and training program.

For some diseases such as ovarian cancer, such screening measures don't exist in the first place. For others, such as Alzheimer's, there's not much doctors can do to alter the course of the disease.

- **What will the fallout be?** A positive result could be psychologically devastating and full of ramifications for you and your family. Even a negative result could cause "survivor guilt" if other family members are found to carry the flawed gene, notes Dr. Kelly.

Moreover, health insurers can and often do cancel insurance coverage by declaring genetic test results to be evidence of a pre-existing condition. (However, it's now illegal to refuse someone a job based on test results.)

Clearly, getting tested isn't a simple matter. That's why medical geneticists recommend extensive counseling before and after any genetic test.

ASK THE EXPERTS

If a specific disease runs in your family, you can ask your doctor, whether a test for it is available. (Doctors and other health professionals who are registered with Helix can find out which tests are available and how to order them.) If a test isn't available, you might want to maintain contact with a medical geneticist so that you can be kept up-to-date on the research.

Even if you decide against being tested, you might want to consult a genetics counselor if you have deep concerns about a particular hereditary disease. These specialists can be located through the genetics clinics of large hospitals, medical centers, or comprehensive cancer centers. They can analyze your family history and assess your risk. In addition, they should be able to offer advice about how to minimize your chances of getting the disease.

The bottom line is, genetic tests aren't for everyone. As each disease-causing gene is discovered, it's understandable that a woman would want to know whether or not she carries that gene. But she should also ask herself some tough questions — and be ready for some equally tough answers.

Female Circumcision Comes to America

Performed by new immigrants, veiled in deference to a cultural tradition of the developing world, female circumcision is becoming an American problem

By Linda Burstyn

It is a late-summer night, nearly midnight in Washington, D.C., when the taxicab comes for Mimi Ramsey. She steps into it with a worried look in her eyes and her mouth firmly set. She is on her way to yet another stranger's house, where she will again — for the umpteenth time in the past year — talk about the most personal and most secret of African customs, offering herself as a sort of human roadblock in the traffic of tradition.

At the house Ramsey is kissed on both of her cheeks by her hostess, an Ethiopian immigrant like herself, and ushered into a dimly lit living room decorated with rugs and cloths from their homeland. There she spends the next several hours huddled together with the young mother, Genat, talking in conspiratorial whispers.

"Mother says she will do it anyway, herself — when I'm out of the house — if I don't agree to get it done soon." Genat confides to the woman she hopes will help her. "She says she will take a razor blade and do it." Ramsey nods. She has heard this story many times before, and responds by reciting a long list of reasons why the older woman must be stopped, trying to give Genat the courage to buck tradition and disobey her mother. "You cannot let her do this to your child. Please. It is wrong. You know how painful it is. How damaging. Your daughter may hate you for life for what you allow to happen to her."

Genat shakes her head. She doesn't want her baby girl, just born in this country, to be circumcised, as is customary in her native land, but her mother is adamant.

"She believes in it so strongly," Genat says. "She said if I don't do these things, the girl will grow up horny. She'll be like American girls. And how will I be able to go back to work if my mother is not here to care for my child?"

It is not until many hours later, after a long, sleepless night and a fruitless morning discussion with the older woman, that Ramsey, discouraged, finally ends this peculiar house call. "Please send your mother home," she advises Genat. ' Go on welfare if you have to, but don't let your mother stay in the house and do this to your baby."

To Mimi Ramsey, a forty-three-year-old nurse who lives in San Jose, California, scenes like this one are increasingly familiar. An activist in a growing movement in this country to halt the practice of female circumcision — also called female genital mutilation, or FGM —she, among others, is trying not only to persuade her compatriots to end the practice but also to persuade America to address FGM as a serious health and human-rights issue. It is not an easy task. Even though the details of some of the extreme yet common forms of the practice are as horrifying to most Americans as Nazi human experimentation or brutal child abuse, documentation is hard to come by, and resistance to infringing upon the traditions and mores of another culture is difficult to overcome.

"We don't warn [immigrant] families that we consider this child abuse," says Catherine Hogan, the founder of the Washington Metropolitan Alliance Against Ritualistic FGM. "When you wrap this issue in the cloth of culture, you just can't see what's inside.

From *The Atlantic Monthly* (October 1995), pp. 28-35. Reprinted by permission of Linda Burstyn, a freelance writer based in Washington, D.C.

This is a clear case of child abuse. It's a form of reverse racism not to protect these girls from barbarous practices that rob them for a lifetime of their God-given right to an intact body."

Americans who are aware of the practice, which has been performed on some 100 million to 130 million women and girls worldwide, assume that it is a fact of life only for girls who live in faraway places — a form of barbarism that doesn't touch American homes, schools, or doctor's offices. This is simply not true. As more and more African immigrants move to this country, bringing with them their food, practices, and traditions, perhaps hundreds more daughters of African parents are circumcised in the United States every year.

Many of the immigrant mothers who are making these decisions about their daughters know little or nothing about their own anatomy. They are told that if the clitoris is left alone, it will grow and drag on the ground; that if their daughters are left uncircumcised, they will be wild, and will crave men; that no man from their home country will marry them uncircumcised (although many African men say that they prefer uncircumcised women for sex and marriage); that circumcision aids in menstruation and childbirth (although the opposite is true in both cases); and that it is a religious — usually Islamic — requirement (although none of the major Islamic texts calls directly for FGM). And so these women and their husbands come to the United States filled with misinformation, and remain blindly dedicated to continuing this torturous tradition.

Azza, an Egyptian immigrant who moved to the United States fifteen years ago and now lives in Louisiana, plans to take her ten-year-old American-born daughter back to Egypt in a few months to have her circumcised. "They say it helps us control our emotions," she says. The thirty-three-year-old mother is confused about whether or not she wants to put her daughter through the procedure, first saying that she and her husband are not sure what they are going to do, and finally saying that it is up to him and the Egyptian doctors to decide.

Frequently families will chip in to bring someone from the homeland to the United States to perform circumcisions, because it's cheaper to import a circumciser than it is to send several girls abroad. A taxi driver in Washington, D.C., who hotly defends the practice says that he recently had his daughters circumcised that way. "I stood over her to make sure she

Frequently families will chip in to bring someone from the homeland to the United States to perform circumcisions, because it's cheaper than sending several girls abroad.

cut enough," he says. "I wasn't going to let my daughters have those things!"

As more and more immigrants from countries that practice FGM come to make their homes in Western countries, these countries are facing the task of confronting a custom that is rigidly adhered to and yet taboo to discuss. The United States has not given FGM the attention or the illegal status that many other nations have given it. The United Kingdom has a full-fledged and longstanding anti-FGM movement that involves the country's social-service agencies. France, Canada, Denmark, Switzerland, Sweden, and Belgium all have outlawed the practice. The first attempt to prohibit FGM here died in the previous Congress. However, the legislation has been reintroduced by its original co-sponsors, Representatives Pat Schroeder, of Colorado, and Barbara-Rose Collins, of Michigan. Senator Harry Reid has proposed similar legislation in the Senate. Three states, New York, Minnesota, and North Dakota, have passed laws making the practice of FGM a felony unless it is medically necessary.

Knowing that federal legislation to deal with FGM is far from a certainty, a growing number of people are joining the battle to stop FGM in America. They want this country to start documenting the extent of the practice here and to use the courts and social services to put an end to it — an aim they're finding it difficult to achieve at a time when so many cities are struggling with other pressing issues.

"It's a serious problem in most urban centers in the United States," Hogan says. "There just hasn't been enough empirical documentation of it. But what we see when we see it, anecdotally or empirically, is just like incest was in its time — or child abuse. It's the tip of the iceberg."

Several recent events have helped to strengthen this movement. Probably the most high-profile of these were the publication of Alice Walker's novel on the subject, *Possessing the Secret of Joy*, and the production of Walker's documentary film, *Warrior Marks*, which was shown in cities throughout the United States. Also significant was the well-publicized court case of a Nigerian woman living in Oregon who won asylum in this country by pleading that her daughters would be in grave danger of being forcibly circumcised if they were sent back to their homeland.

Women's-rights groups such as Population Action International, Equality Now, RAINBOW, the Washington Metropolitan Alliance Against Ritualistic FGM, and the Program for Appropriate Technology and Health (PATH) and other groups form a loose information-and-activist network on FGM. More important, immigrant women who were circumcised as children have joined forces to fight the tradition among compatriots in this country.

Soraya Mire, a thirty-four-year-old Somali film maker who lives in Los Angeles, has been touring the country with her film *Fire Eyes*, which shows African children being circumcised. Asha Mohamud, a Somali who has worked as a pediatrician and who lives in Alexandria, Virginia, now directs several FGM projects in Kenya and the United States for PATH. Mimi Ramsey has made it her avocation to visit African businesses and communities in this country and proselytize against FGM.

Ramsey typifies many who, after hearing about FGM in the media, have finally been able to talk about an experience long suppressed. For years, she had gone to doctors for help with the aftereffects of her radical circumcision. For years doctors, either because they were stunned by what they saw or because they were trying to be culturally sensitive, said nothing to Ramsey about what had been done to her and simply prescribed various topical creams and jellies to ease her pain. But in February of last year all that changed.

"I went to a doctor for the problem I have down there." Ramsey says. "He asked me, 'Why did they do this to you? Why did they remove all your genitalia?' He was in shock." After returning to her apartment, depressed and confused, Ramsey, a devout Christian, prayed for some answers. Later that night she saw a television program about FGM and the Nigerian woman's asylum case in Oregon. It answered many of her questions. "I was angry and still am. The morning after the show I got up and called all the African women from my address book who live in the United States. I asked them, 'Are you a victim too?' And they said yes. I said, 'Let's talk about it. I'm not going to shut up anymore.'"

Most of the talk about circumcision in this country has focused on male circumcision, as people have made the case that it causes physical and psychological pain to infant boys. When it comes to women, "circumcision" is at best a misnomer.

"Cutting off the clitoris is equivalent to cutting off much of the penis," Asha Mohamud says.

This is why opponents and medical leaders use the more descriptive and more accurate term "female genital mutilation." Although in a tiny percentage of cases FGM consists of a small cut to the hood of the clitoris, typically it is much more severe. it usually involves the complete removal of the clitoris, and often the removal of some of the inner and outer labia. In its most extreme form — infibulation— almost all the external genitalia are cut away, the remaining flesh from the outer labia is sewn together, or infibulated, and the girl's legs are bound from ankle to waist for several weeks while scar tissue closes up the vagina almost completely. A small hole, typically about the diameter of a pencil, is left for urination and menstruation. The cutting is usually done with a razor, a kitchen knife, or a pair of scissors. It is rare for any anesthesia to be used. The age at which FGM is performed varies among countries and communities. In some countries it is done on infants in the days or weeks after birth; in others, such as Senegal, it is part of an elaborate rite of passage that comes with puberty. In parts of Nigeria and Burkina Faso, FGM is practiced during the seventh month of a woman's first pregnancy, in the belief that if the baby at birth comes in contact with its mother's clitoris, it will die.

There is no doubt within the medical community that FGM is a brutal, harmful practice. A World Health Organization report on FGM says,

> The immediate physical effects — acute infection, tetanus, bleeding of adjacent organs, shock resulting from violent pain, and hemorrhage — can even cause death. In fact, many such deaths have occurred and continue to occur as a result of this traditional practice. The lifelong physical and psychological debilities resulting from female genital mutilations are manifold: chronic pelvic infections, keloids, vulval abscesses, sterility, incontinence, depression, anxiety and even psychosis, sexual dysfunction and marital disharmony, and obstetric complications with risk to both the infant or fetus and the mother.

The American and British medical professions have in the past practiced FGM to varying degrees. There are reports of clitoridectomies having been performed as recently as the 1950s, to cure nymphomania and melancholia in girls. In the nineteenth century both clitoridectomies and female castration (removal of the ovaries) were practiced by British and American physicians, as cures for melancholia, masturbation, nymphomania, hysteria, lesbianism, and epilepsy. The American medical profession stopped performing clitoridectomies decades ago, only to find itself today confronting the practice in patients from cultures that perform FGM.

The United States is at best ambivalent about its responsibility in preventing and punishing female circumcision. In fact, there is almost no legal protection against it.

It is far easier to convince Americans of the horrors of FGM than it is to persuade them that it is enough of a problem here to warrant action. Proving just how widespread the practice is in the United States is a critical step. The legislation proposed in both the House and the Senate calls for the Department of Health and Human Services to gather data on the number of females living in the United States who have been subjected to FGM. However, the current lack of such data means that opponents can only point to anecdotal evidence to estimate the extent of FGM.

"I think some people leave some traditions behind, but some traditions are stronger than others." Mohamud says. "This is one that is very strong. The community here sees explicit sex on television, they hear a lot of alien things, and so it becomes more urgent for mothers to do this to their daughters so the girls don't fall into loose groups. They think if they don't follow the tradition, they don't know what will happen."

It is estimated that at least 7,000 women and girls immigrate to the United States each year from countries where at least a majority of females, if not all of them, are circumcised. Most of these new immigrants live in California, New York, and the Washington, D.C., area. It is difficult to determine the true circumcision rates in their home countries, because in most the practice is not discussed publicly. Nevertheless, rough estimates of what is common in each country suggest that almost half the women of Africa have been circumcised. The rate of FGM in Somalia is nearly 100 percent, in Ethiopia over 90 percent, in Egypt 50 percent. The list of places where it is traditionally practiced includes twenty-six countries in Africa and various areas of the Middle East, Asia, and South America. Even if only a small percentage of newly arrived families from these countries maintain the tradition of FGM, these figures suggest that hundreds of young girls either brought here or born here are in danger each year.

Mimi Ramsey spent part of the past year trying to track down circumcisers rumored to be living in this country. But not all families depend on finding a circumciser. Last September, Ramsey heard about a man in San Jose who had just circumcised his daughter over the objections of his wife. He had waited until his wife left the house and then locked his three-year-old in the bedroom with him and performed the FGM. 'He said that she was too wild." Ramsey says. She liked to play outside too much. She had friends who were boys. He said this will tame her.'"

If a native-born American father had mutilated his daughter, the action would incontrovertibly constitute child abuse. But this country is at best ambivalent about its role and responsibility in preventing and punishing FGM. In fact, other than in the three states previously mentioned, there is almost no legal protection against FGM for girls in the United States, both because it's difficult to uncover and because, absent a specific law against the practice, courts are unsure about how to punish it. One effort at prosecuting a woman in Georgia who cut off her niece's clitoris failed in part because of the legal confusion surrounding the problem.

Legislating these issues is going to be really crucial." says Leah Sears, a justice on the Supreme Court of Georgia who has been doing research on FGM and legal questions pertaining to it. "Legal issues concerning FGM are complex. Can an adult woman do this to herself? We American women consent to have our breasts enlarged, which is another bizarre thing women do for the pleasure of men. Is that so different? I think we need comprehensive legislation in this area."

In England and Canada — places where people from FGM-practicing countries have immigrated — laws against FGM and against taking a child out of the country to circumcise her have been passed. France has also made FGM illegal, and in 1993 it sentenced a Gambian woman to five years in prison after she paid $70.00 to have her two daughters circumcised. The medical associations in most of the Canadian provinces have passed prohibitions with strict penalties against circumcision and reinfibulation (sewing the vagina nearly shut again after childbirth). They have also begun educational efforts in those communities where FGM is most likely, preferring to discourage the practice rather than punish a parent after a girl has been circumcised. Unlike the United States, these countries take it for granted that FGM is occurring. Even though most U.S. legal experts interpret child-abuse laws broadly to cover FGM, very few preventive measures, such as education and community outreach, have been implemented in this country.

In this legal vacuum doctors and others who provide social services that could educate and inform communities about FGM and protect uncircumcised girls are caught in the ethical bind of trying to show respect for another culture and at the same time guide people away from a harmful practice that is very much a part of that culture. For instance, in response to growing concern about FGM, the American College of Obstetricians and Gynecologist released a statement opposing all medically unnecessary surgical modification of female genitalia (although doctors here continue to perform cosmetic reduction surgery on both the clitoris and the labia), and declared that

FGM should be stopped; but its guidelines end there. Some hospitals and doctors continue to reinfibulate women and to say nothing against parents' plans to circumcise their daughters. An article published in 1993 in the *American Journal of Obstetrics and Gynecology* clinically details one obstetrician's efforts to deliver a child vaginally from an infibulated woman. The article, written as a guide for dealing with such a situation, ends with a recommendation on how to perform reinfibulation and concludes, "The issue of whether the woman will want her own infant daughter circumcised also needs to be discussed so that she can make an individual, culturally appropriate and educated choice."

"My patients say doctors are often shocked when they see them, and don't know how to help them," says Carol Horowitz, an internist who cares for East African immigrants in Seattle. "I try to deal with them with respect and dignity and try to help them with their problems, surgically or nonsurgically.' Horowitz says that she is mindful of the risk of offending her patients when she educates them about the harmful aspects of what was done to them or counsels them against circumcising their children — and that some doctors with whom she has worked will not broach the subject at all. "To many patients, a circumcised vagina is normal. Any change is going to have to come from within that community."

Teachers, nurses, and administrators in elementary schools located in areas with many African students are often ill equipped to detect and help a child at risk for mutilation, or to help a child following this potentially traumatizing experience. "There was a time I got a call from someone in northern Virginia," Asha Mohamud says. "They heard of a girl in a school who was at risk. The teacher was teaching about sex education, and the young girl pointed out the clitoris and said, 'That part is really bad, and my mother is taking me back in the summer to have that cut out.'" Mohamud tried to find the girl, but by the time the story had reached her, it was too late. The girl had already graduated and returned from her trip to Africa.

"If that family-life teacher was aware she could have done something immediately," Mohamud says. "It's something also that made the issue more urgent to us. Things are happening here right under our own noses. Girls are probably being taken back right now."

A desire to educate both the officials in her adopted country and immigrants from her native one drives Mimi Ramsey. The New York–based international women's-rights group Equality Now is raising money to fund Ramsey's efforts so that she will be able to spend more time doing what she does best: taking her message to the streets.

In a dark restaurant in Los Angeles paper placemats are decorated with maps of Ethiopia. Shiny red-vinyl booths are filled with brightly dressed residents of the local immigrant community. Original Ethiopian artwork and African posters cover the walls. The smell of cooked meat and the sound of quiet laughter surround the booth where Ramsey sits, with her just served lunch. Her own conservative dress is more likely to be found in Orange County than in Addis Ababa. She bows her head and prays aloud: "Please, God, save girls from being tortured. Please. God. Please. Thank you."

Just minutes after she begins her meal of traditional Ethiopian bread dipped in a stew of vegetables and meat, she gets up and approaches a table of four Ethiopian men. She exchanges pleasantries in their native language, Amharic, but quickly the conversation turns tense. A few English words are mixed with the foreign ones. A man says, Tradition." Ramsey replies, "Let's talk about it." and squeezes in next to the men.

"In this country you see a lot of young women unmarried, pregnant." Yashanu, an Ethiopian taxi driver in his mid-forties, says, leaning back in his chair. "Maybe if American girls were circumcised, this wouldn't happen. When I was growing up, a girl had to stay within the family. She could be home no later than five or six in the afternoon. But in this country there are no rules." He shakes his head. "When you circumcise a woman, they're less active sexually and more interested in their schoolwork."

Mimi describes the physical pain, the burning and irritation, she still feels from what was done to her when she was six years old. She takes a small tube of cream from her purse and shows it to them. The cream is supposed to soothe her damaged nerve endings. "I can't enjoy sex," she tells them. "I feel nothing. I will never forgive my mother for doing this to me. Will you join me in stopping people from doing this to little girls? We have to help them," she says, smiling, touching one of the young men on his arm.

By the time Mimi stands up, thirty minutes later, the three younger men, all of whom knew vaguely about FGM because they had had sex with women who were circumcised, are horrified. They each promise earnestly to call their families back in Ethiopia to talk with them about the practice. But the older man remains unconvinced.

Across the street, at another African-owned restaurant, Ramsey speaks to a table of very modern-looking young women. One of them, a beautiful twenty-five-year-old in jeans who works for a Hollywood studio, pulls Ramsey aside and hands her a piece of paper. On it is the name of one of her close friends, a Los Angeles resident, who is planning to take her baby daughter back to Ethiopia for a circumcision in a week's time.

In her own community Ramsey patrols the African shops and restaurants like a diligent security guard. Her golden-brown face lights up whenever she sees a person she recognizes as a fellow Ethiopian, and she immediately engages in traditional greetings before turning the subject to that which is taboo.

Was this done to you?" she asks the women. "It was done to me. I'm trying to stop this practice. Will you join me?" These encounters, usually the first time these women have ever discussed the issue, often end with tears, an embrace, and an exchange of phone numbers.

Beletu, a thirty-five-year-old Ethiopian immigrant, lives with her husband and their three daughters just outside Washington, D.C., in Maryland. She has had all three of her daughters circumcised — the youngest, two and a half, just last summer, durring a short trip back to Ethiopia. "People practice without knowing," Beletu says regretfully, now that she has learned about the harmful aspects of the procedure. "Even though I lived here years, I didn't know. Nobody told me. I wouldn't have put my daughters in this situation if I had known." Five months pregnant with another girl, she vows to leave this one uncircumcised.

"My mother told me it's protection for us — from boys," says Azza, the Egyptian immigrant in Louisiana. "It's very bad pain. I don't want my daughter to have it, but it depends on what the doctor tells us." When told that information exists about the medical effects of the procedure, she begs for it to be sent to her. "The more education the better," she says. "It's done from generation to generation by word of mouth. But why is it done?" I'm confused about it."

Soraya Mire. the Somali film maker, is one of a handful of women trying to find the finances and forums to educate an immigrant population that views FGM as a comforting tie to the morality and traditions of its homeland. She uses screenings of her documentary as opportunities to discuss the issue. Like others, Mire is motivated by her own experience as a mutilated woman.

They use vegetable thorns to sew because they are very strong," Mire says, describing the process of infibulation that she experienced. "The stitches stay in until marriage. Then three days before the wedding they ask the groom. Do you want to open her or do you want us to open her? A good man will say, You

go ahead and do it. Others want to tear the woman open themselves.

"I get calls from people within the community asking me if I know someone who will circumcise their children. I of course say no, and try to talk them out of doing it. I got a call last year from a man in L.A. who said he had just performed a circumcision on a girl. He said, 'She had a problem with her clitoris and I corrected it. There's nothing you can do to stop it.'"

Last year Mire went into hiding after receiving death threats from Somalis who were angry about what they saw as her traitorous behavior. She is now cautious when she's out in public and is reluctant to divulge the whereabouts of her secluded Los Angeles-area home.

At the Raleigh Studios, in Los Angeles, she shows her film to an audience of thirty-two people. The viewers cringe as they watch. A young girl is shown being held down. The circumciser reaches for a razor blade. The audience recoils. Mimi Ramsey is part of that audience. She drops her head to her lap and sobs.

After the film is over, Ramsey is asked to speak. She walks to the front of the stage but is still overcome. She simply cries and gasps, unable to talk for several minutes. The theater is perfectly silent except for her crying. Finally she speaks.

"I was struggling and calling my mother," Ramsey says in a hushed and breathless voice, trying not to break down again. "Little did I know that my mother had set me up. She paid for it to be done to me. This is something we all have to struggle with. While we're watching this, more little girls are being cut. My best friend was cut. She was my friend. My buddy. They did her the same day they did me, only she bled to death. What I'm doing now, I'm doing for her. I'm doing it for my buddy. She died for no reason. Please, let's fight it together. Please. Please."

Ramsey is still shaking an hour after the screening. "I need to go home, to face my mother. I need her to say she's sorry. Then I want her to go through Ethiopia with me, talking to women — talking them out of doing this to their daughters. She needs to go ahead of me. I will stand back and let her take the lead. It's only through this that I will forgive her."

Back home in San Jose, sometime later, Ramsey hears again from Genat, in Washington. Genat has sent her mother back to Ethiopia. She happily reports that her daughter is safe. Crying, Ramsey thanks her, returns the phone to its cradle, and bows her head in prayer.

As far as women's hearts are concerned, the road to health may run through a vineyard or two. But nothing is ever simple: Drinking carries considerable risks — breast cancer among them — and moderation is key.

Alcohol and Health: Mixed Messages for Women

Temperance leader Carrie Nation would be appalled: Thanks to findings about alcohol's heart healthy benefits, U.S. dietary guidelines now endorse moderate alcohol consumption. Though early evidence of alcoholic cardiac benefits came from studies on men, several recent studies suggest that the benefits apply to women as well — at least to those women at risk of developing heart disease.

However, this rosy picture is not without thorns. Though the cardiac benefits appear to be real, many physicians are reluctant to endorse a practice that can have such devastating physical, emotional, and social consequences when carried too far.

Says New York cardiologist Marianne Legato, "The incidence of alcoholism is increasing among women. It's a much-underestimated addiction in this country. Alcohol is the last thing I would recommend for coronary artery disease."

And even when alcoholism is excluded, any assessment of alcohol's benefits for women must be balanced against the potential risks. Heavier drinking is associated with an increased risk of breast cancer and with a host of other serious health problems (see "Good Reasons to Cork It"). Moreover, a woman's body is especially vulnerable to alcohol abuse, sustaining damage at lower levels of consumption than a man's.

GOOD IN SMALL DOSES

The sticking point for most critics is the concept of moderation — and how well or poorly it may be applied in the real world (see "How Much is Too Much?").

During the last two years several studies have found lower death rates among light to moderate drinkers (generally defined as one to two drinks per day). The findings point to a "U-shaped curve" — that is, risk is lowest for moderate drinkers, who fall in the middle, and highest for teetotalers and heavy drinkers.

A recent report from the massive Nurses' Health Study supports these findings. In that study, published in the May 11, 1995 *New England Journal of Medicine*, light drinkers (one to three drinks per week) had a 17% lower risk of death than non-drinkers. The risk was 12% lower for moderate drinkers (four drinks per week to about two drinks per day). Heavy drinkers had a 19% higher risk of dying.

The survival advantage of modest drinking was primarily attributable to fewer deaths from heart

---

How Much Is Too Much?

Alcohol researchers define moderate alcohol consumption as one to two drinks per day. That's easy enough. But many of us kid ourselves about how much we drink, especially when it comes to sipping wine from tall goblets or to free-pouring an evening cocktail. Here's what "moderate" alcohol consumption really means on a daily basis:

Beer	Wine	Spirits
one to two 12-ounce cans	one to two five-ounce glasses	one to two 1.5-ounce shots

If your favorite wine glass holds eight ounces of wine, for example, and you drink two glasses a day, you're pushing beyond moderate consumption. By some definitions, you would be considered a heavy drinker.

From *Women's Health Advocate* (February 1996), pp. 4-5, 8. Reprinted with permission from *Women's Health Advocate Newsletter*. For subscriptions call 1-800-829-5876 and ask for the introductory price of $16 per year, a 33% discount.

attacks. However, it applied only to women at risk of heart disease — those who were over 50 or who had other coronary risk factors, such as smoking, high cholesterol, high blood pressure, obesity, or a family history of heart disease. (Much of the increased risk of death among heavy drinkers was due to breast cancer.)

How alcohol protects the heart isn't entirely clear. Several studies have suggested that alcohol discourages clot formation. A key factor, however, appears to be its favorable effects on cholesterol levels.

Specifically, alcohol consumption increases high-density lipoprotein (HDL, the so-called good cholesterol). Before menopause, women have higher HDL levels than men do — a fact that's believed to explain premenopausal women's relative protection from heart disease. When estrogen production declines at menopause, however, HDL levels begin to fall and heart attack rates begin to climb. By the time women reach age 65, we're as likely as men to die of heart attacks.

Estrogen appears to be a key link in the alcohol-HDL connection. Women who drink have higher circulating levels of estrogen than do non-drinkers — a factor that presumably boosts their HDL and reduces the risk of heart disease. But that estrogen upswing might also contribute to the increased incidence of breast cancer seen in heavy drinkers.

Further complicating the picture is the fact that even modest amounts of alcohol raise triglycerides. High triglycerides are a particularly ominous coronary risk factor in women. For a woman whose triglyceride level is on the high side (a level consistently over 200 mg/dl), moderate drinking might do more harm than good.

THE GENDER GAP

In the women and alcohol debate, one thing is clear: women pay a heavy price for heavy drinking. And in research circles, heavy drinking "means as few as three drinks a night."

Because of gender differences in body composition and metabolism, women suffer alcohol-related physical problems at lower levels of consumption than men. And these medical problems may remain hidden longer for several reasons.

For one, many women are closet drinkers. And some doctors may still be reluctant to broach the "indelicate" subject of alcohol abuse with a woman — or when they do, her reported amount of drinking may not raise a red flag.

In reality, however, it takes less alcohol to damage a woman's liver and heart. "There's no question that alcohol has a bigger impact on women than men in

---

Good Reasons to Cork It

Heavy drinking takes a toll on women's health. Liver disease, weakened hearts, damage to unborn children, and accidents are the better-known risks. But heavy alcohol consumption also is believed to aggravate or contribute to the following conditions:

- stroke
- cancers of the liver, head and neck, pancreas, and breast
- osteoporosis
- high blood pressure
- depression
- anxiety
- insomnia
- premenstrual syndrome
- infertility
- nutritional deficiencies

A final — and important — consideration is alcohol's long-term effects on the brain. "The cognitive effects of heavy drinking are greatly underestimated," says New York cardiologist Marianne Legato. "People stop being able to think clearly, they lose their memory, and they have little blackout spells. Though they seem to be 'functional,' they're not if you measure them very carefully in terms of what they once were."

---

terms of cirrhosis, says Dr. Legato, an associate professor of clinical medicine at Columbia Presbyterian College of Physicians and Surgeons.

Moreover, a serious heart condition called alcoholic cardiomyopathy is a problem for both men and women who drink heavily. In this condition, chronic alcohol consumption weakens heart muscles, compromising heart function and leading to heart failure in many patients. According to a report in the July 12, 1995 *Journal of the American Medical Association*, it takes much less alcohol to cause this damage in women than it does in men.

Gender differences in metabolism appear to be to blame for alcohol's exaggerated effects in women. Women have less of an enzyme called alcohol dehydrogenase, which breaks down alcohol first in the stomach and then in the liver. As a result, less alcohol is processed at these sites and more passes to the liver, brain, and other parts of the body.

And the lower fluid content of a woman's body also contributes to their inability to handle alcohol according to a recent report. Less fluid means less opportunity for the alcohol to dissolve and more opportunity for alcohol molecules to reach the brain. In practical terms, a woman may have fewer drinks than a man but end up with a blood alcohol level as high or higher than his.

WEIGHING THE RISKS

So what are women to do? Given the public's proclivity to grab a headline and run with it, many cardiologists are decidedly uncomfortable with stories on alcohol's heart benefits.

For Dr. Legato, the entire issue is at best overblown and at worst potentially dangerous. "Alcohol is such a problem in our society," she emphasizes. Attempts to legitimize alcohol as a medical intervention for heart disease are "like using morphine to treat a migraine."

If you don't drink at all, don't start in hopes of reducing your heart disease risk. Other lifestyle modifications are far more important — stopping smoking, getting regular exercise, losing weight if you're overweight, keeping high blood pressure and diabetes in control, and watching dietary fat intake.

If you do drink, you're best off leaning toward the "light" side of moderation — one drink a day or less.

That level of consumption shouldn't elevate your breast cancer risk, says breast cancer surgeon Laura Esserman, M.D., M.B.A. "Everything has to be put in perspective" says Dr. Esserman, an assistant professor of surgery and co-director of the Breast Cancer Center at Mt. Zion Hospital and the University of California, San Francisco. "Modest amounts of alcohol are associated with improvements in cardiac risk factors, and cardiac problems are a much more significant health risk for women than breast cancer."

However, "heavy drinking — three to four drinks a day — clearly is associated with breast cancer," she continues. "In fact, moderate to heavy alcohol use increases a woman's breast cancer risk as much as family history. But someone who drinks three to five glasses of wine a week should be fine."

If We've Come Such a Long Way, Why Are We Still Smoking?

By Sharon Lerner

Seventy-five years ago, a woman ran for president of the United States on an antismoking platform. Lucy Page Gaston, who ran against known smoker Warren G. Harding, thought that smoking led to drinking, a life of crime, and a condition she called "cigarette face." She objected particularly to smoking by minors and women and, with the support of a substantial turn-of-the-century antismoking movement, she helped restrict smoking in more than 20 states by the mid-1920s. At the time, women accounted for an estimated 5 percent of all tobacco consumers.

We've come a long way since then, of course. Women now make up nearly half of all smokers in the U.S. (48 percent), and researchers predict we will soon be the majority. The number of females who begin smoking during high school and college has risen steadily, while the number of males has declined. And recent studies on smoking trends show that women as a group — in particular women living in poverty and those with less education — are doing worse with smoking than the overall population.

What is perhaps most upsetting about these landmarks is that we reach them in the face of overwhelming evidence that smoking does cause disease — things far worse than "cigarette face." While men have thus far dominated the habit during a period of ignorance about health effects, women are poised to become the majority of smokers at a time when it's absolutely clear that smoking is harmful.

IGNORING THE MEDICAL EVIDENCE

At least part of the problem is that it's still not widely understood just how harmful it is to smoke.

Many people still lump it in with risks like pesticides on fruit or sunbathing. The truth is that smoking kills more women than alcohol, illicit drugs, car accidents, suicide, and homicide — *combined*. It's by far the number one cause of premature death in women, causing approximately 20 percent of *all deaths*, killing roughly one in seven — or 141,832 — women annually. Lung cancer, which has increased over 400 percent in women in the past 30 years, is now the biggest cancer killer of women — bigger even than breast cancer. And together, conditions such as emphysema, heart disease, stroke, and various other cancers are responsible for more smoking-related deaths than lung cancer.

There is now also overwhelming evidence that women are uniquely vulnerable to certain smoking-related health problems. Women smokers are more

The medical news about smoking has had far less impact on women's smoking than on men's.

susceptible to reproductive tract infections and cervical cancer, and those who use oral contraceptives have an especially high risk of stroke and heart disease. Smoking also wreaks havoc on women's hormonal systems — decreasing fertility, increasing the chances of premature menopause and osteoporosis, and disrupting pregnancy. Women smokers have more preterm stillbirths, and their children are more likely to suffer and die from a variety of birth defects.

If the full extent of the above litany is not common knowledge, most of us have gotten the basic message: smoking is bad for you. Nevertheless, the medical news about smoking has had far less impact on women's smoking than on men's. Middle-class white men have stopped smoking in greater number than any other group, while women's smoking has gone down only slightly overall.

STARTING YOUNG

Why have female smokers been so unresponsive to the grim health news? A large part of the answer, according to Jean Forster, a researcher at the University of Minnesota School of Public Health, lies in the fact that most smokers — over 90 percent — take up the habit before age 20. African American girls constitute the one exception to this rule. The smoking rate among black teenagers has dropped in the past 10 to 15 years, but the rate significantly increases for black

> *"Women often smoke as a way of claiming and marking their personal space."*

women later in life. Researchers have yet to reach a consensus as to why African American women often start smoking at a later age.

The average teen smoker begins at age 13. "At that point," says Forster, who has conducted focus groups with teenage smokers, "the public health message means nothing to kids. They're simply too young for it." And the earlier people start, the more likely they are to smoke heavily and the harder it will be for them to quit. But according to Forster, most teenagers are not worried about that. They are confident they will quit before they develop health problems, even before they become addicted. And, for teenage girls especially, concerns such as social acceptance, attractiveness, and body image often far outweigh thoughts of serious illness in the far-off future.

Cigarette marketers' ability to appeal to these concerns has been critical to their success in replacing the two to three million smokers who either quit or die each year. With the industry now spending over $4 billion annually on advertising and promotion (after cars, cigarettes are the second most advertised consumer product in the U.S. — despite the fact that cigarette advertising is banned from broadcast media), marketing techniques have reached a new level of complexity. Lately, many brands have taken to offering products geared to women that can be bought with proofs of purchase from cigarette packs. These incentives are offered with a time limit, so that you have to buy 400 packs of Merits within six months, for example, to get the "Merit Award" of a suede

Helpful Hints for Quitting

- **Be encouraged.** Half of the adult smokers in the U.S. have quit. You can too.

- **Decide.** The first step is to make up your mind that you absolutely want to be a nonsmoker and prepare yourself to withstand some hardship in getting there.

- **Plan.** Set a quit date during a relatively stress-free time and let the people around you know when it is so they can be prepared and supportive. Decide on your method. You may want a prescription for nicotine gum or the "patch," which supply you with nicotine while you kick the habit, since using them is generally more effective than going cold turkey. The patch isn't effective for everyone; some people have allergic reactions, and pregnant women are advised not to use it.

- **Gather your motivational resources.** Write down your most important reasons for quitting so you can refer to them. Keep materials that remind you why you don't want to smoke (photos of tar-stained fingers, abscessed lungs, tobacco executives . . .). Reminders of why you want to quit, such as pictures of you at your most vibrant or an encouraging note from someone who loves you and wants you to quit, may also be helpful.

- **Join a support group if possible.** The American Cancer Society (800-ACS-2345) or the American Lung Association (800-586-4872) can help you locate quitting support groups throughout the country, such as Smokers Anonymous. There are even online quitting support groups (alt.support.stop smoking)

On the appointed day . . .

- **Disguise your ashtrays.** Put plants or nuts in them. Better yet, just throw them out.

- **Avoid smoke-filled settings.** At least at first, it will be extremely hard to be around other people who are smoking, especially if you have anything alcoholic to drink. You'll save yourself much unpleasantness by dodging these situations whenever possible.

- **Reward yourself.** You are doing a wonderful thing for yourself, and this should be acknowledged as much and as often as possible by yourself, and the people around you. Give yourself tokens of your appreciation.

- **Think of yourself as a nonsmoker.** While you are losing a habit, you are gaining an identity as a nonsmoker. This can come with its own set of new rituals, perhaps a long-lost hobby or some sort of exercise, such as a routine after-dinner walk instead of a cigarette.

—S.L.

barn jacket. For the outfit featured in Virginia Slims's V-wear ad, you have to buy about five and a half packs a day for six months, according to the calculations of Dr. Elizabeth Whelan, president of the American Council on Science and Health, who keeps close track of cigarette ads aimed at women.

While cigarette companies regularly devise new marketing gimmicks such as these, the main themes of their ads have remained the same since they began marketing to women and girls about 70 years ago. One longtime favorite, the association of smoking with independence, equality, and, yes, feminism, dates back to when women's smoking was socially unacceptable. Tobacco marketers capitalized on the allure of breaking that taboo, casting cigarettes as a symbol of women's liberation: one public relations agent even arranged for a contingent of women to march in the 1929 New York City Easter parade carrying "little torches of freedom." To this day, variations on the theme that smoking makes women tough, independent, and equal to men surface in ads — especially in Virginia Slims ads, from "You've come a long way, baby" to the recent "You can do it" slogan.

Another recurrent theme of cigarette marketing to women — identifying smoking with being thin — began with Lucky Strikes' 1920s "Reach for a Lucky instead of a sweet" ad, which featured a slim woman with a shadow of a double chin looming behind her. Female models in cigarette ads still conform to standard ideals of beauty, including thinness. And ads often emphasize the words "slim" and "thin," as in the Capri slogan "There is no slimmer way to smoke" and Misty's "slim and sassy." As a result, according to former Surgeon General C. Everett Koop, many young girls are left with the misconception that taking up smoking will actually make them thin. "Most of the adolescent female smokers I have talked with tell me they smoke to prevent gaining weight," says Koop, who has traveled extensively throughout the country interviewing young smokers. "They believe that if women who stop smoking gain weight, smoking must be a preventive to weight gain as well."

But regardless of content, the presence of cigarette ads alone influences women by affecting the editorial policies of the publications that carry them. It's now widely known that magazines that accept cigarette ads are less likely to report on the health effects of smoking, and studies have shown that tobacco ad revenue has an ever greater impact on health reporting in women's magazines than in other publications.

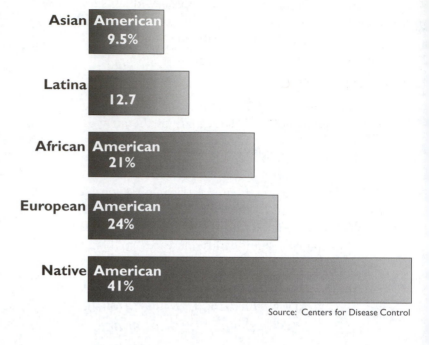

Source: Centers for Disease Control

Tobacco funding also complicates anti-smoking efforts by women's professional and political groups. Unfortunately, the practice is unlikely to change, given the scarcity of funding for women's organizations and the good publicity it affords the tobacco companies. Betty Dooley, president of the Women's Research and Education Institute, says that without the support of the tobacco industry, the organization would be unable to continue its public policy fellowship program — the only one of its kind for women. Spokesman K. Richmond Temple insists that Phillip Morris' motivation for funding women's groups comes from its female employees, who "support women's participation in all aspects of life."

STAYING SMOKING

While the image of smoking has much to do with its initial appeal, the *experience* of smoking is, of course, why people continue to smoke. Smoking is pleasurable. It can relax muscles, increase concentration, and relieve anxiety. Because women are more likely to live in poverty and juggle multiple roles, these physical effects hold particular appeal as ways to reduce stress and to exert control over their environment. Lorraine Greaves, vice president of the International Network of Women Against Tobacco and a sociologist who has analyzed the many ways smoking functions for women, notes that it can provide them with an escape when no others exist. "Women often smoke to claim and mark their personal space," says Greaves. "This allows them to separate or break from partners, children, and workmates whenever desired."

The special social significance of smoking to women may explain the gender differential in quitting success. According to the Centers for Disease Control's 1993 National Health Interview Survey, slightly more women than men want to quit completely (73 percent as opposed to 67 percent, respectively), while slightly fewer female smokers (46.7 percent as opposed to 51.9 percent) are successful in their attempts.

But the reality is that it's extraordinarily difficult for anyone to quit, mostly because tobacco is incredibly physically addictive (despite what some tobacco executives say). As Jack Henningfield, a scientist at the National Institute on Drug Abuse, sees it, although gender-related pressures may add to women's difficulties in quitting, the main problem is simply being exposed to nicotine. "All the advertising in the world wouldn't affect women if nicotine weren't addictive," says Henningfield. "Just having a normal, healthy, functioning brain means that you are prewired to be a nicotine addict."

SLAYING THE GIANT

Many in the antismoking movement look to regulatory possibilities — such as further restricting advertising, tightening youth access, limiting public smoking, and classifying and regulating tobacco as a drug — as their best hopes. But with annual revenues of $48 billion at stake, the industry is a daunting opponent, and so far it has managed to preserve its

Many young women are left with the misconception that smoking will make them thin.

profits by creatively circumventing restrictions. When tobacco ads were banned from radio and TV in 1971, for instance, the industry compensated by stepping up other ad efforts; the relative share of tobacco ad revenue in women's magazines soared after this point — it more than tripled from 1967 to 1986. And many see the current trend of expanding sales into the "developing" world as a direct result of increased restrictions in the "developed" world.

The recent Republican electoral landslide, made possible in part by $1 million in campaign contributions from tobacco companies, seems to have allowed the industry to yet again avoid serious regulation. In addition to the strong antiregulatory tenor of this current Congress, the November election brought a shift in leadership that bodes badly for tobacco regulation. Representative Henry Waxman (D.-Calif.), who oversaw the recent investigation of industry manipulation of nicotine levels, has been deposed — and the investigation halted. The person who now has control over almost all tobacco-related regulation is Representative Thomas Bliley, Jr. (R.-VA), who (until redistricting in 1990) represented a congressional district in which Phillip Morris is the largest employer. During the last election, Bliley received more contributions from tobacco industry political action committees than any other member of the House.

Although a few optimistic health advocates see potential for bipartisan support of tobacco control by casting it as a "pro-family" issue, most have a grimmer outlook, at least for the moment. But while the possibilities may be bleak in Washington, D.C., women are increasingly active and successful in fighting tobacco on other levels. Such organizations as the Berkeley, California-based Women and Girls Against Tobacco, the American Medical Women's Association, and NOW, as well as a growing network of international women's organizations, have recently begun major outreach projects to raise consciousness about the tobacco issue. And people all over the country are fighting the image war, covering cigarette ads with their own antismoking stickers and putting up counter-ads, such as a "Virginia Slime" campaign that recently ran in the New York City subway system. The point, of course, is to heighten women's personal and collective awareness that smoking has more to do with being exploited than with being liberated.

Sharon Lerner is a New York city-based freelance health writer and editor.

PART 6

Medical Matters

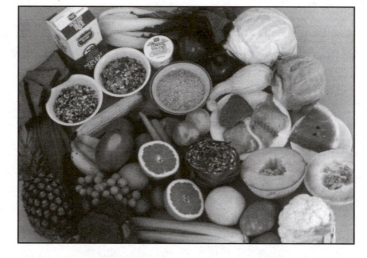

There has been much debate that women's health concerns are not taken seriously by many members of the traditional medical establishment, which has been predominately male. For example, the rate of hysterectomies performed in the United Sates has been a cause for concern of late, and some health professionals and activists think that many of these surgeries are unnecessary. Some women think that physicians take hysterectomies too lightly, minimize the risks that the surgery poses, and leave other options unexplored. The readings in this part deal with very specific medical matters that have potentially serious health consequences. These readings provide more information, and more current information, than is found in standard textbooks on these topics. The more you know on a given topic, the better informed you will be when making health care decisions and consenting to medical tests or procedures. Information is power, and the more one knows, the better equipped one is to get the best possible care.

Pap smears save lives, but what happens when costs are cut at labs that perform these tests? Are patients' lives at risk? Reading 34 discusses this controversial issue. Women trust their doctors and the tests they receive. But Reading 34 ("It's a Crime") emphasizes that a woman must be an advocate on her own behalf, and push doctors to answer questions and concerns. Women are often taught not to challenge the authority of doctors. But learning how to do that is essential for women's lives and health. (Please see the **Quick Reference Guide to Topics/Readings/ WWW Sites** and **Appendix A: WebLinks: A Directory of Annotated World Wide Web Sites** to select WWW sites that coordinate with the readings in this part.)

Karin Smith died of cervical cancer after a lab misread
her Pap smear — three times. Her legacy is that now,
when a doctor, lab, or HMO cuts costs and a patient dies,
it's not just a mistake,

It's a Crime

By Jan DeBlieu

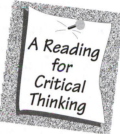

A Reading for Critical Thinking

The wedding of Peter Smith and Karin Knudsen took place on a sunny September Saturday in 1989. They had already been celebrating for two days. On Thursday Karin turned 24; Peter had turned 25 just the day before. "When we picked the date," Peter recalls. "Karin said, 'Boy, you'll never be able to forget our anniversary.'"

After the ceremony in a Catholic church near Milwaukee, about 300 guests attended the reception in a Swiss chalet-style restaurant. Karin, usually careful with money, impetuously tossed out her budget with the bouquet. Let the guests drink as much champagne as they want, she told the caterers. "There was a lot of electricity in the air," Peter says. "Everybody was on the dance floor."

That evening when the revelry wound down, Peter and Karin faced their first disappointment as husband and wife. After they made love, Karin began to bleed profusely. It had happened before, always after sex. "She was upset by it," Peter says. "But by then the problem was so much a part of our lives that we didn't let it bother us too much."

Karin had started bleeding after intercourse two years earlier, when she and Peter were students, deeply in love, at the University of Wisconsin in Milwaukee. She never felt pain; the bleeding came and went without warning or symptoms. Doctors at the university clinic took a Pap smear — a swab of cervical cells that can show early cancer — and said she was fine. But Karin was a health conscious young woman who didn't take chances. When she got her first job after college and joined the company's health maintenance organization, she asked her new doctor for another Pap smear. Over the next three years Karin went to doctors 15 times and had three Pap smears and three biopsies of her cervix, as her doctors searched for some medical clue to her chronic bleeding. Each time, the tests came back from the HMO's lab with the same verdict: no cancer. And every time, the verdict was wrong.

In March 1995, at the age of 29, Karin Smith died of a disease that shouldn't kill any woman receiving routine medical care. Cervical cancer is the greatest success story in the war on cancer. Deaths have decreased 70 percent since women began getting annual Pap smears. Today fewer than 5,000 American women a year die of cervical cancer, and half of those women never had a Pap smear in their lives. Karin, by contrast, did everything right. The athletic, ambitious brunette exercised regularly and ate a healthy diet. She got a Pap smear every year, even before she began bleeding after sex. She asked her doctors smart questions and followed their advice closely.

In the months before her death, wasted to less than 100 pounds from futile treatments begun too late, Karin Smith began a crusade to prove she was being killed by a health care system that encourages doctors — and the laboratories they depend on for diagnoses — to cut corners in the quest to save money. She was dying, she testified before Congress, because her HMO had contracted with a discount lab in an effort to lower costs. In her mind, what had happened to her was criminal.

In April 1995, within a month of her death, an inquest jury agreed with her. In an unprecedented move, the jury recommended that Chem-Bio Corporation be charged with the crime of reckless homicide. Finally Karin's message had been heard. But the real triumph of Karin's crusade is that her case has given good doctors — and the rest of us — a weapon with which to fight back. Now when a health care provider ignores medical standards to save money and a patient dies, it's no longer a matter of malpractice. It could be homicide.

When Karin and Peter met in 1984, she was a serious accounting major who dreamed of a house in the suburbs and he was a business student who liked to play more than study. "I'd stay out partying on Friday night until 4 a.m."

Peter found himself drawn to this determined, quick-witted woman who lived her life as carefully as he lived his care-free. She was someone with a future. "She was driven. Nobody could tell Karin she couldn't do something," he says. "She'd set out to prove them wrong every time." While he admired her mettle, he also loved to tease her. "She helped me focus on my career, and I helped loosen her up a bit."

At first, in 1987, Karin's postcoital bleeding was infrequent and light, a minor annoyance. An athlete, she played volleyball regularly and jogged ten miles at a time. But when the bleeding continued, her concern grew. After she was hired by the Arthur Andersen accounting firm, she went to a clinic run by Family Health Plan Cooperative, the HMO she'd joined. A physician's assistant took a Pap smear and sent it off to Chem-Bio, the lab her HMO had contracted with since 1979. Several days later the results came back normal. A year later another Pap smear came back normal, so the HMO referred Karin to a gynecologist, who did a biopsy, taking a tiny fragment of tissue from Karin's cervix to test it for cancer. That, too, came back negative for cancer. Instead, the lab pathologist suspected Karin had hyperplasia, an excessive growth of normal cells in the cervix — nothing to worry about. In June 1989 the gynecologist froze off the cells, which should have fixed the problem.

But four months later, at the time of Karin's marriage, the bleeding returned. Truly stumped, the doctor took a second biopsy. Like the others, this test was sent to Chem-Bio and came back negative. Searching for some solution, the doctor suggested Karin stop using birth control pills, which might be irritating her cervix. Over the next 12 months, through mid-1990, Karin's bleeding grew more frequent and heavier — sometimes lasting for weeks. In June Karin passed out twice after a volleyball game. She had been bleeding continuously for 21 days. By then Karin knew something was wrong, although she was sure her doctors were right: It couldn't be serious. "She thought she was anemic," Peter says. "She was working so much, we figured she was just worn out."

Karin and Peter had just built a house in the suburb of Sussex for the family they hoped to have. This time she went to the HMO's clinic near her new home, where they recommended another Pap smear and another biopsy, her third in two years. Frustrated, she asked to return to the Milwaukee gynecologist who had been treating her since 1988, but the HMO's rules required her to see the doctor nearest her home. Her new doctor noted she had a red, irritated cervix, one symptom of cervical cancer. But reassured by the repeated negative tests, the doctor told Karin, "Don't worry. I've seen cancer, and this isn't cancer," Peter recalls.

Within a few months Karin felt tired most of the time. She and Peter had all but stopped having sex. Hoping for some sort of resolution, she went yet again to the gynecologist, who again examined her cervix. Afterward, blood poured from Karin. It covered the table; it spilled onto the floor. And she broke down for the first time. "I was crying, and the nurse came in and tried to help me clean it up," she later testified. Figuring that there must be a blood vessel too close to the surface of her cervix, the doctor tried repeatedly to stop the bleeding by cauterizing, or searing, the cervical tissue. It never worked.

After four years of bleeding, three Pap smears, and three biopsies, Karin Smith finally lost faith in her health care plan in 1991. She went to see William Stewart, a highly regarded gynecologist not affiliated with her HMO, prepared to pay his fee out of her own pocket. The moment he looked at her cervix, he knew Karin was in serious trouble. He called David Hoogerland, a specialist in cervical cancer, who conducted an extensive biopsy and sent it to the lab he used (not Chem-Bio). The results were unquestionable: cancer.

Karin, who longed to have children, was scheduled for a radical hysterectomy. When the surgeons opened her they found that the cancer — slow-growing by nature — had penetrated her cervix and was spreading toward her bladder and bowel. It had already entered her lymph nodes, which could carry the disease throughout her body. Karin Smith would have had a 90 percent chance of surviving if the cancer had been detected in one of her early Pap smears, Hoogerland said in a deposition. But the doctors weren't even sure how to treat her at this point. "The doctors told us there was no protocol for treating such advanced cervical cancer — because it's so rare," Peter says. By Christmas 1991 the couple knew Karin was going to die.

Within weeks of her diagnosis, Karin and Peter contacted Patrick Dunphy, a lawyer who specializes in malpractice cases. Over the next 18 months Dunphy put together a chilling picture of mismanaged care. Testimony from Hoogerland and other physicians established that postcoital bleeding is a key sign of cervical cancer and that the appearance of Karin's cervix should have made the HMO's doctors more than a little suspicious. Yet they hadn't once mentioned her bleeding on the orders sent to the lab with the Pap smears and biopsies — a simple note might have caused the lab to examine her tests with extra care.

Karin blamed her doctors and a managed care system that encourages speed and impersonal treatment for condemning her to death. "Due to their gross incompetence and shameful errors, I am now dying," she testified before Congress. "I have spent countless days and nights nauseated and sick from both the radiation and the chemotherapy. . . . I have lain in a hospital bed, isolated from my family, my friends, even my husband, because my immune system was so suppressed that a minor cold could destroy me. . . . An HMO has cost me my life."

In June 1993 the Smiths agreed to accept a $6.3 million malpractice settlement from Family Health Plan Cooperative, the Chem-Bio lab, her doctor, and the technicians who misread her tests. But money provides small comfort to a dying woman. Karin wanted justice. "She wanted her story made public," says her close high school friend Karen Carleton. "She felt the doctors had committed a crime against her, and it was all being swept under the rug."

In the fall of 1994 Karin Smith and Patrick Dunphy asked Milwaukee district attorney Michael McCann to bring criminal charges against her doctors. McCann looked at the evidence and saw a killer, but not the killers Karin blamed. After all, he reasoned, even careful doctors must rely on the crucial information provided by laboratory tests when making their diagnoses. And six separate tests had told Karin's doctors that the one thing she did not have was cancer. To McCann, it was clear that the blame for what had happened to Karin rested with the Chem-Bio lab.

Betty Setum, a soft-spoken woman with a clear, direct gaze, began supervising work at Chem-Bio in 1990, just after it was sold to Damon Clinical Laboratories. The knowledge of what happened there still haunts her. "I used to be proud of what I do," she says. "Now I don't mention it unless I'm asked."

McCann saw a killer when he looked at the evidence, but not the one Karin blamed. The culprit, he said, was the lab.

Reading a Pap smear accurately is difficult for even the best cytotechnologists, as technicians trained to read Pap smears are called. Each slide may contain as many as 300,000 cells; when cancer is present, only a few may have the darkened center or malformed shape indicating the disease. It's like searching for a few odd blossoms in a roomful of flowered wallpaper.

For that reason, cytotechnologists need about five minutes to check a Pap smear slide, according to the College of American Pathologists. The work is so painstaking that professional guidelines have long recommended cytotechnologists read no more than 100 slides a day. In 1990 federal law set the limit at 120 slides, but concerns about accuracy caused the government to cut the limit to 100 slides a day in 1992.

A few days after Setum began work at the lab, June Fricano, a freelance cytotechnologist, told her to be especially careful with slides that had case numbers ending in 2; those were the ones that would be rescreened for quality control. "My jaw hit the floor," Setum says. "Quality control is supposed to be random. If it's not, there's no point doing it."

Then, in January 1991, Setum noticed a stack of 160 slides in Fricano's work area. Half had been marked with the next day's date, making it appear that she hadn't exceeded the legal limit. Setum had the slides rescreened. One, which Fricano had marked as normal, showed clumps of ominous dark cells. Fricano was fired that week.

A month later Setum took a phone call from the medical secretary at a nearby hospital. Doctors performing a hysterectomy on a 39-year-old woman had discovered advanced cervical cancer. Could they check her previous Pap smears? Setum pulled a 1987 Pap smear from the files and had it examined. "There were almost no normal cells on it," she says quietly. "Cancer's ugly. It's black and horrible. It was the worst thing I've ever seen."

That Pap smear belonged to Dolores Geary, a physical therapy aide and mother of three who also belonged to Family Health Plan Cooperative. She would become the second homicide victim in Michael McCann's criminal case. The slide had been read, and reported as normal, by June Fricano.

Fricano, it turned out, had screened more than 48,000 Pap smears in a year — four times the safe caseload. For her speedy work, she was paid $2 a slide, earning $96,000 at a time when top staff cytotechnologists made $33,000. Her mistakes were never detected, perhaps because she knew which slides would be rescreened for quality control.

Robert Lipo, the medical director of the lab, was aware that Fricano screened slides in half the needed time. In a deposition he said, "She prided herself on her speed and accuracy. . . . She'd sit there like a machine, and she'd just work like crazy."

Neither Lipo nor Fricano would agree to an interview for this story. Both had good reputations in the local medical community. But Karin's lawyer alleged that Lipo had a financial incentive to overlook, perhaps even to condone, Fricano's dangerous practices. He hired her to read all of his lab's Pap smears during the years that Karin Smith and Dolores Geary were repeatedly misdiagnosed — a workload that should have been shared by two full-time technicians plus a part-time employee, according to professional standards. Robert Lipo saved his lab between $12,000 and $36,000 a year by contracting with such an extraordinarily fast freelancer.

The ultimate slap in Karin's face: the same woman who had misread all her Pap smears was hired by the HMO's new lab.

To be sure, cytology labs have a troubled history dating back to the 1970s, when so-called Pap smear mills churned out inaccurate results with numbing regularity. Tighter professional standards and tougher federal laws are supposed to have changed that. The more Karin Smith and her lawyer learned about how Chem-Bio operated, the more they became convinced that cost-driven medicine had undone some of the safeguards.

"It was no coincidence that the lab which was contracted by my HMO performed inferior work," Karin told members of Congress. "The owner was on the HMO's board of directors, and in order to retain the HMO's business, he was forced to 'meet or beat' lab prices from the competition. . . . It's a system that encourages the lab to provide services at artificially low prices, which leads to lack of quality control and excessive workloads."

Traditionally, labs have charged health plans for each test they analyze. Under managed care, labs have begun bidding on what is known as a capitated contract. The lab agrees to analyze all of the HMO's tests — regardless of the number — in exchange for a monthly flat fee. The lowest bidder usually wins the contract. For 11 successive years Lipo, who sat on the board of Family Health Plan Cooperative's parent company until 1991, made the lowest bid and won the contract every time.

"How could Lipo make money and still come in as low bidder year after year?" asks Patrick Dunphy. How could Chem-Bio do work at a price no other Milwaukee lab could afford? "He couldn't do it without sacrificing quality," Dunphy says. "And Family Health Plan Cooperative was interested in getting their lab results as cheaply as possible."

Philip Dougherty, a spokesman for Family Health Plan Cooperative, says that's not true. "We are committed to providing quality care, and not just care that's cost efficient," he says. "We have lots of satisfied clients that we've served for a long time."

Yet consider these figures: In 1986 Chem-Bio offered to analyze all of Family Health Plan Cooperative's lab tests for $5.60 a year per HMO member. The cost of analyzing just one Pap smear is about $20. So once Chem-Bio had the contract, the lab may have found itself in the same economic bind that is forcing cytology labs around the country to close their doors. In this era of managed care, if Chem-Bio had asked for more money, it might have lost Family Health Plan Cooperative's contract, which accounted for most of its business.

Working under such financial pressure could easily lead to bad medicine, says Franklin Elevitch, chairman of the management resources committee for the College of American Pathologists. A lab with loose standards might urge technicians to work too fast or might pare costs by hiring the cheapest — and least experienced — technicians. "We're in a period of free-wheeling capitalism right now that the public doesn't understand," Elevitch says. "And the risk is that quality labs might not be able to weather the storm."

Chem-Bio decided to get out of the medical laboratory business altogether in 1990; it sold out to Damon Clinical Laboratories. Meanwhile, Family Health Plan Cooperative decided to open its own, in-house cytology department. In what Karin Smith later considered the ultimate slap in her face, the HMO hired June Fricano — freshly fired from Chem-Bio — to work in its new division. Robert Lipo recommended her work highly.

On April 7 of last year, Michael McCann took his evidence of reckless homicide to a Milwaukee inquest jury. Karin had died nine days earlier, so cold and thin, her friend Karen Carleton says, that Peter would lie in the bed to warm it for Karin before she got in.

This case wasn't about malpractice, McCann told the jury. It was about a recklessness so excessive that the perpetrators should have known their actions would kill someone. The case, McCann said, was no different from that of a driver who kills a child while speeding through a school zone. Such recklessness, he said, turns an accident into a crime.

The inquest jury came back with its unprecedented recommendation: Charge Chem-Bio, June Fricano, and Robert Lipo with reckless homicide. But McCann decided against prosecuting Fricano and Lipo. "There was no criminal intent on any individual's part," he says. "It was a confluence of people and conditions at the lab that led to these deaths." Instead, McCann charged Chem-Bio, as a corporation, with two counts of reckless homicide. Then he struck a deal he hoped would protect the public: Lipo agreed not to work as a laboratory director for six years and never again to supervise cytotechnologists or quality control. Fricano agreed never to work more than 42 hours a week and never to analyze more than 100 Pap smears a day.

Last December Chem-Bio pleaded no contest to the charges and paid the maximum legally allowable fine of $20,000, which the judge called "absolutely inadequate." The case marks the first time that a managed care health provider has been convicted of reckless homicide.

Chem-Bio's lawyer, Martin Kohler, believes it was wrong to prosecute the lab. "To commit a crime, you have to have criminal intent," he says. Kohler says Robert Lipo was devastated by the deaths of the two women. "He did not set out to do wrong," Kohler says. "He did not stab anyone. He did not give anyone cancer. The malpractice settlement should have been enough."

But others observing from afar believe this is a classic case of criminal medicine, in which concerns about costs clouded the judgment of people responsible for life-saving tests. A malpractice suit is brought for simple breach of medical standards, says George Annas, a medical ethicist at Boston University. "The question in a criminal case of this kind," he says, "is whether the doctor is putting the bottom line — cost — ahead of patient treatment."

Managed care does not *have* to put cost ahead of care, Annas and Franklin Elevitch agree. Many HMOS don't. But some do, Annas says, and he hopes this case will make those HMOs more cautious. Equally important, he expects doctors, lab technicians — health workers of all types — to cite this case when they feel a health plan is ordering them to take on too many cases for patient safety.

Many health care professionals working with HMOs feel damned if they do and damned if they don't. If they follow the HMO's guidelines — see more patients, spend less time with them, order fewer tests — they expose themselves to malpractice suits. If they ignore the guidelines, they may lose the HMO contracts on which their livelihood depends. This case, Annas predicts, could help health care professionals take a stand. They could refuse to lower their standards of care on the grounds that they, and the health plan, could be charged with homicide. "Criminal prosecution is a pretty blunt regulatory tool," Annas says. "But managed care can be a blunt way of doing medicine."

The home Peter and Karin Smith last shared is on a small lake west of Milwaukee. Beautifully decorated

Pap Smear Warning

An estimated 10 to 20 percent of Pap smears taken from women with cancerous or precancerous cells are wrongly reported as normal. Pap smears are most accurate when analyzed slowly and repeatedly — special care that some pathologists say is at odds with managed care's demands for low costs and efficient work. Are you protected? Here are answers that could save your life.

COULD WHAT HAPPENED TO KARIN SMITH HAPPEN TO YOU?

Not legally. Since 1992 federal law has prohibited cytotechnologists from reading more than 100 Pap smears a day. Labs must also review the statistical records of their employees and rescreen the work of any who report a high number of normal results. Slides that contain too few cells for an accurate diagnosis must be turned back to doctors. Still, an inexperienced or poorly trained cytotechnologist probably couldn't analyze 100 slides a day. Indeed, California limits cytotechnologists to 80 slides a day. And, despite federal regulations calling for annual proficiency exams, there's still no regular testing of cytotechnologists' skills.

SO WHAT CAN YOU DO TO IMPROVE YOUR ODDS?

Get a Pap smear every year if you smoke, have had genital warts, or have been sexually active from an early age — all risk factors for cervical cancer. This cancer is caused by the human papilloma virus, transmitted sexually, and grows very slowly. Some health plans now pay for Pap smears only every two or three years. But with the test's high error rate, consider paying for it yourself if you have any extra risk.

Ask your doctor if the lab uses a computer to rescreen smears that showed no abnormal cells. Last fall the Food and Drug Administration approved two computer systems that recognize tiny deviations in cell patterns. If the lab does not, and you have symptoms such as postcoital or unpredictable bleeding, ask your doctor to send your latest slide to a rescreening company. The standard fee is about $20.

Schedule your Pap smear for 12 to 14 days after you begin menstruation, when results are most accurate. Do not use douches or vaginal medications for three days before the test. These can rinse away or hide abnormal cells. — J.D.

with bright modern paintings, a large fireplace, and a cozy sunroom, it is a house they bought with money from their civil lawsuit — a home purchased with pain. Today Peter Smith seems light-years away from the devil-may-care college student who once courted a vibrant but no-nonsense accounting major. In her last months Karin worried ceaselessly about leaving him alone.

"We decided we were going to enjoy our time together and try not to be bitter about what had happened," he says softly. "I'll never meet anyone else like her."

Does he think Karin would be at peace with the conviction?

He pauses. "Yeah, I think she would. We didn't hit a home run, but we hit a solid double. Articles about this case are on the bulletin board in every cytotech lab in the country. I truly believe something like this will not happen again."

Jan DeBlieu is a writer in Manteo, North Carolina. This is the second article in a series on managed care.

HARVARD WOMEN'S HEALTH WATCH

Fibroids

Uterine fibroids, known to scientists as *leiomyomas, myomas,* or *fibromas,* are more common than blue eyes. They affect at least one-fourth of women in their 30s and 40s and half of African-American women in that age group. The solid tumors are usually benign and often produce no symptoms. Yet they are still the leading cause of hysterectomy in the United States.

HOW FIBROIDS FORM

Fibroids are rubbery nodules that may be pink, gray, or pale yellow. Surgeons who have removed the tumors have described them as "potatolike" in form and diversity.

Fibroids begin as irregular cells in the muscular layers of the uterus. They grow slowly and erratically into bundles of smooth muscle bound by fibrous tissue. Most are somewhere between the size of a walnut and the size of an orange; the largest reported weighed 140 pounds. Gynecologists often discuss fibroid disease by comparing the size of a fibroid distended uterus to that of a woman at a certain point in a pregnancy. For example, a "12-weeker" is about the size of a uterus holding a 3-month fetus.

The causes of fibroid growth and development still elude scientists. One theory, which suggests that the tumors are the result of an abnormal response to estrogen, is based on several observations: they do not occur before puberty; they grow larger with oral contraceptive use and during pregnancy; and they shrink after menopause but increase with hormone-replacement therapy (HRT). In other words, they wax and wane in tandem with estrogen levels. There is also evidence that progesterone stimulates fibroid growth as well.

However, because women with fibroids do not have higher circulating levels of estrogen, scientists believe that genetic factors may also play a role. Some researchers cite a lower incidence among African women than among African-American women as evidence that environment may be important. There is also speculation that the rapid growth of fibroids during pregnancy is due to the increased blood supply to the uterus.

TYPES OF FIBROIDS

Fibroids are categorized according to their location. *Submucous* fibroids grow just beneath the endometrium, or lining of the uterus. *Intramural* fibroids expand within the wall of the uterus, and *subserous* fibroids grow out from the outer wall of the uterus. Very rarely, fibroids are found in other parts of the body.

Some fibroids develop a thin stalk called a *pedicle.* The stalk remains attached to the uterine wall, allowing the tumor to swing inside the uterus or into the abdominal cavity. As the uterus contracts in an effort to rid itself of this "foreign body," the pedicle may become twisted, causing bleeding, pain, and sometimes infection. Occasionally, a pedunculated fibroid may protrude through the cervix into the vagina.

SYMPTOMS

The most commonly reported symptom of fibroids is excessive bleeding, often severe enough to cause anemia. It is usually caused by submucous tumors, which do not bleed themselves, but rather stimulate excessive endometrial bleeding, usually during and sometimes between menstrual periods.

Rapidly growing fibroids are cause for concern because they may indicate a malignancy — especially in postmenopausal women, whose fibroids usually shrink. In other cases, the sheer bulk of the fibroid is enough to cause problems. When fibroids grow large enough to push against a ureter, they may affect kidney function; those encroaching on the bladder or bowel can cause urinary frequency or constipation. They can also be the source of abdominal bloating.

The location of a fibroid often has more to do with the trouble it generates than its size does. Small tumors that block the fallopian tubes or distort the cervix may cause infertility; they can also be responsible for miscarriage or preterm delivery. Fibroids pressing on a pelvic nerve may be a source of chronic hip or back pain.

DIAGNOSIS

Clinicians often detect fibroids during a routine pelvic exam; the uterus feels enlarged and irregular. If your clinician has detected fibroids, he or she may recommend an additional examination with ultrasound to determine their number and location. In ultrasound images, fibroids usually appear as discrete, irregular masses attached to the uterus, though, occasionally, it is difficult to distinguish them from ovarian masses. If a subsequent MRI is taken and is also uninformative, a diagnostic laparoscopy, in which a miniaturized video camera is inserted into the abdomen through a tiny incision, may be necessary to determine the nature of the tumors.

TREATMENT

Most fibroids require no treatment at all. If the tumors are small, your clinician may simply follow them through pelvic exam and ultrasound. Fibroids are almost always benign tumors; women with fibroids rarely develop a sarcomatous (cancerous) change, typified by a rapidly growing mass. Nonetheless, an increase in the growth rate of fibroids is always cause for concern, especially in postmenopausal women.

The pain associated with fibroids can usually be relieved with over-the-counter analgesics such as aspirin, ibuprofen (Motrin, Advil), naprosyn (Aleve), or acetaminophen (Tylenol); most cases of anemia from excessive bleeding are corrected by iron supplements. Even fibroids that degenerate during pregnancy and can be very painful are usually relieved by medication within a day. However, when fibroids are responsible for persistent anemia, constipation, or bladder problems — or when they appear to be the cause of infertility or a threat to future pregnancies — more aggressive therapy is usually recommended. Women may also elect to undergo further treatment because they find the pain, pressure, or bleeding intolerable. If you are considering treatments for fibroids you may want to discuss the following options with your clinician:

- *Myomectomy* is a surgical procedure in which fibroids are removed from the uterus. It is usually performed through an abdominal incision; however, some submucous fibroids can be removed through the vagina in hysteriscopic procedures. Both require general anesthesia. The fibroids are removed one at a time, and surgery may take several hours. To minimize scarring and thus better preserve uterine function, the surgeon will try to limit the number of incisions. Thus, women who have only a few fibroids are the best candidates for myomectomy. Unfortunately fibroids often grow again; about 25% of women who have had this surgery require additional myomectomies and may ultimately need a hysterectomy.

- *Hysterectomy* is a simpler procedure than myomectomy. When the uterus is removed, the fibroids go with it. The ovaries are usually left in, so a woman is not automatically plunged into menopause. There has been much criticism of the high rate of hysterectomy in the United States; fibroids are the reason for an estimated 30% of hysterectomies performed. However, many women who have completed their families choose hysterectomy because it eliminates the problem entirely.

In the past, any fibroid larger than a "12-weeker" was considered reason for hysterectomy, but recent opinion is that size alone, even when the fibroid is very large, may not absolutely necessitate that surgery.

- *Medical treatments.* Drugs to manipulate hormones, including oral contraceptives and progestins, have been used. The most successful are drugs termed gonadotropin-releasing hormone (GnRH) agonists, which eliminate the mid-cycle surge of hormones responsible for menstruation. They are effective in shrinking fibroids and reducing symptoms, and, because they bring periods to a halt, they can raise blood counts for women who are anemic. GnRH agonists can also produce menopausal symptoms like hot flashes, vaginal dryness, and reduced bone density.

The two principal GnRH analogues are Depo-Lupron (leuprolide acetate), a long-acting preparation that is usually given by monthly injection, and Synarel (nafarelin), a nasal spray. Because Synarel's effects wear off quickly, some physicians begin with Synarel to determine how well the side effects are tolerated, then switch to the longer-acting Depo-Lupron.

Unfortunately, the GnRH agonists — which promote bone loss by suppressing estrogen — can't be used indefinitely, and fibroids begin to grow again 4–6 months after treatment is discontinued. To counteract bone loss and other menopausal effects of the

GnRH agonists, some physicians prescribe doses of estrogen and progestins similar to those used in hormone-replacement therapy. This "add-back" approach seems to eliminate most of the side effects of the GnRH agonists without stimulating the growth of the fibroids. However, scientists are still studying these regimens to find the best combinations and doses of drugs and hormones, as well as to determine their long-term side effects.

These drug therapies are sometimes used to shrink fibroids before myomectomy, thus reducing incision size and blood loss. If you're in your 40s, they may enable you to avoid surgery and buy time until menopause, when your fibroids should shrink.

Obviously there is no single prescription for managing fibroids. If you have fibroid disease, you and your clinician will want to consider the size and location of the tumors, the pros and cons of the options for therapy, and your lifestyle in deciding on a course of treatment.

Incontinence: Breaking the Silence

Many women mistakenly assume that incontinence affects
only older women — and that nothing can be done. In fact,
it affects women of all ages, and there's no reason to suffer silently.

It's rare today to find women unwilling to speak
their minds or ask for what they need on just
about any health issue. But that's exactly the situation huge numbers of women find themselves in
when faced with bladder control problems.

It's true that many doctors don't ask about incontinence, although they should. And instead of broach-
ing the subject themselves, millions of women suffer
silently, enduring embarrassment and self-imposed
isolation. According to one survey, women wait an
average of seven years before seeking help.

One factor that contributes to the silence is the
misguided notion that surgery is the only solution. In
the not-so-distant past, some of the few women who
mentioned bladder control problems to their gynecologists may have been offered a decidedly unsavory
option: We can do a bladder suspension and a hysterectomy at the same time." And older women may
have friends who underwent major surgery for incontinence years ago but found little relief.

No wonder so many women have convinced
themselves that a little leaky urine isn't so bad after
all. But in truth, surgery is a last resort for most
women with mild bladder control problems.

START WITH SELF-HELP

The cheery advertising for adult diapers makes
them sound like the ideal solution to incontinence.

In fact, there are other, less-expensive — and more
effective — options to consider:

- **Kegels.** Kegel exercises, which strengthen the
pelvic-floor muscles, are a mainstay of treatment for
stress incontinence, and they may help with urge
incontinence as well. (For a description of the various
kinds of incontinence, see "Which Incontinence?")
Kegels are easy to learn — though many women do
them incorrectly — and easy to perform (see "Love
Those Kegels").

- **Dietary modifications.** Irritating substances can
contribute to urge incontinence. Try reducing or

Which Incontinence?

There are four primary types of incontinence:

- **Stress.** You lose urine when you exercise, laugh,
cough, sneeze, run, stand up, or get out of bed.
Women with stress incontinence typically use the
bathroom many times during the day.

- **Urge.** You lose urine as soon as you feel the need
to go to the bathroom, drink even a small amount of
liquid or hear water running. People with urge incontinence may get up several times during the night or
wet the bed.

- **Mixed.** It's not uncommon for some women to have
symptoms of both stress and urge incontinence.

- **Overflow.** You feel as if you can never fully empty
your bladder. You may dribble small amounts of urine
all day long and go to the bathroom several times
during the night. You may produce only a tiny amount
when you try to urinate.

If you're unsure about which type of incontinence
you have, keep a seven-day diary of your symptoms. That
can help you — and your physician — zero in on the
problem.

From *Women's Health Advocate* (March 1996), pp. 4-6. Reprinted with permission from *Women's Health Advocate Newsletter*. For subscriptions call 1-800-829-5876 and ask for the introductory price of $16 per year, a 33% discount.

eliminating acidic beverages (such as orange juice), alcohol, caffeine, chocolate, diet drinks and other products sweetened with aspartame, nicotine, spicy foods, and tomatoes.

In addition, drinking plenty of water — at intervals throughout the day — may help by diluting your urine and keeping it less irritating. (Don't try this if you have overflow incontinence.)

● **Tampons.** For mild stress incontinence, try a tampon. (If vaginal dryness is a problem, moisten the tampon with a little water before inserting it.)

Tampons help support the pelvic organs, pushing against the urethra and helping to keep it closed. "Tampons are very good for mild incontinence," says Kristene Whitmore, M.D., clinical associate professor of urology at the University of Pennsylvania. "Certainly, if you put a tampon in before you go for a jog and it does the trick, then it's an inexpensive and easy-to-use option."

● **Bladder training.** If you have mild urge or stress incontinence, bladder retraining or timed voiding can help.

In timed voiding you go to the bathroom on a set schedule — at one-hour intervals, for example — whether you feel the urge or not.

In bladder retraining, the goal is to learn to resist the urge to urinate. Learning to "hold it" for longer and longer periods of time actually improves your bladder capacity by expanding and strengthening bladder muscles.

Begin by trying to resist the urge to urinate for one hour. (Relaxation techniques such as deep breathing can help you resist the urge to run to the bathroom.) As you gain confidence in your ability to wait and as your bladder capacity improves, expand the time intervals. Your goal is to be able to wait three to four hours.

Try as many self-help measures as you can, as they can have a cumulative effect. And don't sell yourself short by giving up too soon: It often takes weeks, sometimes months, to see significant improvement.

THE NEXT STEP

If self-help measures don't work or your problem is a severe one, you may need to consult a physician and consider the following medical interventions:

● **Muscle-strengthening devices.** One way to strengthen the pelvic floor muscles is to "work out" with a series of graduated weights. In what amounts to a "super" Kegel, the user places a weighted cone in the vagina and attempts to retain it through muscle contraction for a set amount of time — usually 15 minutes. Over the course of several weeks, increasingly heavier cones are used. (The cones are used primarily for stress incontinence.)

Alternatively, an electronic device can be used. The device delivers a minute shock directly to the pelvic floor muscles, which causes the muscles to contract and builds muscle strength.

● **Support devices.** Pessaries — rubber or soft plastic ring-like devices — can be inserted into the vagina. They support the bladder and uterus, but they don't support the bladder neck, which makes them less effective than other measures for stress incontinence.

A newly approved device called Introl addresses that problem. Introl has two prongs that support the bladder neck (*WHA*, July 1995). The device can't be worn during sex, but otherwise can remain in for a day or so and then taken out for cleaning.

● **Collagen.** Collagen, Teflon, and even body fat have been used to build up the area around the urinary sphincter and help keep the bladder opening closed. Of all these materials, collagen is the most useful.

However, only a small percentage of women are candidates for collagen therapy — those with severe

Love Those Kegels

Most women, incontinent or not, can benefit from doing Kegel exercises. For one thing, the exercises may help prevent bladder control problems from ever developing. For another, many women find that their sex life is enhanced by doing Kegels.

Performed correctly, Kegels strengthen the pelvic-floor muscles that support the uterus and bladder. If done improperly, however, they may make the problem worse.

The trick is to identify the correct set of muscles and then to make sure that you are contracting only those muscles — and not those in the abdomen, buttocks, or thighs.

You can identify the correct muscles by stopping your urine flow in mid-stream as you sit on the toilet — or by inserting a finger into your vagina and squeezing around it. (At the same time, place your hand on your abdomen to ensure that you aren't inadvertently contracting those muscles.) If you aren't sure whether you're doing Kegels correctly, biofeedback monitoring can answer this question for you. In addition, it can quantify the strength of the contractions.

Once you've isolated the correct muscles you can begin a daily program of Kegels. Contract the muscles and hold the contraction for as long as possible working up to 10 seconds. Then relax your muscles for 10 seconds. In the beginning, do a set of 10 Kegels three times a day. Your goal should be to work up to 60 to 80 repetitions each day. You should begin to see results in about six weeks.

When done correctly and consistently, Kegels have a reported success rate of up to 87%. And not only are they free and safe, they're completely private — you can literally do them anytime, anywhere.

---

stress incontinence from intrinsic sphincter deficiency (*WHA*, April 1995).

If you fall into this category, you can receive collagen injections on an outpatient basis without anesthesia. "The upside of collagen is that the patient can go right back to her normal activities, and there is minimal invasiveness," says Dr. Whitmore. "The downside is that collagen costs about $300 per syringe. Two to four syringes are needed per treatment and patients usually need more than one treatment — usually two."

● **Plugs.** Silicone devices that temporarily plug or seal the urethra are currently being studied but they aren't on the market yet. The devices prevent urine leakage for several hours at a time and are reportedly comfortable and fairly easy to use, although you need good manual dexterity to put the tiny devices in and take them out.

With all of these options, there's no need for any woman to suffer in silence or to undergo unnecessary surgery. Help is available — and with persistence, most bladder control problems can be overcome.

RESOURCES:

Overcoming Bladder Disorders by Rebecca Chalker and Kristene Whitmore, M.D. (New York: Harper & Row, 1990).

Help for Incontinent People. Call (800) BLADDER or write Box 8310 Spartanburg, S.C. 29305.

The Simon Foundation for Continence. Call (800) 23-SIMON or write Box 835, Wilmette, Ill. 60091.

Urinary Tract Infections

By Paula Dranov

NEW TACTICS MAKE RECURRENT INFECTIONS EASIER TO TREAT THAN EVER BEFORE

My first urinary tract infection (UTI) came as a shock. Why was I racing back and forth to the bathroom just about every other minute? Why was the urge to urinate so insistent and yet so unproductive? I didn't know what had hit me. I just knew I wanted relief. Immediately!

Sooner or later, one in five women develops a bladder infection. (Men are far less susceptible, until they reach the age of prostate problems.) A few days on antibiotics will usually knock out the infection, but some UTI's can be maddeningly persistent. And now urologists suspect that frequent recurrences are not caused by infections at all. Instead they might be a form of interstitial cystitis, a mysterious inflammation that may be much more common than doctors once believed (see "A Puzzling Condition").

Both disorders make you feel as though your bladder is about to burst; other common symptoms include urinary frequency with or without burning and an ache in the general area of the pubic bone. You may not get all the symptoms. I never had burning or pain, but take my word for it, the urge alone is bad enough. I was reduced to tears of frustration more than once.

When you're in the throes of UTI misery, it's small comfort to remember that most of these infections are easy to diagnose, simple to treat and worrisome only if neglected. Untreated infections can wend their way from the bladder up the urinary tract through the tubelike ureters to the kidneys. Once there, the symptoms generally escalate to fever, chills, pain in the small of the back, headaches and nausea or vomiting.

A kidney infection (pyelonephritis) is curable with antibiotics, but a severe one can cause permanent damage and, in rare cases, kidney failure, which can be life threatening. For this reason, the symptoms should never be ignored. The sooner treatment begins, the better.

Today, uncomplicated UTI's are easier to diagnose and treat than in the past. Increasingly, doctors are likely to entrust the management of stubborn cases to patients themselves, a strategy that seems to work well. Patients are much better at diagnosing recurrences than doctors are because they know their own bodies, says Dr. Kristine Whitmore, a urologist at the University of Pennsylvania and the author of *Overcoming Bladder Disorders*. Other new tactics emphasize prevention. At present, this means, getting the jump on recurrent infections with antibiotic treatment before symptoms appear. But if a vaccine now being tested pans out, the age-old battle against recurrent UTI's may soon be won.

Blame the female anatomy for the fact that women are much more prone to UTI's than men. The problem is the proximity of the urinary tract to the vagina and rectum. In 80% of all cases, the bacterium that causes UTI's is *Escherichia coli*, an organism that lives in the bowel and is present in stool. "Bacterial spread may be unavoidable, no matter how excellent your hygiene," says Whitmore. The bacteria can easily migrate from the rectal area to the entrance of the vagina and into the urethra, the tube through which urine flows from the bladder out of the body.

The other 15% to 20% of UTI's are harder to account for, since they're caused by *Staphylococcus*

From *American Health* (May 1995), pp. 66-69. Reprinted by permission of *American Health*. © 1995 by Paula Dranov.

A Puzzling Condition

An estimated 500,000 women — and perhaps many more — are affected by a mystifying bladder ailment called interstitial cystitis. Though many of its symptoms, including urinary frequency, urgency and burning, resemble those of a urinary tract infection (UTI), IC is a bladder irritation or an inflammation of unknown cause. "I think IC is often underdiagnosed," says Dr. C. Lowell Parsons, a urologist at the University of California at San Diego. "The women I thought had recurrent infections turned out to have IC."

Only a decade ago, urologists tended to dismiss IC symptoms in younger women, blaming stress rather than examining the bladder for the telltale signs of the disorder. That was before Dr. Vicki Ratner, an orthopedic surgeon in San Jose, Calif., developed excruciating pelvic pain that none of the 14 physicians she consulted could explain. After she finally learned she had IC, Ratner founded the Interstitial Cystitis Association, an activist organization that has been singularly successful at raising consciousness and spurring research into the long-neglected disorder. As a result, most urologists now recognize that IC can affect younger as well as older women. Although there's no cure, there is a widening range of treatments that can control all but the most severe cases.

The cause of IC remains a mystery, but a few clues have emerged. One points to leaks in the bladder's inner lining that may allow irritating substances such as the salt in urine to seep through and injure the underlying wall. Another suggests bacteria may play a role after all. Researchers at Tulane University in New Orleans have found fragments of bacterial DNA in the bladder tissue of IC patients. Even if bacteria are not a direct cause of IC, their presence may trigger an inflammatory response that could contribute to the problem, says research director Dr. Gerald Domingue. Another theory holds that IC might be an autoimmune disorder, in which antibodies attack the body they're supposed to protect.

Diagnosing IC isn't easy. "If a woman has frequent UTI recurrences — say, six or more a year — that typically occur after sex or in the week before her period and she has a negative urine culture, she probably has mild IC, not a recurrent UTI," says Parsons. Sometimes the urologist may prefer to view the fully distended bladder (under anesthesia) and examine its inner surface via a cystoscope inserted through the urethra. Doctors look for tiny hemorrhages dotting the bladder lining. In severe cases, they discover bleeding ulcers that scar and shrink the bladder. "IC usually gets as bad as it's going to get early on," says Dr. Philip Hanno, chairman of urology at Temple University in Philadelphia. He reassures patients that the disorder often goes into remission, sometimes for years, that it won't cause cancer and that surgery is required in less than 5% of cases.

Since about half of all IC cases go into remission for no reason, says Hanno, treatment depends on how uncomfortable the patient feels. Those who can tolerate the symptoms need no treatment at all, since the disease usually doesn't worsen. Then too, the bladder distension procedure done to diagnose the disorder may bring temporary relief. If not, doctors may prescribe the antidepressant amitriptyline (Elavil) to reduce pain and bladder spasms. The only drug approved by the FDA specifically to treat IC is DMSO (dimethyl sulfoxide), which must be instilled into the bladder.

Other drugs for IC are in development. One medication, sodium pentosanpolysulfate (Elmiron), which may help repair the bladder lining, is awaiting FDA approval for IC.

Finally, avoiding alcohol, carbonated drinks, caffeinated beverages and irritating acidic foods such as tomatoes and citrus fruits and juices can help.

saprophyticus, a bacterium that does not live in the body. Doctors know neither how nor why this bug shows up in the urinary tract, though for some unknown reason these infections tend to be more common in spring and summer.

Most of the time, bacteria in the urethra are washed out with urine before they can cause trouble. But if the bladder's defenses are less than optimal, a bacterial invasion can prove hard to flush away. As the bacteria multiply, the chance of infection increases.

Urinary tract abnormalities, which are rare, can increase one's susceptibility to UTI's (as can diabetes), but doctors estimate that 90% of recurrences are due to genetic factors that compromise the bladder's ability to rid itself of harmful bacteria. For example, the urine of infection-prone women tends to be less acidic than normal and thus more hospitable to bacteria. Then too, genetic defects in the membrane structure of the cells lining the urinary tract may permit bacteria to adhere more easily.

Sex and diaphragm use also increase the risk of infection. During intercourse, bacteria lurking in the genital area are easily introduced into the urethra. Using a diaphragm doubles the likelihood of repeated infections, although how it does so is less clear. It's possible that pressure from a diaphragm's spring rim may bruise the tissues surrounding the urethra, causing inflammation and somehow obstructing urinary flow.

Risk also increases with age. When estrogen levels fall after menopause, bacteria called lactobacilli, which maintain the vaginal acidity that holds *E. coli* in check, begin to disappear. This change, says Dr. Jill Maura Rabin, head of urogynecology at Long Island Jewish Medical Center in New Hyde Park, N.Y., correlates with a rise in UTI's. Estrogen replacement therapy restores lactobacilli and cuts down on infections.

Luckily. diagnosing UTI's isn't difficult. I found out what was wrong with me by phoning my brother, a doctor, to ask whether the unrelenting urge I was experiencing was treatable or terminal. As in my case, the symptoms alone usually tell the tale, although before beginning treatment doctors usually do a simple urine dip-stick test to confirm an infection. (Most doctors do not order a urine culture for a first UTI unless the dipstick test is negative.) Recurrences are another matter. A urine culture is considered positive when the lab counts 100,000 bacteria per milliliter of urine, but at least half of all women with persistent symptoms have much lower counts.

In theory, the infections are easy to treat: Most cases can be cured by taking an antibiotic for three days. Unfortunately, antibiotics can bring on unpleasant side effects, including headaches, nausea, diarrhea, dizziness and fatigue. Although these symptoms vanish as soon as the drugs are stopped, another common side effect, vaginal yeast infections, can be more persistent and almost as bothersome as the cystitis symptoms themselves. Yeast infections develop when antibiotics wipe out the protective vaginal bacteria that limit the population of *Candida albicans*, the fungus responsible for the infections (see "The Other Infections,").

For doctors, the trick to treating UTI's is to prescribe an antibiotic that works, is least likely to cause side effects and is inexpensive. In a recent comparison of the four drugs most commonly used, researchers at the University of Washington School of Medicine found that a combination of trimethoprim and sulfamethoxazole (found in Bactrim. Septra and Cotrim, for example) was the most effective and least expensive. Six weeks after completing treatment, 82% of the women who took the drug were infection free, compared with 61% of those treated with nitrofurantoin, 66% of those who took cefadroxil and 67% of the women on amoxicillin.

Antibiotics work so fast that symptoms can disappear within hours of swallowing the first pill, but you can get some relief even before you fill your prescription: An over-the-counter drug called Azo-Standard eases the sting and maddening sense of urgency. Two prescription drugs, Pyridium and Urised, provide more potent relief for people prone to recurrent bouts of infection. None of these drugs fights the actual infection, however, so you still need to take antibiotics as your doctor directs.

Most women (80%) develop only one or two recurrences, usually within a year of the first bout. But an unlucky 20% get far more than their share. In such cases, infections tend to recur for six months to a year and then disappear for a year or two.

Sometimes you can head off a recurrence simply by drinking lots of water — about two to three quarts

I found out what was wrong by calling my doctor-brother to ask whether the urge was terminal or treatable.

a day. With luck, the water will flush the troublesome bacteria out of the body. As for the old wives' tale about drinking cranberry juice, it does help. An Israeli study reported in *The New England Journal of Medicine* showed that both cranberries and blueberries (but no other fruit) contain compounds that prevent *E. coli* from sticking to the lining of the bladder. And a Harvard University study showed that drinking 10 ounces (oz.) of cranberry juice a day reduced bacteria counts in a group of older, symptom-free women. "The only harm in drinking cranberry juice," cautions internist Jerry Avorn, who heads the Harvard team, "would be in thinking it's a substitute for taking an antibiotic when you do have an infection." A two-year follow-up study at Harvard will determine whether drinking 20 oz. of cranberry juice a day can reduce the rate of recurrences in a group of young women who have acute infections.

In the meantime, there are other things women can do to head off recurrent infections. Some women take a prescription antibiotic immediately before or after sex. Others test their own urine with a dipstick, available at most drugstores without a prescription, as soon as they sense a UTI brewing — a single distinctive chill while urinating may be a tip-off — and begin taking antibiotics if the test confirms an infection. A small study in the *Annals of Internal Medicine* found that women correctly diagnosed UTI's 90% of the time and successfully treated 85% of their infections.

When recurrences are very frequent, a doctor may recommend taking a low dose antibiotic daily for six

Preventing Urinary Tract Infections

There's no surefire way to prevent urinary tract infections (UTI's), but urologists advise the following:

- Drink lots of fluids, preferably water, to help flush bacteria out of the bladder.
- Drink cranberry juice, especially if you feel a UTI coming on.
- Urinate as soon as you feel the urge; empty your bladder completely.
- Urinate after having sex.
- Wipe from front to back after a bowel movement.
- If possible, substitute another form of contraception for a diaphragm.

Take showers, not baths, to keep bacteria from migrating to the bladder.

The Other Infections

Although bladder-related symptoms are usually the sign of an ordinary urinary tract infection, other organisms are sometimes to blame. Some types of vaginitis, including yeast infections and even chlamydia, a sexually transmitted disease, can cause burning upon urinating and may be mistaken for a UTI.

Such infections are common. About one-third of all women eventually develop a yeast infection or other form of vaginitis. In most cases, characteristic discharges are the main symptoms, but burning, if present, can confuse matters. Ironically, yeast infections can be the by-product of antibiotic treatment for a UTI. *Candida albicans*, the fungus that causes yeast infections, is naturally present in the vagina and is held in check by other microorganisms. But antibiotics can upset the vagina's normal bacterial balance, allowing candida to flourish. Symptoms include redness, itching and burning in the vagina and the surrounding vulva; the discharge is usually white and odorless. The infections almost always clear up when treated with over-the-counter vaginal creams and gels, such as Gyne-lotrimin and Monistat 7.

A vaginal infection called trichomoniasis can cause burning during urination. Other symptoms may include a yellow-gray vaginal discharge with an unpleasant odor and sometimes redness and swelling of the vulva. Trichomoniasis is treated with prescription metronidazole (Flagyl). Since the infection can be sexually transmitted, both partners should be treated.

Although chlamydia usually doesn't cause symptoms in women, burning during urination may occur. Unfortunately the organisms responsible won't show up in a urine culture or respond to the antibiotics that banish UTI's. Since an unchecked infection can lead to pelvic inflammatory disease and even infertility, it's vital to test for chlamydia if a urine culture is negative. Infections are treated with antibiotics such as azithromycin or doxycycline, and partners should be checked.

---

months, or even indefinitely with periodic breaks, to see whether the infection returns. At low doses, the drugs are generally well tolerated, and even if resistance develops, doctors can usually switch to a different antibiotic.

On the horizon is a vaccine called SolcoUrovac that would provide simple and effective protection against UTI's. Researchers at the University of Wisconsin in Madison have completed safety studies and launched a two-year trial to determine whether the vaccine is effective. If it works, chief researcher Dr. David Uehling estimates the vaccine could become available in two to three years.

In my case, I don't think I'll need the vaccine, although it would be nice to know it's available — just in case. After my first UTI flare-up, I had a succession of recurrences for about four months. I drank enough water to float a battleship. I gratefully took Pyridium and antibiotics as my doctor directed. I was beginning to think I was doomed to a lifetime of this crazy routine when, for no apparent reason, the infections ceased, and they haven't come back. Knock on wood!

Paula Dranov is a New York City-based writer who reports frequently on women's health issues.

Medical | Report | **BY DEBORAH SHIPPEY**

Ovarian cysts: What's normal, what's not

Any woman who ovulates can develop an ovarian cyst. Here, when to wait, when to act

It was in the heat of passion that I first noticed the pain. It began as a dull ache on the right side of my abdomen and persisted the next three times I had intercourse. Worried, I called my gynecologist. "Sounds like an ovarian cyst," she said. "See me tomorrow."

The next day my doctor performed a bimanual exam, inserting two fingers into my vagina and pressing on my abdomen with her other hand. Her suspicion had been correct: A tiny sac was growing on my right ovary. Probably nothing to be concerned about, she reassured me; most cysts are a normal consequence of ovulation and nearly always go away on their own. Sure enough, when I returned for a check-up immediately after my next period, the cyst was gone.

Nearly every woman will have an ovarian cyst at some time in her life. And like me, most women will find that this condition clears up without medical intervention. But some cysts are more worrisome. A small percentage of women develop non-functional ovarian cysts, larger growths that can cause severe pain and are associated with infertility and, in rare cases, cancer. Here is what you need to know about the various kinds of cysts and how they're treated.

Why do ovarian cysts form?

Functional cysts can form before or after ovulation. A follicular cyst forms when the follicle that houses the ovum continues to grow instead of rupturing and releasing the egg. This may occur as a result of abnormal hormonal signals caused by stress or illness, or simply because the surface of the ovary tends to become thickened and scarred after years of ovulation. Corpus luteum cysts form after the egg has passed through the follicle, usually when there is bleeding at the site of rupture. Like follicular cysts, corpus luteum

cysts, which are fluid or blood filled, usually disappear on their own.

The origin of non-functional cysts is less clear. Some may result from hormone imbalances, others as a side effect of endometriosis, a condition in which endometrial tissue is found outside the uterus, usually on the ovaries, bowel, bladder and fallopian tubes.

Who's at risk for developing cysts?

Any woman who ovulates. Also, women taking fertility drugs are especially likely to develop several

---

Functional Cysts

TYPE: Follicular (Fluid filled)

SYMPTOMS: Often none, but sometimes lower abdominal pain

OCCURS IN: Nearly all ovulating women at some point in their lives

HEALTH RISK: Always benign

SIZE: Rarely grows larger than five centimeters in diameter

TREATMENT: Usually none because these cysts rupture or shrink after one or two menstrual cycles. Oral contraceptives may be prescribed to shrink a large cyst or prevent future ones. Surgery for large cysts (five centimeters or bigger)

TYPE: Corpus luteum (blood or fluid filled)

SYMPTOMS: May cause pain on one side of the abdomen and menstrual changes

OCCURS IN: Same as follicular cysts

HEALTH RISK: Always benign

SIZE: Can grow from the size of an egg to the size of a softball

TREATMENT: Same as follicular cysts

From *Glamour* (May 1996), pp. 74-75. Reprinted with permission from Deborah Pike, Body/Mind editor, *Self* magazine.

(not necessarily painful) functional cysts at one time because their ovaries are being stimulated to produce more eggs than usual.

About 20 percent of women have a condition that causes many tiny, harmless cysts to form on the ovaries. About half of women with polycystic ovaries, as these are called, have polycystic ovary syndrome (PCOS). Women with PCOS have higher-than-normal levels of the male hormone testosterone, which interferes with ovulation and increases their risk of developing heart disease and diabetes later in life.

Nonfunctional Cysts

TYPE: Endometrioma (blood filled)

SYMPTOMS: Sometimes none, though severe menstrual cramps, pain during intercourse or pain during bowel movements can occur

OCCURS IN: Half of women with endometriosis (roughly 7 to 8 percent of all women)

HEALTH RISK: Nearly always benign but can cause infertility

SIZE: Can grow as large as a grapefruit

TREATMENT: Surgical removal

TYPE: Polycystic ovary syndrome (fluid filled)

SYMPTOMS: Irregular periods, excess body hair, acne, loss of hair from top of scalp, obesity

OCCURS IN: 10 percent of women (onset during teens and early twenties)

HEALTH RISK: Benign, but increased risk of infertility, diabetes and heart disease

SIZE: Tiny (generally two to four millimeters in diameter)

TREATMENT: Oral contraceptives or progesterone alone to restore ovulation; fertility drugs to interfere with the body's production of testosterone

---

TYPE: Dermoid (filled with skin, hair, bone and fluid because they derive from the ovary's germ cells, which give rise to these body parts early in fetal development)

SYMPTOMS: Usually none, although can grow large enough to press on internal organs

OCCURS IN: One percent of women

HEALTH RISK: One percent chance of malignancy

SIZE: About that of a golf ball

TREATMENT: Surgical removal

TYPE: Cystadenoma (either serous, filled with a watery fluid; or mucinous, filled with a thick gelatinous material)

SYMPTOMS: Usually none. Large cysts (bigger than five centimeters) may press on internal organs and cause constipation and pain

OCCURS IN: Less than 5 percent of women

HEALTH RISK: 5 to 10 percent are malignant

SIZE: Can range from one pound to even larger — orange to grapefruit size — with isolated cases of excessive growth

TREATMENT: Surgical removal

What are the symptoms of a cyst?

Eighty to 90 percent of cysts produce no symptoms at all. When they do, a woman may feel a dull ache on one side of her abdomen, particularly during intercourse. Large cysts can press on internal organs, resulting in pain, constipation and bloating. The hormonal imbalance that causes PCOS may make menstrual cycles irregular, and corpus luteum cysts can cause bleeding during the last half of the cycle or longer-than-normal periods.

Occasionally a large cyst can rupture, producing intense abdominal pain along with weakness, nausea and vomiting. The pain usually subsides within 24 hours, and the fluid from the cyst is absorbed back into the body. The exception is a ruptured dermoid cyst; the solid material that remains can irritate surrounding tissue and should be removed. Cysts that twist on their stems and stop blood flow into and out of the ovary can also cause intense bursts of pain.

In general, experts say, you should consider surgical removal of any cyst that causes severe, consistent pain.

How are cysts diagnosed?

Usually via a bimanual exam. If a doctor detects a small cyst when examining a woman in the middle of her menstrual cycle, she will ask her to return after her next period. If the cyst remains or has grown, an abdominal or transvaginal ultrasound will reveal its consistency (an important clue in determining malignancy), as well as the number of cysts present, according to Patricia Braly, M.D., chief of gynecologic oncology at Louisiana State University Medical Center in New Orleans.

How often are cysts malignant?

Five to 10 percent of women will undergo surgery for a suspected ovarian growth at some point in their lives, according to the 1994 National Institutes of Health consensus statement on ovarian cancer. Of those, 13 to 20 percent will have cancer. But we don't know whether cancer starts as a cyst or whether a cell in the ovary becomes malignant." says Dr. Braly.

Malignant growths tend to be solid rather than fluid filled, larger than five centimeters in size and to contain wartlike structures. Ovarian cancer is most common among postmenopausal women: The lifetime risk of developing the disease is one in 70.

A cyst is always surgically removed if blood or other fluid (independent of the growth) is detected in the pelvis, as this is a sign of cancer. If a woman between the ages of 50 and 60 develops a nonfunctional ovarian cyst, surgeons generally remove both ovaries — even the healthy one. This reduces cancer risk to nearly zero.

What happens if a cyst forms when I'm pregnant?

The likelihood of developing a cyst during pregnancy is less than one percent, says Frank W. Ling, M.D., chairman of the department of obstetrics and Gynecology at the University of Tennessee College of Medicine in Memphis. If one *does* develop, it should be closely monitored by your doctor (it's likely to be nonfunctional because you're no longer ovulating. If surgery is necessary, it should be postponed until your second trimester, when the risk of miscarriage is low.

Can a cyst cause infertility?

It depends on the type. Functional cysts can temporarily interfere with your ability to conceive because they disrupt ovulation. A large cyst— about ten to 15 centimeters (around grapefruit size) — can cause infertility by compressing and destroying ovarian tissue. Cysts that twist can block blood supply to the ovary, effectively killing it. But even women with only one functioning ovary can continue to ovulate monthly.

Any scar tissue or adhesions on the ovary may impair ovulation to some degree. Unfortunately,

The majority of cysts produce no symptoms at all. When they do, a woman may feel a dull ache on one side of her abdomen, particularly during intercourse.

surgery to remove a cyst can exacerbate this problem: Studies show that 30 to 50 percent of women who undergo surgery will have scarring around the ovary or fallopian tubes. It may also be technically difficult to save these organs when removing a large cyst. Consequently, unless a woman is over 40, has a history of ovarian cancer or is in pain, doctors will often monitor a cyst that appears benign with ultrasound and try to reduce its size with medication before making a decision to remove it.

Can the Pill treat or prevent cysts?

The Pill prevents cysts from forming by suppressing ovulation (which may also be why the Pill cuts ovarian cancer risk by up to 80 percent). Oral contraceptives may be prescribed to shrink a persistent functional ovarian cyst.

Do cysts recur?

Any woman who has had a functional cyst is likely to get another because her ovaries may be slightly thickened or scarred. Nonfunctional cysts also may recur, perhaps because one or two of its cells may remain after surgery. Endometriomas often recur because the condition that causes them — endometriosis — is ongoing. Finally, a non-functional cyst can recur if it ruptures and is not entirely removed.

Deborah Shippey is a freelance health writer living in New York.

The Live Longer Diet

By Ilene Springer

"I was always on the go and **continuously ate fast food** in my car. **I never ate sitting down** at a table," says Jan Croft, 54, a real estate agent from Jackson, Miss. "I later found out I was eating 8,000 to 10,000 calories a day." After a **10 a.m. burger** one day, Croft finally admitted that she had a **terrible problem**. It was time for professional help. Croft checked herself into the Duke University Diet and Fitness Center in Durham, N.C., and learned how to change her eating habits for the better — and for good. When she first entered the program, she was so overweight she had trouble walking up a single flight of stairs. "I would be panting by the time I got to the top of the flight," she says. Croft's cholesterol level was too high, and her self-esteem was nearly nonexistent. But the Duke program helped her change all that. Since October 1993, Croft — who at one time carried 225 pounds on her 5-foot, 3-inch body — has lost and kept off more than 60 pounds. Her blood pressure is better than normal, her cholesterol level has come down significantly, and she feels good about herself again.

Like many of us, Croft had let her eating patterns veer dangerously out of control. By making one poor food choice after another, she gained weight, lost her good health and self-respect, and enjoyed life less and less. Not a pretty picture — and, unfortunately, not an unfamiliar one, either. But this grayest of gray clouds has a silver lining: Even after a lifetime of unhealthful eating, you can change your habits and make a difference in your long-term health, well-being, and appearance. Even small changes can increase your "healthspan" — the time you live disease free — and may even add years to your life. High cholesterol levels, excess weight, high blood pressure, brittle bones, and greater-than-normal risk of disease can, for the most part, be reversed or at least reduced by changing the way you eat. It's as simple — and as difficult — as that. Croft changed her life by relearning how to eat healthfully, and you can, too.

TAKING CONTROL

Change can be frightening, especially when it involves habits you've built up over a lifetime. But what's most exciting about changing your diet is that the tiniest improvements can go a very long way. For example, every 1% drop in your total blood cholesterol level results in a 2% drop in your risk for a heart attack. And every 1% increase in your HDL (good cholesterol) level equals a 3% decrease in heart disease risk. With numbers like those, change is within reach.

> Even small changes can increase your "healthspan"—the time you live disease-free — and may add years to your life.

Take a look at Croft's before-and-after health profile: Before she altered her lifestyle, she was obese; because of this, her risk for a heart attack was greater than that of a non-obese person. But now that she's lost weight, her risk has been reduced. "She has eliminated one risk factor for heart disease," says Michael Hamilton, M.D., director of the Duke University Diet and Fitness Center. And there's more: As Croft lowered her total cholesterol level from 264 to 189, her risk of heart disease plummeted, says Hamilton. Eating too little can be as dangerous as eating too much. But, again, change is possible. A visit with Julie Yakov proves this. Osteoporosis runs in Yakov's family, but it was her 10-year struggle with bulimia that left her with the bone density of an old woman. At the time, the New York singer was 29. "A 12-step program

helped me recover from bulimia," says Yakov. However, her doctors told her that her bones were still in trouble due to a chronic lack of nutrients.

Yakov consulted the osteoporosis center at the Hospital for Special Surgery in New York. To improve her bone density, she began taking Tums and started drinking a specially formulated milk that had 500 mg. of calcium per serving. And she continued to exercise. Her actions may have saved her bones: "We were pleased to see that in four years' time, Julie had increased her bone mass by approximately 5% in the hip and spine," says Theresa D. Galsworthy, R.N., O.N.C., director of the hospital's osteoporosis prevention program.

> "It's important to build pleasure into a meal. Be experimental and have some fun."

LEARNING NEW TRICKS

Convincing yourself that you should modify the way you eat is fairly easy, but actually altering your diet is much harder. It requires educating yourself, taking control, and making some sacrifices. And it requires changing what's in your head — how you think about food — as much as changing what you put on your dinner plate. How do you do all this? Experts offer this advice:

1. Think before you change. "Assess the situation," recommends Stephanie Sturiale, a registered dietitian in New York City. Before you eliminate even a single peanut butter cup from your diet, think about your long-term goals. Do you want to lower your blood pressure? Lose weight? Eat more whole foods and fewer processed foods? Figure out your goals, then decide how you need to change your diet.

2. Set concrete goals, and tackle them one at a time. Say you want to replace the junk food in your diet with whole foods. Elizabeth Ward, a registered dietitian who practices in Boston, recommends making a list of specific strategies (i.e., eat three vegetables a day, eat three fruits a day, replace white bread with whole-wheat bread, etc.) Begin with the vegetable goal. Then, when you're in the habit of eating your vegetables, add the fruits. "Get solid on one change before making the next," Ward advises.

3. Accept that change will take time. A change in your diet may take weeks, months, even years, depending on how much you change and the source of your motivation. "I tell my clients to give up to a full year before you expect your diet to change permanently," Ward says, "It depends on the person, of

A How-To Guide

Each person has to find his or her own best way to change eating habits. But experts agree that the following steps offer a successful framework for change:

1. **Write down everything you eat.**

"People forget that donut in the office or that they finished off someone's cake," says Georgia Kostas, nutrition director of the Cooper Clinic in Dallas. By keeping track of your food intake, you remain aware of exactly what you're eating — and that awareness helps prevent unconscious eating. "Writing down what you eat also helps you see a connection between your emotions and eating," says Ronette L. Kolotkin, Ph.D., of the Duke University Diet and Fitness Center. "For example, you may begin to notice the pattern of reaching for something right after a fight with your mother."

2. **Evaluate what you need to change.**

Perhaps it's the quantity — the portions — of food you need to change. Or it may be the type of food, says Kostas. You may have to lower your fat intake or increase your fruit and vegetable servings to the recommended five per day. Maybe you need more calcium to prevent osteoporosis, and you need to find a way to work in 1,000 mg to 1,500 mg. of calcium painlessly into your diet. Figure out exactly what you need to do, and then design a specific eating plan.

3. **Individualize your eating plan.**

If you make your own ground rules based on your personality, lifestyle, and food preferences, you're most likely to be successful. For example, counting your total daily fat grams gives you the most control over your food choices. But if you're too busy, you can rely on predesigned menus or choose items from preselected food groups.

4. **Seek help if you need it.**

If you have trouble changing on your own or don't really know which direction to go, seek assistance. A registered dietitian or a quality weight-loss and fitness program will help you devise an eating plan and support your efforts.

5. **Enlist the support of your family.**

Because eating is a social activity, it's much easier if you get all of your family members involved in the changes that you want to make, says preventive cardiologist Harvey Simon, of the Harvard Medical School. "It's easier to have one kind of milk in the refrigerator than three."

Put Your Diet to the Test

Is your diet on the right track? This quiz, developed by Elizabeth Ward, R.D., will give you an idea of how well you eat by exposing problem areas and strong points. For each question, circle the number of the answer that best describes how you eat most days.

1. How many servings of grain foods do you eat each day? (Sample serving sizes: 1 slice bread; ½ cup cooked cereal, pasta, or grain; 1 ounce ready-to-eat cereal; 3–4 small crackers)

1. three or fewer
2. four
3. five
4. six or more

2. How many servings of fruit do you eat daily? (Sample serving sizes: 1 medium-size piece of fruit; ¾ cup juice; ½ cup cubed fresh fruit; ¼ cup dried fruit)

1. fewer than one
2. one
3. two or three
4. four or more

3. How many servings of vegetables do you consume each day? (Sample serving sizes: ½ cup chopped raw or cooked vegetables; 1 cup raw leafy vegetables; ¾ cup vegetable juice)

1. fewer than one
2. one
3. two
4. three to five

4. How many servings of protein foods do you eat daily? (Sample serving sizes; 1 oz. cooked meat, fish, or poultry; 1 egg; ½ cup cooked legumes; 2 Tbs. peanut butter; ½ cup nuts)

1. two or fewer
2. more than seven
3. three to five
4. five to seven

5. How many dairy products do you eat daily? (Sample serving sizes: 8 oz. milk or yogurt; 1½ oz. hard cheese; 2 cups cottage cheese; 1 cup frozen yogurt)

1. less than one
2. one
3. two
4. three or more

6. In a typical day, how much total fat do you add to food, in preparation and at the table, including butter, margarine, oil, cream, full-fat salad dressing and mayonnaise, and cream cheese?

1. more than 4 Tbs.
2. 4 Tbs.
3. 3 Tbs.
4. 2 Tbs.
5. 5 Tbs. or less

7. How many times a week do you eat seafood?

1. less than once
2. once
3. twice
4. three times or more

8. How many times a week do you consume dinners containing no meat, poultry, or seafood?

1. never
2. once
3. twice
4. three times or more

9. How many times each week do you eat meat (beef, pork, and lamb)?

1. four times or more
2. three times
3. twice
4. once
5. rarely or never

10. How many times a week do you eat fried food?

1. three times or more
2. twice
3. once
4. once every two weeks
5. rarely or never

11. How often do you remove the skin from poultry before eating?

1. never
2. sometimes
3. most of the time
4. always

12. How often do you bake, broil, grill, or microwave meat, poultry, and seafood without adding additional fat?

1. never
2. sometimes
3. most of the time
4. always

13. How many times a week do you consume vitamin C-rich fruits or vegetables, such as oranges, tomatoes, or green peppers?

1. twice or less
2. three or four times
3. five or six times
4. seven or more times

14. How many times a week do you eat at fast-food restaurants?

1. four or more times
2. three times
3. twice
4. once
5. rarely or never

15. How many days a week do you eat breakfast?

1. once or less
2. two or three
3. four or five
4. six or seven

16. How often do you choose lowfat milk (1% or skim) or other low- and nonfat dairy products rather than full-fat dairy products?

1. never
2. sometimes
3. most of the time
4. always

17. How much water do you drink daily?

1. 16 oz. or less
2. 16 to 32 oz.
3. 32 to 48 oz.
4. more than 48 oz.

18. How many ounces of sweetened soft drinks do you drink each day?

1. 48 oz. or more
2. 36 oz.
3. 24 oz.
4. 12 oz. or less

19. Which describes your typical daily meal pattern?

1. one meal
2. two meals
3. two moderate meals and one or two snacks
4. three meals, or three moderate meals and one to two snacks

20. How many times a week do you munch on foods like cookies, candy, chips, donuts, and cake?

1. seven or more
2. six
3. two to five
4. fewer than two

SCORING:

Add up the numbers corresponding to your choices.

61 to 84 points: Very good. Chances are you meet nearly all the requirements of a well-balanced, lowfat diet.

41 to 60 points: Good, but could be better. You probably don't eat the recommended number of servings from each food group. Also, you may need to eat a smaller amount of fat and fewer processed foods.

21 to 40 Points: Fair. There's a lot of room for improvement. You shortchange yourself by not eating enough fruits and vegetables and be feasting on too much high-fat fare.

20 points or fewer: Critical. You're in need of professional help. You consume dangerously small amounts of critical vitamins and minerals from food, way too much fat, and possibly too many calories. See a registered dietitian for a major overhaul.

course. I've seen people change their diets overnight because of fear" after a heart attack or other dramatic event. What matters is not how quickly you change, but whether your changes are permanent.

4. **Look at the emotional side of food.** "Understand why you're eating, and look at your hunger" says Sturiale. People eat because they're bored or lonely, they need comfort or a reward, they enjoy the ritual, and for many other emotional reasons. To control emotional eating, figure out what your food/emotion danger zones are, and avoid them. Try to find something else that gives you a similar pleasure. Sturiale offers this suggestion: If you eat when you're lonely, and you like to shop, then go shopping when

Who Wins, the Hare or the Tortoise?

Is it better to change your habits cold turkey or one step at a time? Although the answer is, ultimately, an individual one, authorities differ in opinion.

One view comes from Dean Ornish, M.D., director of the Preventive Medicine Research Institute in Sausalito, Calif., and author of several books on heart disease and diet, including *Eat More, Weigh Less* (HarperCollins, 1993). Ornish proposes comprehensive lifestyle changes to prevent or reverse heart disease. According to Ornish, if you make only moderate changes, you'll feel deprived because you're not eating everything you want and you're also not changing enough to benefit your health. Dropping immediately, he says, to a vegetarian diet of 10% or less of calories from fat will make you feel so much better so quickly that you won't experience lingering pangs of deprivation or hunger.

But Michael Hamilton, M.D., director of the Duke University Diet and Fitness Center, offers a completely different opinion. While Hamilton says he agrees with the value of the Ornish diet, he disagrees with the method. "We operate toward modification rather than revolution. The object of our program is a permanent lifestyle change. But we think if you modify what you eat and still enjoy it, you're more likely to stick with it."

Harvey Simon, M.D., of Harvard Medical School and author of *Conquering Heart Disease*, (Little Brown & Co., 1994) also believes in going easy. "Start by changing breakfast. Go from a donut to a muffin to bran cereal. Then, when you've got that under control, move on to other meals." The drastic-change approach works best, he says, if people have had a jolt — like a heart attack.

Simon knows firsthand about changing his diet. At 34, he weighed 200 pounds and was at high risk for heart disease. his first step was to exercise; later he changed his diet. Now 52, Simon has slimmed down to 165 pounds and has normal blood pressure and cholesterol levels. "I changed my eating gradually. But each person has to find his own sequence of change."

you're lonely instead of eating. Does that mean you have to spend $150 on a new dress whenever you feel blue? Certainly not. Shop for a greeting card for a friend or something else that is inexpensive and that will boost your spirits at the same time.

How do you know if you're eating for emotional reasons? "If you can't seem to fill yourself with food, food may not be what you really want," says Ronette L. Kolotkin, Ph.D., director of the behavioral program at Duke. "Maybe you really need to take a nap, stop procrastinating on a project, or talk something out with someone. Don't use food as a tranquilizer."

5. **Find substitutes for favorite foods.** "One of the most painful things is having to give up foods you like," says Susan M. Lark, M.D., author of *Women's Health Companion* (Celestial Arts, 1995). "Work in substitutions so you don't have a big hole in your diet," she advises. For example, if your goal is to cut down on saturated fats, replace ice cream with nonfat frozen yogurt and full-fat cheese with lowfat substitutes. "It's important not to take a meat cleaver to your diet and end up with nothing but fruits and vegetables and a little lean chicken," Lark says.

6. **Believe that your tastes will change.** Anyone who has switched from whole milk to skim is familiar with the I'll-never-be-able-to-do-it principle. Whole milk drinkers think they can't switch to skim, force themselves to make the change, then contort their faces in disgust when they sip whole milk again. "It tastes like *cream*!" they cry. As skim milk drinkers know, tastes change — you actually can train yourself to prefer healthful foods. "You lose your preference for many high-fat foods," Ward says. "You may even get an upset stomach eating the things you used to eat."

> "Unfortunately, the body is not naturally drawn to nutritious foods."

7. **Accept that you must change your diet permanently.** Most diets are geared toward temporary change — and we try them, hoping they'll help us squeeze into a dress or look better for a family reunion. Croft says she had tried every crazy diet that came her way before accepting the fact that what she needed was permanent change, not gimmicks. Once she learned not to diet but to change the way she lived, ate, and cooked, "the weight just naturally came off." Success comes when you learn to make the right choices — not just until you fit into that little black dress, but forever.

Why do Americans Have Such Lousy Diets?

Grab a danish and coffee for breakfast. Munch a burger and fries for lunch. Dive into a juicy steak for dinner. Devour a piece of gooey chocolate cheese cake for dessert.

Despite all of the warnings, many of us still eat poorly. We stuff ourselves at restaurants, grab candy bars when we skip lunch, and plow through pillow-size bags of chips in a single sitting. If we're supposed to know better, why do we still cave in to bad foods?

Blame it on a fast-paced society, the convenience of bad-for-you foods, powerful advertising, and brains that are eager to be tempted, says Elizabeth Ward, a registered dietitian with the Harvard Community Health Plan and a spokeswoman for the American Dietetic Association. Most people simply don't have time to plan, much less prepare, a healthy meal. Pressed for time, they're likely to opt for fattening convenience foods. "I had one patient tell me he doesn't even have time to peel an orange," Ward says.

Add to that the relentless mouth-watering ads for gooey desserts, cheesy pizzas, and fattening beers. To make matters worse, these foods taste wonderful. "Unfortunately, the body is not naturally drawn to nutritious foods," says Liz Marr, a registered dietitian in Denver.

The same brain that tells us vegetables are good for us also remembers ice cream tastes better than broccoli. In other words, eating bad foods is a learned behavior, reinforced by the memory of a good taste. "When you're faced with a Big Mac and french fries, a salad doesn't sound so appetizing," Marr says.

— Winifred Yu

8. **Leave room for fun.** Eating is a sensual experience, and, if you take all the fun out of it, you'll feel empty. So look for ways to keep your diet interesting: Try exotic recipes from a lowfat cookbook, eat a wide variety of foods, and select nutritious, enjoyable snacks and treats that fit into your healthful diet. "Food is pleasurable; meals are pleasurable," Lark says. "It's important to build pleasure into a meal. Be experimental, and have some fun rather than making it painful."

9. **Find ways to compromise.** You don't have to give up every food you love, you simply have to work them into a healthful diet. Dallas resident Lillian Sills proves this point. Thirty-four pounds overweight, Sills knew she was at risk for a heart attack. (A recent study in the *Journal of the American Medical Association* showed that a woman who gains 18 to 24 pounds may increase her heart attack risk by more than 65%.) Sills wanted to lose weight, but she didn't want to give up all of her favorite foods. So she worked one-on-one with a nutritionist and found a compromise that satisfied her taste and reflected an improvement in her diet. "I don't deprive myself," she says. "For breakfast, I still have my two slices of crisp bacon, an egg, and a thick piece of whole-wheat bread with jam." But she balances her breakfast with a day of sensible eating: The rest of her meals are very low in fat, adding up to only 20 fat grams per day. "I also allow myself a big chocolate bar every six weeks. Actually, I've had it only once in a year and a half, but just knowing that I can occasionally do it means I don't feel compelled to."

SMALL CHANGES, BIG RESULTS

If you worry you'll need to revamp your diet completely, take heart: You may need to change less than you realize. "You can make little changes in your eating habits that add up to big differences," says Georgia Kostas, M.P.H., R.D., nutrition director of the Cooper Clinic and author of *The Balancing Act — Nutrition and Weight Guide* (Balancing Act Nutrition Books, 1994). "People often fear that to change their eating habits they have to start with big changes."

Changes You Can Make Today

Just as a journey of a thousand miles begins with a single step, overhauling your diet begins with a single meal. Some very small adjustments in what you eat can bring about some big results, so start by making some of the following easy changes.

Maintain a healthy weight.
Eat what you eat now — simply reduce all portion sizes by 10% to 25%

Increase calcium intake.
Drink a tall glass of skim milk with every meal, and you'll get all the calcium you need.

Cut cholesterol.
Eat vegetarian dinners on Tuesdays and Thursdays.

Cut fat.
Limit butter use to only one meal a day. Switch to non-fat dairy products.

Eat more fruits and vegetables.
Start every meal or snack with a piece of fruit or a serving of fresh vegetables. Aim for a least five a day.

Increase fiber intake.
Have a high-fiber cereal, such as raisin bran, every weekday morning. Switch exclusively to whole-wheat bread.

Up your intake of antioxidants.
Drink citrus juice at breakfast, eat a raw carrot at lunch, and prepare a leafy green vegetable for dinner every day.

To prove her point, Kostas talks about one of her new clients. He has typically eater an extra-large hamburger and a large order of french fries five days a week for lunch. Instead, she's encouraging him to eat a small hamburger and a small order of fries twice a week and turkey sandwiches on the other days. "He'll end up saving a total of 3,500 calories and 125 grams of fat per week," Kostas says. "At this rate, he'll lose about a pound a week, which is just fine. In about 10 weeks his total cholesterol should come down, his blood pressure should normalize, and his percentage of body fat should decrease. And, if he regularly exercises in addition to changing his eating habits, his HDL should go up." Kostas's client can lose weight and reduce his risk of disease — just by changing his lunches.

Sometimes a poor diet is simply a symptom of a larger problem. That was the situation for Hazel Merz, 62, of Richardson, Texas, who realized she needed to change her life, not just her eating habits. Forty-five pounds overweight, she found herself reaching for what she calls "feel-good foods" when she felt stressed or depressed. Her blood pressure, cholesterol level, and blood sugar were too high. Merz consulted with Kostas at Cooper for an eating plan. She learned how to cut fat, reduce calories, and so on. But she learned something else: "I have to feed my spirit," she says. "I find that when I surround myself with upbeat people, go to church, listen to good music with my husband, and stay active, I handle food better. When I end up in front of the TV, I start reaching for my old feel-good foods." The result? Merz has lost weight, lowered her blood pressure, cholesterol, and blood sugar, and reduced her reliance on medication. And she enjoys herself more.

By changing the way she eats, Merz has changed her life for the better. She has increased her chances of living a long, happy life, and, at the same time, she's decreased her risk of life-threatening diseases. While there are no guarantees for Merz or anyone else — we've all heard stories of healthy people dying young, and of overeating, hard-drinking smokers who flaunt their bad habits well into their 90s — the best we can do is to try to improve our odds. It requires educating ourselves, taking control, and making some sacrifices. But if you ask Croft, Merz, Sills, and all of the other people who have changed their diets whether the sacrifices were worth it, they'll say yes. Without a moment's hesitation.

Ilene Springer is a freelance health and nutrition writer based in Brookline, Mass. She's written for Ladies' Home Journal, Cosmopolitan, *and* Family Circle.

PART 7

Women as We Age

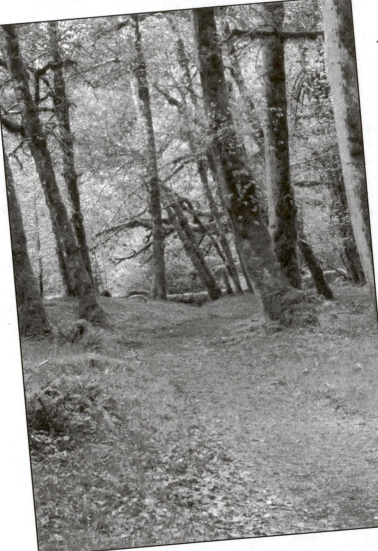

Many social observers and commentators have pointed out that the Baby Boom generation has just begun to reach middle age. Generally speaking, women in this population have expected more of life and health than women of previous generations, and, consequently, some social scientists and health care practitioners are wondering how this generation of women will confront menopause. Women today can expect to live twenty to forty years or more after menopause. That is not a short period of time! What impact will this have on the health care system?

Every reading in this section focuses on topics women face as they age. And remember, forewarned is forearmed, so even if you have some time yet before you will be dealing with these issues personally, it is never to early to start learning and preparing.

The controversial reading in this section (Reading 40) looks at the role that mammograms play in cancer detection. Mammograms offer some protection, but they are not a cure-all for breast cancer detection. This reading illustrates that we are a long way from conquering breast cancer.

Many women may have negative ideas about menopause, and the last reading in this section (Reading 45, "Positive Passage") puts menopause in its proper context. (Please see the **Quick Reference Guide to Topics/Readings/WWW Sites** and **Appendix A: WebLinks: A Directory of Annotated World Wide Web Sites** to select WWW sites that coordinate with the readings in this part.)

Are You Too Young For a Mammogram?

By Martha Burk

Breast cancer has become the number two cause of all cancer deaths in women in the U.S. It's probably the number one cause of anxiety. Most women have seen the statistics: one in eight will get breast cancer in her lifetime, and rates have been steadily climbing in the last 35 years. Recent data on risk factors such as family history have upped the worry quotient even more: 70 percent of women who get the disease have *none* of the recognized risk factors. And working out the best strategy for breast cancer detection is far from simple.

Mammography guidelines have shifted often in a research tug-of-war. When the issue became politicized last year during the national debate over health care reform, there was heated disagreement over when women should begin getting mammograms (and when insurance companies should begin paying for them). At the heart of the debate was whether mammograms provide any health benefit to women under 50. The National Cancer Institute (NCI) and 11 other national health organizations first recommended age 40 for a baseline mammogram. But the NCI changed its recommendation to age 50 on the basis of a major 1992 Canadian study that found no advantage for women in their forties. Adding to the discord, the Canadian study was widely criticized as flawed, and some charged that the NCI's switch had more to do with concerns about cost-cutting than women's health.

Last April a new analysis published in the journal *Cancer* shifted the ground once more. Researchers took a comprehensive look at eight studies of mammography — including the Canadian study — and found a 14 percent reduction in breast cancer

There is heated debate over whether regular mammograms provide any benefit to women under 50.

deaths among women ages 40 to 49 who were screened. When the data from the Canadian study were not included, deaths were reduced by 23 percent.

At the time of the Canadian study, the National Women's Health Network (NWHN) also came out for later mammography (see *Ms.*, May/June 1993), saying that no benefits had been shown for premenopausal women (who are usually under 50). According to NWHN program director Cindy Pearson, the organization will not change its position based on the new data: "The false-positive rate for mammography on premenopausal women is unacceptably high, around 38 percent, because their breast tissue is denser, and the new study hasn't changed that. Being told you have cancer when you don't carries a huge emotional cost." But what about the women whom early mammography does help — not to mention the freedom from fear that comes from knowing you've been checked? "We just don't think the evidence is there that younger women benefit that much unless they have undergone early menopause," Pearson says. "Early diagnosis might not go that far in saving their lives." Dr. Judith Jacobson, a researcher in epidemiology at the Columbia University School of Public Health, agrees: "I don't think the Canadian study was aberrant in the first place." Even taking the data from the new study into account, she says: "Mammography can only provide early detection, not prevent breast cancer. The fundamental question is: Does it save lives? And the weight of the evidence makes me doubtful that there is a benefit in terms of survival for women under 50." Pearson and other critics of early mammography also stress the dangers of unnecessary biopsies and the cumulative effect of radiation from the mammography X rays. Says breast cancer researcher Devra Lee Davis: "The damage from repeated radiation far outweighs any gains from screening for women in their twenties and thirties, and for many women in their forties."

Not all women's health organizations agree. The National Black Women's Health Project (NBWHP) recommends beginning annual mammograms at age 35, stressing that African American women get breast cancer earlier and that the strains they get may be more deadly. "Whatever the cost of false positives, it is nothing compared to stress levels later if cancer goes undetected due to lack of screening," maintains Julia Scott, director of public education and policy. "Does earlier screening save lives? We don't know. That's why we err on the side of not waiting for data that says it definitely does or doesn't." The National Coalition of Hispanic Health and Human Services Organizations also comes down on the side of earlier mammography, beginning at age 40. The group, which is conducting a national breast and cervical cancer prevention program in Latino communities for the Centers for Disease Control, bases its recommendation on a rationale similar to that of the NBWHP — that Latinas, while having lower breast cancer rates overall, have higher mortality rates and more aggressive forms of the disease.

It could be argued that "protecting" women from false positives is no better than the condescending, patriarchal medical model still pushed on women by many practitioners after all, the core of feminist philosophy is that women should be empowered to make their own choices after weighing all the information available. Pearson does not disagree. "We respect the right of women to make informed choices," she says. "It really comes down to whether you're the type who wants to leave no stone unturned regardless, or whether you would see lack of evidence that there are benefits as a reason to avoid unnecessary tests and possibly biopsies. Our position is that you shouldn't have mammograms until after menopause, although we do tell premenopausal women that other people recommend mammography if breast cancer runs in your family. And if you weigh all the evidence and opt for an early mammogram — if the risks are acceptable to you — that's an informed choice."

So what's the bottom line? The answer may turn on what scares you most and whether you're a skeptic. Lining up with the National Cancer Institute, the NWHN wants clear proof that mammograms help younger women. It doesn't see that evidence yet — even going so far as to discount some of the data in the new study. The NBWHP and the majority of national health organizations take the other view — research suggests that benefits may be there, so caution dictates earlier mammograms.

The uncertainty for women is not likely to change until we get better technology — such as imaging techniques that are more accurate for dense breast tissue — or different methods of detection altogether. And unfortunately, the current budget-cutting fever on Capitol Hill will likely set back government funding of the large-scale research that brings much of our advanced technology. We see ads on television describing a simple, painless blood test for prostate cancer. Why not for breast cancer?

Martha Burk is director of the Center for Advancement of Public Policy, which runs the Washington Feminist Faxnet.

Profile

Zen and the Art of Breast Maintenance

I can walk into a room or walk down the street and pick out the women who have had breast surgery," says Pamela Ferguson. "They hold their arms protectively over their scars as if sheltering injured birds." She believes that the main reason behind this almost ritualized habit is inadequate physical therapy after surgery. Ferguson has spent the eight years since her own mastectomy trying to remedy that situation. Expanding on her work as a Shiatsu instructor and her knowledge of yoga and tai chi, she developed a series of upper-body exercises she calls "drawing circles" that enable women to regain full range of motion after breast surgery and avoid lymphedema, a common but serious arm swelling caused by congestion of the lymph nodes.

By increasing the diameter of the circles every day, Ferguson was able both to gauge her rehabilitation and to move gracefully again after surgery. Now a breast cancer activist promoting prevention *and* rehabilitation, she teaches the exercises to mastectomy survivors, physical therapists, and health care providers worldwide. But, she cautions, attention to breast health (through good upper-body exercises as well as sensitivity to breast changes) should be a priority all the time — not just after something goes wrong. Besides, adds Ferguson, if women were encouraged to develop knowledge of and appreciation for their breast physiology, perhaps they would rebel against the whims of fashion that promote unnecessary surgeries and elaborate undergarments to "fix" their bodies.

Jennifer Baumgardner

Ferguson's book of post-mastectomy exercises, "The Self-Shiatsu Handbook," is available from Putnam.

Physical Activity and Health

A Report of the Surgeon General/Executive Summary

Message from Donna E. Shalala
Secretary of Health and Human Services

The United States has led the world in under-standing and promoting the benefits of physical activity. In the 1950s, we launched the first national effort to encourage young Americans to be physically active, with a strong emphasis on participation in team sports. In the 1970s, we embarked on a national effort to educate Americans about the cardiovascular benefits of vigorous activity, such as running and playing basketball. And in the 1980s and 1990s, we made break-through findings about the health benefits of moderate-intensity activities, such as walking, gardening, and dancing.

Now, with the publication of this first Surgeon General's report on physical activity and health, which I commissioned in 1994, we are poised to take another bold step forward. This landmark review of the research on physical activity and health — the most comprehensive ever — has the potential to catalyze a new physical activity and fitness movement in the United States. It is a work of real significance, on par with the Surgeon General's historic first report on smoking and health published in 1964.

This report is a passport to good health for all Americans. Its key finding is that people of all ages can improve the quality of their lives through a life-long practice of moderate physical activity. You don't have to be training for the Boston Marathon to derive real health benefits from physical activity. A regular, preferably daily regimen of at least 30–45 minutes of brisk walking, bicycling, or even working around the house or yard will reduce your risks of developing coronary heart disease, hypertension, colon cancer, and diabetes. And if you're already doing that, you should consider picking up the pace: this report says that people who are already physically active will benefit even more by increasing the intensity or dura-tion of their activity.

This watershed report comes not a moment too soon. We have found that 60 percent — well over half — of Americans are not regularly active. Worse yet, 25 percent of Americans are not active at all. For young people — the future of our country — physical activity declines dramatically during adolescence. These are dangerous trends. We need to turn them around quickly, for the health of our citizens and our country.

We will do so only with a massive national com-mitment. . . . Families need to weave physical activity into the fabric of their daily lives. Health profession-als, in addition to being role models for healthy behaviors, need to encourage their patients to get out of their chairs and start fitness programs tailored to their individual needs. Businesses need to learn from what has worked in the past and promote worksite fitness, an easy option for workers. Community lead-ers need to reexamine whether enough resources have been devoted to the maintenance of parks, play-grounds, community centers, and physical education. Schools and universities need to reintroduce daily, quality physical activity as a key component of a comprehensive education. And the media and enter-tainment industries need to use their vast creative abilities to show all Americans that physical activity is healthful and fun — in other words, that it is attractive, maybe even glamorous! . . .

★ ★ ★ ★ ★

INTRODUCTION

This is the first Surgeon General's report to ad-dress physical activity and health. The main message of this report is that Americans can substantially improve their health and quality of life by including moderate amounts of physical activity in their daily lives. Health benefits from physical activity are thus achievable for most Americans, including those who may dislike vigorous exercise and those who may have been previously discouraged by the difficulty of

From Physical Activity and Health: A Report of the Surgeon General/Executive Summary (July 1996), pp. 9-14.

adhering to a program of vigorous exercise. For those who are already achieving regular moderate amounts of activity, additional benefits can be gained by further increases in activity level.

This report grew out of an emerging consensus among epidemiologists, experts in exercise science, and health professionals that physical activity need not be of vigorous intensity for it to improve health. Moreover, health benefits appear to be proportional to amount of activity; thus, every increase in activity adds some benefit. Emphasizing the amount rather than the intensity of physical activity offers more options for people to select from in incorporating physical activity into their daily lives. Thus, a moderate amount of activity can be obtained in a 30-minute brisk walk, 30 minutes of lawn mowing or raking leaves, a 15-minute run, or 45 minutes of playing volleyball, and these activities can be varied from day to day. It is hoped that this different emphasis on moderate amounts of activity, and the flexibility to vary activities according to personal preference and life circumstances, will encourage more people to make physical activity a regular and sustainable part of their lives.

The information in this report summarizes a diverse literature from the fields of epidemiology, exercise physiology, medicine, and the behavioral sciences. The report highlights what is known about physical activity and health, as well as what is being learned about promoting physical activity among adults and young people.

The major purpose of this report is to summarize the existing literature on the role of physical activity in preventing disease and on the status of interventions to increase physical activity. Any report on a topic this broad must restrict its scope to keep its message clear. This report focuses on disease prevention and therefore does not include the considerable body of evidence on the benefits of physical activity for treatment or rehabilitation after disease has developed. This report concentrates on endurance-type physical activity (activity involving repeated use of large muscles, such as in walking or bicycling) because the health benefits of this type of activity have been extensively studied. The importance of resistance exercise (to increase muscle strength, such as by lifting weights) is increasingly being recognized as a means to preserve and enhance muscular strength and endurance and to prevent falls and improve mobility in the elderly. Some promising findings on resistance exercise are presented here, but a comprehensive review of resistance training is beyond the scope of this report. In addition, a review of the special concerns regarding physical activity for pregnant

women and for people with disabilities is not undertaken here, although these important topics deserve more research and attention.

Finally, physical activity is only one of many everyday behaviors that affect health. In particular, nutritional habits are linked to some of the same aspects of health as physical activity, and the two may be related lifestyle characteristics. This report deals solely with physical activity; a Surgeon General's Report on Nutrition and Health was published in 1988. . . .

MAJOR CONCLUSIONS

1. People of all ages, both male and female, benefit from regular physical activity.

2. Significant health benefits can be obtained by including a moderate amount of physical activity (e.g., 30 minutes of brisk walking or raking leaves, 15 minutes of running, or 45 minutes of playing volleyball) on most, if not all, days of the week. Through a modest increase in daily activity, most Americans can improve their health and quality of life.

3. Additional health benefits can be gained through greater amounts of physical activity. People who can maintain a regular regimen of activity that is of longer duration or of more vigorous intensity are likely to derive greater benefit.

4. Physical activity reduces the risk of premature mortality in general, and of coronary heart disease, hypertension, colon cancer, and diabetes mellitus in particular. Physical activity also improves mental health and is important for the health of muscles, bones, and joints.

5. More than 60 percent of American adults are not regularly physically active. In fact, 25 percent of all adults are not active at all.

6. Nearly half of American youths 12–21 years of age are not vigorously active on a regular basis. Moreover, physical activity declines dramatically during adolescence.

7. Daily enrollment in physical education classes has declined among high school students from 42 percent in 1991 to 25 percent in 1995.

8. Research on understanding and promoting physical activity is at an early stage, but some interventions to promote physical activity through schools, worksites, and health care settings have been evaluated and found to be successful.

SUMMARY

The benefits of physical activity have been extolled throughout western history, but it was not until the second half of this century that scientific evidence supporting these beliefs began to accumulate. By the 1970s, enough information was available about the beneficial effects of vigorous exercise on cardiorespiratory fitness that the American College of Sports Medicine (ACSM), the American Heart Association (AHA), and other national organizations began issuing physical activity recommendations to the public. These recommendations generally focused on cardiorespiratory endurance and specified sustained periods of vigorous physical activity involving large muscle groups and lasting at least 20 minutes on 3 or more days per week. As understanding of the benefits of less vigorous activity grew, recommendations followed suit. During the past few years, the ACSM, the CDC, the AHA, the PCPFS, and the NIH have all recommended regular, moderate-intensity physical activity as an option for those who get little or no exercise. The *Healthy People 2000* goals for the nation's health have recognized the importance of physical activity and have included physical activity goals. The 1995 *Dietary Guidelines for Americans*, the basis of the federal government's nutrition-related programs, included physical activity guidance to maintain and improve weight — 30 minutes or more of moderate-intensity physical activity on all, or most, days of the week.

Underpinning such recommendations is a growing understanding of how physical activity affects physiologic function. The body responds to physical activity in ways that have important positive effects on musculoskeletal, cardiovascular, respiratory, and endocrine systems. These changes are consistent with a number of health benefits, including a reduced risk of premature mortality and reduced risks of coronary heart disease, hypertension, colon cancer, and diabetes mellitus. Regular participation in physical activity also appears to reduce depression and anxiety, improve mood, and enhance ability to perform daily tasks throughout the life span.

The risks associated with physical activity must also be considered. The most common health problems that have been associated with physical activity are musculoskeletal injuries, which can occur with excessive amounts of activity or with suddenly beginning an activity for which the body is not conditioned. Much more serious associated health problems (i.e., myocardial infarction, sudden death) are also much rarer, occurring primarily among sedentary people with advanced atherosclerotic disease who engage in strenuous activity to which they are unaccustomed. Sedentary people, especially those with pre-existing health conditions, who wish to increase their physical activity should therefore gradually build up to the desired level of activity. Even among people who are regularly active, the risk of myocardial infarction or sudden death is somewhat increased during physical exertion, but their overall risk of these outcomes is lower than that among people who are sedentary.

Research on physical activity continues to evolve. This report includes both well-established findings and newer research results that await replication and amplification. Interest has been developing in ways to differentiate between the various characteristics of physical activity that improve health. It remains to be determined how the interrelated characteristics of amount, intensity, duration, frequency, type, and pattern of physical activity are related to specific health or disease outcomes.

Despite common knowledge that exercise is healthful, more than 60 percent of American adults are not regularly active, and 25 percent of the adult population are not active at all. Moreover, although many people have enthusiastically embarked on vigorous exercise programs at one time or another, most do not sustain their participation. Clearly, the processes of developing and maintaining healthier habits are as important to study as the health effects of these habits.

The effort to understand how to promote more active lifestyles is of great importance to the health of this nation. Although the study of physical activity determinants and interventions is at an early stage, effective programs to increase physical activity have been carried out in a variety of settings, such as schools, physicians' offices, and worksites. Determining the most effective and cost-effective intervention approaches is a challenge for the future. Fortunately, the United States has skilled leadership and institutions to support efforts to encourage and assist Americans to become more physically active. Schools, community agencies, parks, recreational facilities, and health clubs are available in most communities and can be more effectively used in these efforts.

School-based interventions for youth are particularly promising, not only for their potential scope — almost all young people between the ages of 6 and 16 years attend school — but also for their potential impact. Nearly half of young people 12–21 years of age are not vigorously active; moreover, physical activity sharply declines during adolescence. Childhood and adolescence may thus be pivotal times for preventing sedentary behavior among adults by maintaining the habit of physical activity throughout the school years. School-based interventions have been shown to be successful in increasing physical activity levels. With evidence that success in this arena is possible, every effort should be made to encourage schools to require daily physical education in each grade and to promote physical activities that can be enjoyed throughout life.

Outside the school, physical activity programs and initiatives face the challenge of a highly technological society that makes it increasingly convenient to remain sedentary and that discourages physical activity in both obvious and subtle ways. To increase physical activity in the general population, it may be necessary to go beyond traditional efforts. This report highlights some concepts from community initiatives that are being implemented around the country. It is hoped that these examples will spark new public policies and programs in other places as well. Special efforts will also be required to meet the needs of special populations, such as people with disabilities, racial and ethnic minorities, people with low income, and the elderly. Much more information about these important groups will be necessary to develop a truly comprehensive national initiative for better health through physical activity. Challenges for the future include identifying key determinants of physically active lifestyles among the diverse populations that characterize the United States (including special populations, women, and young people) and using this information to design and disseminate effective programs. . . .

★ ★ ★ ★ ★

Historical Background and Evolution of Physical Activity Recommendations

1. Physical activity for better health and well-being has been an important theme throughout much of western history.

2. Public health recommendations have evolved from emphasizing vigorous activity for cardiorespiratory fitness to including the option of moderate levels of activity for numerous health benefits.

3. Recommendations from experts agree that for better health, physical activity should be performed regularly. The most recent recommendations advise people of all ages to include a minimum of 30 minutes of physical activity of moderate intensity (such as brisk walking) on most, if not all, days of the week. It is also acknowledged that for most people, greater health benefits can be obtained by engaging in physical activity of more vigorous intensity or of longer duration.

4. Experts advise previously sedentary people embarking on a physical activity program to start with short durations of moderate-intensity activity

and gradually increase the duration or intensity until the goal is reached.

5. Experts advise consulting with a physician before beginning a new physical activity program for people with chronic diseases, such as cardiovascular disease and diabetes mellitus, or for those who are at high risk for these diseases. Experts also advise men over age 40 and women over age 50 to consult a physician before they begin a vigorous activity program.

6. Recent recommendations from experts also suggest that cardiorespiratory endurance activity should be supplemented with strength-developing exercises at least twice per week for adults, in order to improve musculoskeletal health, maintain independence in performing the activities of daily life, and reduce the risk of falling. . . .

Physiologic Responses and Long Term Adaptations to Exercise

1. Physical activity has numerous beneficial physiologic effects. Most widely appreciated are its effects on the cardiovascular and musculoskeletal systems, but benefits on the functioning of metabolic, endocrine, and immune systems are also considerable.

2. Many of the beneficial effects of exercise training — from both endurance and resistance activities — diminish within 2 weeks if physical activity is substantially reduced, and effects disappear within 2 to 8 months if physical activity is not resumed.

3. People of all ages, both male and female, undergo beneficial physiologic adaptations to physical activity. . . .

The Effects of Physical Activity on Health and Disease

Overall Mortality

1. Higher levels of regular physical activity are associated with lower mortality rates for both older and younger adults.

2. Even those who are moderately active on a regular basis have lower mortality rates than those who are least active.

Cardiovascular Diseases

1. Regular physical activity or cardiorespiratory fitness decreases the risk of cardiovascular disease mortality in general and of coronary heart disease mortality in particular. Existing data are not conclusive regarding a relationship between physical activity and stroke.

2. The level of decreased risk of coronary heart disease attributable to regular physical activity is similar to that of other lifestyle factors, such as keeping free from cigarette smoking.

3. Regular physical activity prevents or delays the development of high blood pressure, and exercise reduces blood pressure in people with hypertension.

Cancer

1. Regular physical activity is associated with a decreased risk of colon cancer.

2. There is no association between physical activity and rectal cancer. Data are too sparse to draw conclusions regarding a relationship between physical activity and endometrial, ovarian, or testicular cancers.

3. Despite numerous studies on the subject, existing data are inconsistent regarding an association between physical activity and breast or prostate cancers.

Non-Insulin-Dependent Diabetes Mellitus

1. Regular physical activity lowers the risk of developing non-insulin-dependent diabetes mellitus.

Osteoarthritis

1. Regular physical activity is necessary for maintaining normal muscle strength, joint structure, and joint function. In the range recommended for health, physical activity is not associated with joint damage or development of osteoarthritis and may be beneficial for many people with arthritis.

2. Competitive athletics may be associated with the development of osteoarthritis later in life, but sports-related injuries are the likely cause.

Osteoporosis

1. Weight-bearing physical activity is essential for normal skeletal development during childhood and adolescence and for achieving and maintaining peak bone mass in young adults.

2. It is unclear whether resistance- or endurance-type physical activity can reduce the accelerated rate of bone loss in postmenopausal women in the absence of estrogen replacement therapy.

Falling

1. There is promising evidence that strength training and other forms of exercise in older adults preserve the ability to maintain independent living status and reduce the risk of falling.

Obesity

1. Low levels of activity, resulting in fewer kilocalories used than consumed, contribute to the high prevalence of obesity in the United States.

2. Physical activity may favorably affect body fat distribution.

Mental Health

1. Physical activity appears to relieve symptoms of depression and anxiety and improve mood.

2. Regular physical activity may reduce the risk of developing depression, although further research is needed on this topic.

Health-Related Quality of Life

1. Physical activity appears to improve health-related quality of life by enhancing psychological well-being and by improving physical functioning in persons compromised by poor health.

Adverse Effects

1. Most musculoskeletal injuries related to physical activity are believed to be preventable by gradually working up to a desired level of activity and by avoiding excessive amounts of activity.

2. Serious cardiovascular events can occur with physical exertion, but the net effect of regular physical activity is a lower risk of mortality from cardiovascular disease. . . .

Patterns and Trends in Physical Activity

Adults

1. Approximately 15 percent of U.S. adults engage regularly (3 times a week for at least 20 minutes) in vigorous physical activity during leisure time.

2. Approximately 22 percent of adults engage regularly (5 times a week for at least 30 minutes) in sustained physical activity of any intensity during leisure time.

3. About 25 percent of adults report no physical activity at all in their leisure time.

4. Physical inactivity is more prevalent among women than men, among blacks and Hispanics than whites, among older than younger adults, and among the less affluent than the more affluent.

5. The most popular leisure-time physical activities among adults are walking and gardening or yard work.

Adolescents and Young Adults

1. Only about one-half of U.S. young people (ages 12–21 years) regularly participate in vigorous physical activity. One-fourth report no vigorous physical activity.

2. Approximately one-fourth of young people walk or bicycle (i.e., engage in light to moderate activity) nearly every day.

3. About 14 percent of young people report no recent vigorous or light-to-moderate physical activity. This indicator of inactivity is higher among females than males and among black females than white females.

4. Males are more likely than females to participate in vigorous physical activity, strengthening activities, and walking or bicycling.

5. Participation in all types of physical activity declines strikingly as age or grade in school increases.

6. Among high school students, enrollment in physical education remained unchanged during the first half of the 1990s. However, daily attendance in physical education declined from approximately 42 percent to 25 percent.

7. The percentage of high school students who were enrolled in physical education and who reported being physically active for at least 20 minutes in physical education classes declined from approximately 81 percent to 70 percent during the first half of this decade.

8. Only 19 percent of all high school students report being physically active for 20 minutes or more in daily physical education classes. . . .

Understanding and Promoting Physical Activity

1. Consistent influences on physical activity patterns among adults and young people include confidence in one's ability to engage in regular physical activity (e.g., self-efficacy), enjoyment of physical activity, support from others, positive beliefs concerning the benefits of physical activity, and lack of perceived barriers to being physically active.

2. For adults, some interventions have been successful in increasing physical activity in communities, worksites, and health care settings, and at home.

3. Interventions targeting physical education in elementary school can substantially increase the amount of time students spend being physically active in physical education class.

Women and Heart Disease

The myth that heart disease is something that happens only to men — especially busy executives — seems to be at last on its way to oblivion. There's a growing awareness that the prevention of cardiovascular disease is — or ought to be — a pressing personal concern not only for men but for women, too. It's true that before menopause, few women suffer from cardiovascular disease. But after age 50, women begin to develop cardiovascular disease at an increasing rate. By the time they reach 60, women develop cardiovascular disease at the same rate as men at 50 — and this 10-year gap prevails until about the age of 75 or 80, when the differences disappear and the rates become similar. At age 65, as many women die of heart disease as of cancer, and after age 75 heart disease is the chief killer of women. Typically American women can now expect to live 25 to 30 years past menopause — about one-third of their lives — at significant risk for cardiovascular disease.

The performance of doctors in preventing and treating cardiovascular disease in women has recently come under fire not only from women but also from many doctors. For example:

- Since scientists have tended to treat cardiovascular disease as if it affected "men only," most of the major studies have dealt with men. One exception is the ongoing Framingham Heart Study, which includes both sexes.

- According to Dr. Bernadine Healy, Director of the National Institutes of Health, medical treatments for women are all too often based on a "male model."

- A large study published last July in the *New England Journal of Medicine* showed that despite "greater cardiac disability in women" — that is, the women in the study were, on average, sicker than the men — physicians treated coronary artery disease (CAD) less aggressively in the women. Of patients with positive stress tests, 40% of the men but only 4% of the women were referred for angiograms (an advanced diagnostic test for determining the degree of arterial blockage). Another study in the same issue showed that only after a woman actually had a heart attack did she receive the same treatment as a man. The *Journal* called these findings a demonstration of the "Yentl" syndrome, the name of a heroine in an Isaac Bashevis Singer story who has to pretend to be male in order to study the Talmud.

- Perhaps because CAD is rare — though not unknown — in women under 50, doctors are less likely to pay attention to such symptoms as chest pain when a younger woman has them.

It's true that the medical profession has sat up and taken notice recently, and important new studies have already appeared while others are underway. But it's essential for women to understand how to guard their cardiovascular health, and to refuse to settle for unequal care.

THE ESTROGEN PUZZLE

Estrogen, one of two major female hormones, plays a role not only in ovulation, menstruation, and pregnancy but in heart disease as well. Estrogen appears to protect premenopausal women from CAD and heart attack, but no one is sure how it works. Estrogen does have a positive effect on blood cholesterol, raising the good element (high-density lipoprotein, or HDL) and lowering the bad (low-density lipoprotein, or LDL), and some experts think it may also lower blood pressure. Oral contraceptives, which usually contain estrogen. actually increase heart attack risk slightly, but this is significant only for smokers or women who already have some form of cardiovascular disease.

When estrogen production declines at menopause, a woman's blood cholesterol may rise. However, this is by no means uniform or universal, so other factors are also clearly at work.

HORMONE TREATMENT FOR EVERY WOMAN?

It's always been a good guess that estrogen replacement therapy will reduce the risk of heart disease in postmenopausal women, and many studies have supported this hypothesis, but the evidence remains controversial. Last September, however, the *New England Journal of Medicine* published the results of a large scale 10-year study of almost 50,000 nurses who had taken estrogen since the onset of menopause. The results were clear: these women had reduced their risk of heart disease by half. Their risk for stroke, however, was not affected. Some experts hailed the study, declaring that the benefits of taking estrogen had now been conclusively shown to outweigh the risks. Another widely publicized study published a month later in the *Journal* found that low-dose estrogen raises HDL and lowers LDL, thus protecting against arterial disease. Thus estrogen therapy might be appropriate for postmenopausal women with elevated cholesterol levels, but controlled studies will be required to verify the effectiveness of this preventive measure.

But some concerns cannot be brushed aside. Estrogen therapy is suspected of increasing the risk for cancers of both the uterine lining (endometrium) and the breast. Secondly, according to Dr. Elizabeth Barrett-Connor of the University of California at San Diego, estrogen therapy may not be the only factor reducing cardiac risk in the women studied so far.

Postmenopausal women who take estrogen are usually relatively well-educated, upscale women with better access to health care and high motivation to take care of themselves. These factors might be just as protective as estrogen.

Finally, estrogen therapy is increasingly being replaced by a combination of low-dose estrogen and progestin (a synthetic form of progesterone, the second major female hormone). This therapy is just as effective against hot flashes and other postmenopausal symptoms and is less likely to cause endometrial cancer. But no one knows whether it will have the same protective effect against heart disease that estrogen alone appears to have. The only way to find out is by clinical study — and while some work is underway, much remains to be done.

THE RISK LIST FOR WOMEN

Though the risk factors for CAD and heart attack are similar for women and men, some items on the list appear to need qualifying for women.

Smoking. This is about the worst thing a woman can do to her heart. Among young and middle-aged women, who seldom have CAD, an estimated 65% of all heart attacks that do occur are attributed to: cigarette smoking. No level of smoking is safe, and the risk of having chest pains and heart attack rises with every cigarette smoked daily. Birth control pills, as we've said, won't put a healthy woman at risk for CAD or other cardiovascular disorders unless she smokes.

Family history. If heart attacks, strokes, and other forms of cardiovascular disease run in a woman's family, she should pay special attention to her other risk factors.

Elevated blood cholesterol. Most studies have shown that high blood cholesterol levels — above 200 milligrams per deciliter — put women at risk for CAD just as much as men, especially when the HDL reading is below 35 milligrams per deciliter. However, triglycerides (fats in the blood that are transported with the cholesterol) in women may be more directly connected to heart disease than in men.

Obesity. Being overweight is bad for anybody's health, but more women are obese than men. Obesity is hard for scientists to explain, hard for doctors to treat, and hard to cure by diet. But women should understand that if their weight is creeping up year by year, it's important to cut calories and develop good exercise habits.

Sedentary life. It's well known that lack of exercise is bad for the heart. It's also true that most of the studies that demonstrate this have been done on men. Nevertheless, a large-scale, long-term study several

Terms of the Heart

Heart disease is a general, vague term that covers all ailments of the heart, from heart attacks to congenital defects.

Cardiovascular disease is a broad term referring to disorders of the heart and circulatory system ("cardio" means heart, "vascular" means blood vessels). This includes hypertension, atherosclerosis, stroke, rheumatic heart disease, and other disorders.

Coronary artery disease (CAD) refers to the conditions that cause narrowing of the coronary arteries (atherosclerosis) so that blood flow to the heart is reduced. This results in *coronary heart disease (CHD)*, damage to heart muscle caused by insufficient blood supply from obstructed coronary arteries. Permanent damage to, or death of, heart muscle is called a *heart attack* (myocardial infarction). When there is an insufficient supply of blood to the brain, a *stroke* can result.

What a Woman Can Do

- Know your family history. If close relatives have CAD or have had a heart attack, especially if they had it before the age of 50, you may be at high risk and should be sure to have routine screenings at regular intervals. If you are black, you may also be at greater risk.

- Follow a low-fat diet. Keep your cholesterol consumption below 300 milligrams daily (one egg, for instance, has on average 215 milligrams). Rely primarily on fruits, vegetables, grains, and low-fat dairy products. Look upon meat and cheese as side dishes or condiments.

- Keep your weight at recommended levels for your height and build. A low-fat diet and exercise will help.

- Don't smoke. Quit smoking if you do smoke — your risk of CAD will drop to that of a nonsmoker within two years.

- Make regular aerobic exercise (walking, running, cycling, swimming) and other kinds of physical activity (gardening, dancing, tennis, or whatever you enjoy) a part of your daily and weekly routine.

- Have your blood pressure checked regularly, as well as your blood cholesterol levels.

years ago at the Cooper Institute for Aerobics Research in Dallas showed that high levels of physical fitness (as determined by treadmill tests) were associated with a low risk of heart disease in women under 65, just as in men.

Hypertension. Nobody knows precisely what causes it, but chronically elevated blood pressure is a major risk factor for heart disease and stroke. Levels above 140/90 are generally thought to require medical treatment. However, a caucus of women physicians last year reviewed all current studies and published their work in the *Annals of Internal Medicine.* They found that "treatment guidelines are primarily based on studies of men." Since then a large-scale national study has shown that hypertensive women benefit from treatment (drugs and life-style changes) as much as men: the treated women in the study showed a marked decrease in death from stroke. Black women who develop hypertension tend to get it about 10 years earlier than white women, and in this study black women showed the most benefits from treatment.

ASPIRIN: GOOD FOR WOMEN, TOO?

In 1988, as was widely reported, the Physicians' Health Study conducted by researchers at Harvard University demonstrated that taking one adult-size aspirin (325 milligrams) every other day reduced the risk of heart attack by half. One problem was that all the subjects in this rigorously scientific investigation were men. As we pointed out at the time, it was impossible to say whether aspirin would have the same effects for women. Last summer, however, a six-year study of almost 90,000 female nurses showed that taking one to six aspirins weekly reduced their risk of heart attack by 30%. Dr. JoAnn Manson, who directed the study, noted that the evidence was inconclusive because the women were not following a strict protocol of aspirin doses as in the Physicians' Health Study. However, the news was encouraging. And a study published last year — this time including both women and men who were already heart patients — showed that half a baby aspirin daily (30 milligrams) was as effective at warding off heart attacks as a larger dose. No one should start an aspirin regimen on her own, but women at risk for heart attack should certainly discuss aspirin with their doctor.

HIGHER RISK FOR WORKING WOMEN?

Women in the workplace have never been shown to have higher rates of CAD than women who stay home — in spite of occasional scary articles claiming that women who work like men will have heart attacks like men. As one researcher put it, "remunerative employment does not in itself increase coronary risk." However, some aspects of working women's lives raise a few concerns. It's now accepted that working at jobs with high levels of demand and little room for decision-making can contribute to hypertension and ill-health in men (see *Wellness Letter,* June 1990). Women tend to hold a disproportionate number of these jobs — such as waitresses, computer operators, and clerks. The Framingham Heart Study did show that women in clerical jobs have more heart attacks than women who stay at home. Furthermore, for many employed women, even highly paid professionals, a job at work is followed by a job at home. But data on the consequences of work overload for women have yet to be gathered and analyzed.

HRT:
Frequently Asked Questions

At menopause, which occurs around age 50 for most women, the body gradually reduces its production of estrogen and progesterone, the principal female hormones. Ovulation, the monthly release of an egg from the ovary, declines and stops: menstrual periods cease. If the uterus is surgically removed before menopause, menstruation stops, but hormone production remains the same and menopause occurs naturally. If both the uterus and ovaries are removed, an abrupt menopause results. The definition of menopause (for women who have not had hysterectomies) is going a year without menstrual periods.

The declining level of estrogen is what produces the unpleasant symptoms of menopause that most women experience to some degree — hot flashes and sleep disturbances, plus the vaginal dryness that can make intercourse painful or impossible. Estrogen and progesterone, of course, control the reproductive cycle in women. They also play important roles in many other functions and tissues: in blood cholesterol levels and the health of the heart, in building bone and other aspects of growth, in the condition of the skin and hair, and in behavior and brain function. As hormone production declines at menopause, bone thinning (osteoporosis) occurs, but usually not so rapidly as to cause fractures at this stage. And, as the years pass, women lose their "resistance" to heart disease: by age 65 the risk of heart attack is as great in women as in men.

Thus many women and their physicians have come to believe it is a good idea to replace these hormones at menopause. The average woman in the U.S. and Canada can expect to live almost 30 years past menopause — a span of years that she wants to make as healthy and productive as possible.

Why take hormones at all?

Hormone therapy has two purposes: the first is to allay menopausal symptoms such as hot flashes and vaginal dryness. The second is to prevent or postpone heart disease as well as osteoporosis and fractures. Heart disease — though few people are aware of it — kills more women every year than all cancers combined (360,000 American women died of heart disease in 1992, as opposed to 43,000 of breast cancer). Hormone therapy may postpone or even prevent some of these heart disease deaths, as well as the disability caused by fractures in some older women.

Is menopause a medical condition?

Menopause is a gradual rather than dramatic change (except when surgically induced), and the lower levels of hormones characteristic of the menopausal and postmenopausal years are normal and in no sense a medical "disorder." Many women have few or mild menopausal symptoms and no compelling risk factors for heart disease or osteoporosis (see box). If you fall into this category, you may well decide to manage menopause without drugs. Exercise and a good diet can help keep you healthy and are essential with or without hormone therapy.

What's the difference between estrogen replacement therapy (ERT) and hormone replacement therapy (HRT)? Do you have to take a pill every day?

ERT uses estrogen alone; HRT is estrogen combined with progestin (a synthetic that acts like progesterone).

From *UC Berkeley Wellness Letter* (October 1995), pp. 4-5. Reprinted with permission by the *University of California at Berkeley Wellness Letter*. © Health Letter Associates, 1995.

Sometimes this combined treatment is also called PERT (progestin-estrogen replacement therapy). ERT is now usually prescribed only for women who've had hysterectomies. This is because estrogen alone has been shown to increase the risk of cancer of the uterine lining (endometrial cancer) — not a possibility when the uterus has been removed. But adding progestin helps prevent endometrial cancer, so women who have not had hysterectomies take it in addition to estrogen. Because it is newer, HRT has been less intensively studied (and used) than ERT. Hormone therapy comes in two forms: pills (taken daily or on a cyclic basis) or estrogen patches. The standard dosages have been reduced over the years.

Is it wise to take hormones simply to combat such menopausal symptoms as hot flashes and vaginal dryness and then stop therapy after the symptoms go away?

There's no reason not to take hormones for a few years to combat severe menopausal symptoms, if you wish. But before you discontinue therapy, think about your risk factors for heart disease and osteoporosis, as well as other factors discussed below.

My doctor is urging me to try HRT because my mother died of a heart attack when she was only 60. Can hormones help protect me?

Yes. There is good evidence that ERT raises a woman's blood level of HDL ("good") cholesterol and lowers LDL ("bad") cholesterol. High levels of HDL are protective against heart disease. Until recently it wasn't known if HRT was as effective against heart disease. However, a large new study, the "Post menopausal Estrogen/Progestin Interventions Trial," known as PEPI, from the National Heart, Lung, and Blood Institute showed that *although estrogen alone gives HDL levels the biggest boost, all forms of hormone therapy raise HDL and lower LDL cholesterol. In addition, hormone therapy decreases the clotting tendencies of the blood, thus reducing heart attack risk. Yet the therapy does not cause weight gain.*

Hypertension and stroke run in my family, and my blood pressure is already slightly elevated, will HRT increase my stroke risk?

No, on the contrary. There's strong evidence (from PEPI as well as other studies, notably one involving more than 23,000 women in Sweden) that HRT reduces the risk of stroke and does not raise blood pressure. This is a particularly interesting finding because it suggests that hormone therapy does more against heart disease than simply boost HDL.

Will HRT increase my risk of breast cancer?

This remains one of the most troubling questions about ERT and HRT. Your risk for developing heart disease as you grow older far outweighs your risk of breast cancer. But women so fear breast cancer that many are unwilling to do anything that might increase their risk. Short-term use of hormones (five years or less) does not raise breast cancer risk, but the evidence about long-term use remains inconclusive. And the fact that one large well-conducted study *did* show a significant increase in risk is not to be ignored.

Doctors usually do not prescribe HRT for women who've had breast cancer, and sometimes not for those whose first-degree relatives (mother or sister) have had breast cancer. See below for more details on determining your risks.

What about other cancers?

A study begun in 1982 and recently published in the *Journal of the National Cancer Institute* suggested that ERT reduces the risk of dying of colon cancer. Then this July yet another study that included HRT had similar results. Another study from a recent issue of the *American Journal of Epidemiology* suggested that long-term users of ERT (not HRT) might increase the risk of ovarian cancer. Again researchers were cautious. The women studied had begun therapy in the 1970s and 1980s, when much higher doses were prescribed. In any case, this is the only study that has found such an association.

Can HRT prevent bone fractures and other symptoms of osteoporosis?

Yes, for as long as you take it. Many factors influence bone density, but the most important of these are the sex hormones (estrogen in women, testosterone in men), diet (particularly your intake of calcium and vitamin D), and physical activity. Bones respond to physical stress (weight-bearing activities like walking and running) by becoming stronger. At about age 35, in most women, bone density begins to decline, and the decline becomes significant during and after menopause. As a woman grows older, she becomes more susceptible to fractures, "dowager's hump," and the disabilities (and sometimes fatalities) resulting from hip fractures.

There's no question that HRT as well as ERT can slow bone loss and prevent fractures. However, hormone therapy alone is not enough. A healthy diet and weight-bearing exercise are critical. If you have multiple risk factors for osteoporosis, you should consider HRT. But HRT won't prevent bone loss forever. If they live long enough, all men and women will experience some bone loss. Hormone therapy has beneficial effects on bones right after menopause and up into the seventies, but bone mass will still begin to decline in women older than 75. Nevertheless, you'll be better off at 75 for having taken it — your bones will be stronger and thus bone loss should affect you less.

Does HRT keep you looking young and attractive?

No. But it can combat vaginal dryness and thus make sexual intercourse more pleasurable — which might make you feel younger — and it can slow the thinning of the skin that results from lower estrogen levels. It would be a mistake to think of hormone therapy as some kind of "fountain of youth." Both men and women show the effects of aging: there's no therapy yet that can prevent wrinkling, graying hair, or other signs that you are growing older.

Can HRT protect you from Alzheimer's?

No one knows. Two recent population studies of ERT and Alzheimer's had opposite results: one study found that therapy might prevent or delay the onset of the disease, while the other found no evidence that ERT had any impact. But this, of course, remains an interesting avenue of investigation.

What are the immediate side effects of HRT?

Some women experience breast soreness, bloating, fatigue, and depression. Monthly bleeding may continue with some kinds of hormone therapy. Sometimes these symptoms subside; often they can be alleviated by changing dosages or types of therapy.

So should I take HRT or not?
When should I begin?

There is no clear answer to either question. Many women remain in good health for many years after menopause without taking hormones. Much depends on how you feel about the treatment — and on your personal risk factors for heart disease, breast cancer, and osteoporosis (see below). Most doctors think you should begin HRT at menopause and continue for the rest of your life in order to get the greatest protection against heart disease and osteoporosis. You certainly get your greatest gains if you start at menopause, though there's some evidence that HRT can also be beneficial if started later.

A Risk Checklist For Women

You'll need medical advice on whether to start hormone therapy and how long to continue it. But it will be helpful if you yourself understand your risk factors for heart disease, osteoporosis, and breast cancer. If you have multiple risk factors for heart disease and osteoporosis, you should strongly consider hormone therapy. On the other hand, if you have multiple risks for breast cancer, you should consider not taking it.

Growing older is, in and of itself, a risk factor for heart disease, osteoporosis, and breast cancer.

HEART DISEASE RISK FACTORS

- Smoking.
- Family history of heart attack, stroke and high blood pressure in close relatives.
- Elevated total blood cholesterol (above 240 mg/dl is "high"; 200 to 239, "borderline-high"). HDL ("good") cholesterol below 35.
- Obesity.
- Distribution of body fat around the waist and abdomen rather than the hips.
- Sedentary life-style.
- High blood pressure (levels above 140/90).
- Diabetes.

OSTEOPOROSIS RISK FACTORS

- Being of European or Asian origin. African-American women are at lower risk.
- Family history.
- Poor diet, especially one high in sodium and low in vitamins and minerals, particularly vitamin D and calcium.
- Sedentary life-style, especially the lack of weight-bearing exercise.
- Obesity.
- Smoking.
- Heavy alcohol use.
- Long-term use of certain medications, such as cortisone or thyroid hormones.

BREAST CANCER RISK FACTORS

- A first-degree relative (mother or sister) with breast cancer.
- Early onset of menstruation (before 13) or late menopause (after 50).
- Not having had children, or having a first child after 35.
- Not having breast-fed.
- Obesity.
- A breast biopsy that suggested increased risk.

BONE Medicine

By Burkhard Bilger

Liz Meryman grew up believing her mom to be indestructible.

Tall, trim, and well-knit, Sylva came from a line of Swiss women as capable as they were uncomplaining. Although she is 85 now, to her daughter she only truly began to age last year. That was when Liz first noticed the faint slope to Sylva's shoulders, the nervous way she had of clutching a stair rail. "I have this sudden sense that she's diminishing," Liz says. "And her world is shrinking along with her."

Sylva's bent back suggests she has suffered at least one spinal fracture; she noticed recently that she's become shorter than her daughter. "I don't want to fall, I definitely don't want to fall," she says, thinking of the bedridden folk that share her building in Westchester County, New York. "I am afraid if I don't make some changes I'll end up incompetent. That is not a very nice prospect."

Hers is a common fear, and one that, until recently, doctors could do little to comfort. Like skin, bone constantly regenerates itself: Cells known as osteoclasts eat away old bone, while cells called osteoblasts build the skeleton back up. That's fine so long as the osteoblasts have the upper hand, but after the age of 35, the osteoclasts start gaining. Eventually, bone can become so weak that it crumbles at the mildest of jolts. Some 25 million Americans have dangerously thin bones; osteoporosis causes 1.5 million fractures, runs up $10 billion in health care costs, and ends the independence of tens of thousands of elderly people every year.

Yet women like Sylva have long been offered only two troublesome options. Calcitonin had to be injected in the thigh daily, so it had few takers. Estrogen helps prevent heart disease as well as osteoporosis, but it can also cause menstruation to resume (when taken with progestin), and it may encourage cancer.

For Liz, who resembles her mother in her olive skin, dark eyebrows, and willowy frame, Sylva's helpless decline has seemed like a frightening omen. "We all think we're invulnerable," Liz says. "But now that I'm 50, maybe I should get my head turned around differently." Two years ago, Liz had her bone density measured, thereby joining a farsighted minority. According to a recent Gallup poll, three out of four women between 45 and 75 years of age have never spoken to their doctors about osteoporosis. As long as the news was so bad, maybe they were afraid to ask.

Well, the news just got better. This fall, in a rare medical moment worthy of its hype, two new osteoporosis drugs were approved by the Food and Drug Administration, and a third was recommended for approval by the administration's advisory committee. The two that have been approved — alendronate and calcitonin in nasal-spray form — stop bone loss, reduce the risk of fracture by as much as 50 percent, and cause few side effects. The third drug — slow-release sodium fluoride — can actually rebuild bones dramatically, though perhaps at some risk. "It's a very exciting time," says researcher Robert Lindsay, president of the National Osteoporosis Foundation. "For someone like me, who's been in this field for 20 years, it's great to be here right now."

As welcome as they are, the new drugs have turned what was a simple decision into a complex calculus. Like estrogen, alendronate and calcitonin nasal spray have to be taken for life if their benefits are to last. For women Sylva's age, who suffer by far the most fractures, long-term drug use may be a small price to pay. But what about a woman like Liz? According to the bone scan two years ago, she's in the normal range for a woman her age. But as she heads into menopause she can expect to start losing one percent of her bone or more each year — and for every 10 percent lost, her risk of fracture will double. Should she take one of the new drugs? Or are lifestyle changes enough? "I'm not crazy about putting anything into my body," Liz says, "but I keep saying I'll go to the gym and I never do."

For many women, the new drugs are the fulfillment of a dream long deferred. But dreams, as the poet Delmore Schwartz wrote, begin with responsibilities.

WHAT'S THE FIRST STEP?

Have your bone density measured. Less than 20 years ago, osteoporosis was called the hidden epidemic: Regular X-rays could reveal nothing less than a 25 to 40 percent drop in bone density — at which point the disease is well advanced. Today, machines called densitometers can show a one percent bone loss. (The most accurate densitometer uses a technique called dual energy X-ray absorptiometry, and exposes the body to one fiftieth the radiation as in a chest X-ray.) Yet most women find out their bones are weakening only when they start to get fractures.

That's because when treatment options were so limited, doctors tended not to push women to get scans. Unfortunately, doctors still don't, in part because there are only about 1,500 densitometers in the country, some of them reserved for research. Density measurements cost between $150 and $250, and are covered by some insurance plans and by Medicare in some states. "It's hard for me to recommend screening 30 million women over 50," says Robert Recker, director of the Osteoporosis Research Center in Omaha. "There aren't enough machines, and if there were it would bankrupt the health care system."

All the more important, then, that *you* know when to request a bone scan. Ideally, a woman should have her bone density measured at menopause, when bone loss sharply accelerates. If her bones are healthy, she should have them measured again every four years. If she's losing more bone than average, or if her density is low to begin with, she should have it measured again as often as every year. Even if a woman has osteoporosis and has gone on one of the new drugs, she should continue with yearly scans until her bones are out of danger.

Given the cost and effort involved, you may want to know just how closely you need to stick to such a schedule. Start by reviewing your family history, the best predictor for your own risk. Then see if you fit any of the high-risk groups: Have you been through menopause? Did you go through menopause before the age of 45? Are you white or Asian, thin or sedentary? Do you smoke, drink a lot of alcohol, get very

little calcium, or suffer from an eating disorder? Do you take cortisone or other similar medicines, called glucocorticoids? The more of these groups you belong to, the more closely you ought to watch your bone density as you get older.

If local densitometers are drawing more crowds than the pope, ask your doctor about a new alternative. Thanks to new analysis techniques, a simple X-ray of the hand can now provide accurate bone density measurements. Any radiology department that has taken the time to get some rudimentary equipment can take the X- ray; it's sent to OsteoGram Analysis Center in Manhattan Beach, California, which uses computer analysis to reveal as little as one percent bone loss. The cost is about $100, but design improvements are expected to bring it down to $50 or less.

CAN THE NEW DRUGS HELP ME?

The answer is a definite yes if you already suffer from osteoporosis. For an elderly woman, the risk of a hip fracture is as high as her chances of getting breast, uterine, or ovarian cancer combined — and if she's frail, the inactivity that follows such a fracture can lead to fatal complications. The new drugs cut the risk of fracture in half, preventing crippling injuries and disabling fears. And although alendronate and calcitonin nasal spray were approved for patients with osteoporosis, the drugs may also be useful for elderly women on the verge of the disorder.

What about a younger woman who has thinning bones or who simply wants to take out some insurance? In hopes of getting approval for *preventive* use of alendronate, Merck and Company, Inc., which is marketing the drug under the name Fosamax, recently presented the FDA with the results of a study in which newly menopausal women successfully used the drug to prevent the rapid bone loss that occurs in those years. But many experts think it's a bad idea for a menopausal woman to use the new medications unless her bones are very fragile indeed. For one thing, experts lack answers about alendronate's long-term safety. While research on thousands of women worldwide indicates that the drug is extremely safe, the studies have lasted only three years. Alendronate binds to bone in order to obstruct osteoclasts, the cells with the task of breaking bone down for routine rebuilding. At least some of the drug stays in the bone forever. "We don't have a clue as to its long-term safety," says Bruce Ettinger, a senior researcher at the Kaiser Permanente Medical Care Program in northern California, who has studied and written extensively on osteoporosis. "I would be extremely cautious before giving it to a 50-year-old who hasn't started to experience fractures."

As for calcitonin, it flushes out of the body within an hour or so, and years of research (as well as more than a decade of experience with the injectable form) have shown it to have very few side effects. But any nasal spray may irritate the nose with long-term use, leading to pain, nosebleeds, or sinus inflammation.

Another consideration for the younger woman is that the drugs are expensive: Taken for 20 years or more, alendronate or nasal-spray calcitonin would cost as much as a new car. Prudence and the pocketbook dictate that a younger woman not take the new drugs unless a scan ws her bones are so weak they've started to fracture.

WHICH DRUG IS BEST FOR ME?

"Estrogen still makes the most sense," Ettinger says. "It's still the gold standard." Only estrogen treats hot flashes and other symptoms of menopause,

---

How the New Drugs Stack Up

Medicine has had little to offer women facing osteoporosis until now. Two new osteoporosis drugs are the first practical alternatives to estrogen ever approved in this country. Both work, but the new drugs — and others in the pipeline — vary in terms of cost, convenience, safety, and efficacy.

ALENDRONATE is the first nonhormonal osteoporosis drug. Sold by Merck and Company, Inc., under the name Fosamax, it binds to bone that has been targeted by bone-eating osteoclasts, protecting it from being broken down.

DOSAGE: One 10 milligram tablet a day, taken with a full glass of water on an empty stomach, at least half an hour before eating.

COST: $1.75 per tablet.

PROS: Shown to be safe and effective in unusually large studies. In one, women using alendronate thickened their spines by 3 percent a year for three years, lost a third less height, and suffered half as many fractures as women on placebos.

CONS: Side effects of long-term use are unknown. Inconvenient to take.

CALCITONIN is a hormone that slows down osteoclasts. A synthetic version is sold as a nasal spray by Sandoz Pharmaceuticals under the name Miacalcin.

DOSAGE: A spritz a day.

COST: About $1.80 a spritz.

PROS: In an injectable form, calcitonin has been shown to be safe and effective in millions of users worldwide. The spray can be used any time of day, and has few side effects.

CONS: Thickens bones by only one and a half percent per year for two years.

ON THE HORIZON

SLOW-RELEASE SODIUM FLUORIDE is a mineral encapsulated in a wax tablet. In the formulation under development by the Mission Pharmacal Company, the drug seems to slow down osteoclasts and rev up osteoblasts, which build bone. In a small, four-year study, women on sodium fluoride thickened their spines by 5 percent and their hips by 2.4 percent each year; they lost two-thirds less height and suffered a third fewer fractures than those on a placebo. But high doses of sodium fluoride in an older formulation (not slow-release) caused peptic ulcers and built brittle bone. While the slow-release formula seems to avoid side effects, many doctors remain suspicious and say they will demand larger studies before they trust the new formula. If it's approved, patients will need to have their blood fluoride checked once a year to insure it stays below toxic levels.

CALCITRIOL is a hormone that helps in the absorption of calcium and stimulates osteoblasts. It is one of the most popular osteoporosis drugs in the world, but has never been approved for the treatment of osteoporosis in this country. In high doses, it can cause kidney stones if patients also take more than 800 mg of calcium a day. Roche Pharmaceuticals has a synthetic version, called Rocaltrol, used to treat a bone disorder that can result from kidney dialysis. The company is attempting to get approval for its use for osteoporosis.

RALOXIFENE is a compound that attaches to estrogen receptors in the body. The hope is that it will offer estrogen's benefits to bone and the rest of the body without the hormone's negatives. Raloxifene's safety and efficacy are being tested by Eli Lilly and Company; if it works, it is unlikely to be available until the end of the century.

— B.B.

as well as preventing bone loss and heart disease — all for less than $200 a year. Even women who start taking estrogen in their seventies can increase their bone density by 10 percent and reduce the odds of a fracture by up to half. Still, those facts have yet to sway many women, who may worry about the increased risk of uterine cancer or fear estrogen's possible link to breast cancer. In fact, only one in eight women who could benefit from estrogen actually take it.

For now, alendronate is the next best choice. Short term studies indicate it's as safe as its rival, calcitonin, and its cost is comparable, as well. But alendronate builds more bone.

The choice may get tougher if the FDA approves slow-release sodium fluoride. A recent study showed that this medication thickens a patient's spine by 5 percent every year — nearly twice as much as alendronate — with no sign of letup after three years. Slow-release sodium fluoride should cost about half as much as alendronate or calcitonin.

But FDA approval is far from a sure thing. Sodium fluoride has a checkered past: Given in high doses in studies in the late 1980s, the drug did build bone, but the structure of the new bone was weak, leaving it prone to stress fractures. Also troubling is the fact that sodium fluoride caused peptic ulcers in some women. In a small four-year study, the new, slow-release formulation seemed to be free of those problems. Women on the drug had nearly a third fewer fractures than women taking a placebo, and they suffered few side effects. Still, many researchers won't be convinced until they see more studies.

CAN I STRENGTHEN MY BONES WITHOUT DRUGS?

Yes: weight-lifting, calcium, and vitamin D can all strengthen bones, even if they're already frail. "Osteoporosis has to be approached with nutrition and lifestyle as front line tactics," says Recker, director of the Osteoporosis Research Center. "Then, when you can't avoid it, intervene with something more." Healthy habits can help prevent osteoporosis for most women — even when it runs in the family.

After the age of 30, the body hangs on to less of the calcium it takes in. All the more reason to keep the pipeline full. As recently as 1989, the recommended

daily calcium allowance for adult women was 800 milligrams per day. In 1994, the National Institutes of Health upped that recommendation to 1,500 mg for post-menopausal women not taking estrogen. Now some doctors don't hesitate to recommend as much as 2,500 mg — close to five times as much as most adult women get. And don't stint on the calcium if you're taking one of the new drugs; you still need 1,500 to 2,500 mg a day of the mineral to get the drug's full benefit.

In order to absorb that calcium, you also need vitamin D. Your body can make its own if you're exposed to adequate sunlight, but that may be impossible during winter months. Besides, your body's ability to make vitamin D slows with age. Most multivitamins include the 400 mg recommended by bone experts.

No amount of calcium will build a healthy skeleton on its own. Think of it, rather, as the raw material that osteoporosis drugs can forge into bone. Exercise, too, can turn mere minerals into skeletal support: The more you bend or pull bones, the stronger they grow. (And the increases in strength and balance that come with exercise further reduce the risk of a bone breaking fall.) Aerobics and running have long been touted as ways to stave off bone loss, but bone researchers increasingly emphasize the benefits of lifting weights to prevent bone loss at any age. In a study published in 1994 in the *Journal of the American Medical Association*, for example, women as old as 70 who lifted weights twice a week for a year avoided the expected loss of bone and actually increased their bone density slightly.

Weight-lifting to prevent bone loss need not be daunting, says Fredrick S. Hahn, director of clinical exercise for New York Methodist Hospital. Hahn recommends 30-minute sessions, twice a week, with at least two days' rest between sessions. To prevent injuries, he has his patients lift weights slowly and smoothly, increasing the amount of weight gradually over many months. "It's possible to make elderly people phenomenally strong," he says. "It might take six or eight months, but so what? We have a lifetime."

Burkhard Bilger is a senior editor at The Sciences.

positive passage

Menopause is inevitable,
but it's possible to modulate the symptoms.

By Lonnie Barbach, PhD

Just a month before my forty-third birthday, I suddenly could not get through the day without napping. Normally energetic and healthy, I began to catch a cold nearly every month. I felt a fatigue I hadn't known since I was three months pregnant. Whenever I lay down to sleep I got heart palpitations and woke up three times a night to urinate. A vertebra in my neck was suspiciously tender, and one fingernail tingled with cold as if it had just been polished. I blamed my impatience and irritability on fatigue. I also was having pain during intercourse, but this seemed minor. Besides, I was too tired for sex anyway.

I consulted doctor after doctor. One gave me medication for what he thought was a thyroid condition, which made me feel as if I had mainlined coffee. Still exhausted, I couldn't sleep at all. Another doctor said I had chronic fatigue syndrome, for which there is no known cure. A third proffered a diagnosis of systemic Candida (a yeast infection), so I went on a drastic diet for it and lost fifteen pounds. I looked gaunt and awful and still didn't feel much better.

Finally, a Marin County homeopath made me a remedy from a highly diluted substance found in cuttlefish. Except for the irritability, all of my symptoms disappeared. But I still didn't know what had been wrong with me. A year later, an older friend announced that all of the irregular bleeding she had been having for years was the early stages of menopause.

Suddenly, the three short menstrual cycles I had experienced — which I considered to be the result, not the cause, of my mysterious illness — made sense.

Since I was only forty-three and had never had a hot flash (the only symptom I knew to be associated with menopause), I hadn't made the connection. Neither had the doctors — although it turns out that my symptoms were classic.

Other symptoms that signal the beginning of menopause include headaches, mental fuzziness, joint and muscle pain, flatulence and gastric upset, skin sensitivities, acne, mood swings, anxiety, mild depression, exaggerated PMS, heavy menstrual bleeding, and sexual effects such as reduced lubrication, painful intercourse, or a lack of sexual desire. It's hard to believe that such a wide range of symptoms can accompany this transition. But our balance of estrogen, progesterone, and even testosterone directly affects our cardiovascular, digestive, and nervous systems; in fact, it has some effect on almost every part of our body.

For most women, menopause begins in their forties and is over between the ages of forty-five and fifty-five, taking from one to ten years to complete (although in some cases it can take longer). Many women will complete the transition around the same age their mothers did, but several factors, such as smoking's toxic effects on the ovaries, can result in early menopause. At some point, a new hormonal equilibrium is reached, and symptoms cease — generally within two years after menstrual periods have stopped.

Why some women respond to this period of hormonal disequilibrium with one set of symptoms and others respond with another is not known. Fifteen

From *San Francisco Focus* (September 1993), pp. 83-86. This article has been adapted from *The Pause: Positive Approaches to Menopause* (Dutton). © 1993 by Lonnie Barbach. Reprinted with permission granted by the Rhoda Weyr Agency, New York.

percent will experience no discomfort whatsoever. Another fifteen percent will experience symptoms so severe that they will be incapacitated. The rest will fall somewhere in between.

I have to admit, I was horrified at first to realize I was beginning menopause. I believed the notion that a woman is all washed up after menopause. I imagined my years of productivity were over. However, a quick calculation made me realize that I was at the height of my career, not at the end of it; that the years until retirement equaled the time since I had begun working. Consequently, I wanted to rename this transition to reflect its positive aspects.

I now call it "The Pause" because this word suggests a break — like hitting the pause button on your VCR. You may get up for a few minutes, but when you return you expect to continue where you left off. The same is true of The Pause. You may experience symptoms during this transition, but when it's over, most women tend to feel more energetic with the cessation of monthly hormonal ups and downs. Anthropologist Margaret Mead termed this phenomenon "post menopausal zest."

Women also tend to shift their focus at this time from spouse and children to self-fulfillment. They start jobs, become more powerful and self-defined, even more assertive. The problem of menopause, therefore, becomes one of handling uncomfortable symptoms during the turbulent time of hormonal flux.

I discovered that there is a range of effective solutions — acupuncture, homeopathy, herbs, or hormones — to relieve uncomfortable symptoms, but that each of us will respond to these treatments differently. There's no single answer or starting point for all women. You may have to experiment — even mix and match treatments. But relief is possible. With knowledge, the process need no longer be an uncomfortable or scary one.

I ruled out estrogen therapy for myself because of the link between supplementary hormones and breast cancer. I began researching holistic remedies instead. A few acupuncture treatments with a nurse practitioner in Sausalito accompanied by some Chinese herbs quieted my feelings of irritability and anxiety. I was relieved of the pain I had been experiencing during intercourse by drinking a tincture made from the herb Vitex (or chasteberry), which can be found in most health food stores. (My sexual interest returned once my fatigue abated.) I was feeling energetic and in control of my emotions and my life again.

Exercise, vitamins, and diet are also crucial when it comes to symptom relief. For example, exercise raises estrogen levels and can cut the frequency and intensity of hot flashes by 50 percent. It also helps control mood swings, as do vitamin B-6 and magnesium. Vitamin E can reduce hot flashes and relieve breast tenderness. Soy products such as tofu, which are high in plant estrogens, may diminish menopausal symptoms as well.

As we continue through this transition, our hormone balance keeps changing, which means we may have to make subtle adjustments in our chosen remedies. For example, I ended up adding estrogen to my arsenal of solutions once I completed research for my book *The Pause: Positive Approaches to Menopause*. I discovered that the risk of developing breast cancer from estrogen was not as great as I had originally believed. All the data are not in yet, but the current medical thinking is that estrogen does not *cause* breast cancer but can accelerate the growth of an existing cancer. The few studies that do find an increased risk of breast cancer among women taking hormones show that the risk increases by about one in one thousand women per year. Many studies show no increased risk at all.

I now take Estrace, a form of estrogen, during the few days before I ovulate and the week before my period. Estrogen levels are at their lowest during those days, and the herbs are no longer sufficient for some of my mental and emotional symptoms.

Many physicians automatically advise their patients to go on hormones once they have stopped cycling, especially since increased breast-cancer risk appears small. However, this is like saying that all pregnant women should have a cesarean delivery because some may have problems during childbirth. I strongly believe that postmenopause, like pregnancy, is a natural state. If we take care of ourselves through diet and exercise, most of us can get through both quite nicely on our own.

For some of us, however, hormones, like a cesarean section, can be lifesaving. With the aid of a knowledgeable physician, you can determine your own individual risk factors and decide whether you should take hormones.

Hormone-replacement therapy for the prevention of osteoporosis and heart disease *after* menopause is the question to ponder. Estrogen helps prevent cardiovascular disease. But the key to cardiovascular health is diet, exercise, and no smoking — with or without hormones. A minimum of three hours of aerobic exercise a week is essential. In fact, one study showed that an unfit woman of any age can reduce her risk of dying by almost 50 percent if she becomes fit. Next, stop smoking, because smoking alone accounts for 50 percent of all heart attacks. Finally, change to a diet low in cholesterol and saturated fats and relatively high in fiber. In one major study, no one with a cholesterol level below 150 died of cardiovascular disease.

You can retard the course of osteoporosis (porous bones) by taking estrogen after menopause. (Diet and exercise are also effective.) To determine whether you need estrogen to fight this disease, get the density of your bones measured to see if you are within the normal range for a woman your age. If your bone density is below average, you are in a high-risk group, and you should consider estrogen therapy.

But remember that hormones are no panacea: Even if they are advisable, not every woman can adapt to them. The progestin that must be taken with the estrogen once you stop cycling (if you have a uterus) can cause depression and irritability. Estrogen can have a negative effect on some women's emotions. Uncomfortable menstrual cramping is another side effect. Some women who were relieved when their periods finally ended dislike the monthly bleeding that often resumes with hormone-replacement therapy.

Some women tell me that while they didn't enjoy the symptoms they experienced during The Pause, it caused them to change their diet, increase their exercise, and reduce their stress. As a result, they felt better than they had in many years, and looked forward to a longer, healthier life.

This article has been adapted from The Pause: Positive Approaches to Menopause, *by Lonnie Barbach, Ph.D. (Dutton, 1993), which describes medical and holistic approaches to the treatment of menopausal symptoms.*

Menopause Symptoms and Treatments

Premenstrual syndrome, mood swings, irritability, depression:

- Diet — Avoid alcohol, sugar, dairy products, salt
- Exercise — Daily
- Behavior — Prepare family members and colleagues, don't smoke, undergo psychotherapy as needed
- Supplements — Vitamin B-6 (50 to 500 mg per day); magnesium (150 to 400 mg per day)
- Homeopathy — Individual remedies
- Acupuncture and Chinese herbs — Individual treatment
- Herbs — Chasteberry (Vitex)
- Hormones — Estrogen is particularly effective

Hot flashes:

- Diet — Avoid coffee, chocolate, alcohol, spicy foods, and fruits high in acid; keep cold liquids nearby
- Exercise — Daily
- Behavior — Dress in layers, carry a fan
- Supplements — Vitamin E (400 to 600 international units per day); hesperidin (1000 mg per day); vitamin C (500 to 1000 mg three times daily)
- Homeopathy — Individual remedies
- Acupuncture and Chinese herbs — Individual treatment
- Herbs — Chasteberry (Vitex), Black cohosh, Dong Quai
- Hormones — Estrogen, progesterone (for women who cannot take estrogen)

Heavy bleeding:

- Homeopathy — Individual remedies
- Acupuncture and Chinese herbs — Particularly effective
- Herbs — Chasteberry (Vitex), shepherd's purse, blessed thistle
- Hormones — Progesterone
- Medical — D&C; ablation or burning of uterine lining; hysterectomy as a last resort

Sleep disturbance:

- Diet — Avoid caffeine, alcohol, large evening meals; drink warm milk before bedtime
- Exercise — Daily
- Behavior — White noise, hot baths, reading, relaxation exercises
- Homeopathy — Individual remedies
- Acupuncture and Chinese herbs — Individual treatment
- Herbs — Motherwort, passionflower, valerian
- Hormones — Estrogen

— From *The Pause*, by Lonnie Barbach

WebLinks:
A Directory of Annotated Web Sites

A

American Civil Liberties Union (ACLU)　　No. 1

🌐 http://www.choice.org/2.norplant.aclu.html

Maintained by the ACLU, this site presents a fact sheet on Norplant and discusses the potential for abuse, particularly in terms of court ordered use.

American Heart Association　　No. 2

🌐 http://www.amhrt.org/

Site includes information on heart disease and strokes. It is a good site for research and has a searchable database of articles.

The American Medical Women's Association　　No. 3

🌐 http://www.amwa-doc.org/index.html

Description of the AMWA and its activities. Site also has online health information and good links to other sites.

American Society for Clinical Nutrition　　No. 4

🌐 http://faseb.org/ascn/

Provides press releases on new findings, a job page with employment opportunities, information from the Food and Nutrition Science Alliance, and more. Look for position papers on nutrition and weight control. National Institutes on Health links and other related links provided. Also features the highly regarded *American Journal of Clinical Nutrition*.

American Society for Reproductive Medicine　　No. 5

🌐 http://www.asrm.com/

Site maintained by the American Society for Reproductive Medicine (ASRM), which is a nonprofit medical organization devoted to advancing knowledge in the areas of reproductive medicine and infertility. Site offers services to patients, including fact sheets, general information, and recent press releases.

Ann Rose's Ultimate Birth Control Links　　No. 6

🌐 http://gynpages.com/ultimate/

This site was put together by a birth control educator. It includes information on informed decision making on birth control and child bearing, and information on all types of birth control methods.

Ask a Woman Doctor　　No. 7

🌐 http://www.healthwire.com/women/ask.htm

This site is interactive. You ask a question and a woman doctor answers it online. Also contains brief articles on various women's health topics.

Ask the Dietitian　　No. 8

🌐 http://www.hoptechno.com/rdindex.htm

While there are no fancy graphics here, you will find this site chock-full of nutrition information from registered dietitians. There are sections on eating habits, fad diets, fast foods, fiber, food fallacies, junk foods, minerals, sports nutrition, and many other topics. Great resource on nutrition.

Atlanta Reproductive Health Centre WWW: Infertility, IVF, Endometriosis　　No. 9

🌐 http://www.ivf.com/index.html

Maintained by the Atlanta Reproductive Health Centre, this site is for women with concerns about their reproductive health. It is directed primarily at women who are having difficulty conceiving. Site offers advice, resources, case studies, and links.

B

The Best of WWWomen Sites!　　No. 10

🌐 http://www.wwwomen.com/feature/bestwww.shtml

A special page that selects and indexes sites that are outstanding for their content, inspiration, explorations, or presentation, according to the WWWomen organizers. This is an interesting, information packed and even fun page with an extremely inclusive variety of links for and about women.

Birth and Midwifery　　No. 11

🌐 http://www.efn.org/~djz/birth/birthindex.html

This site provides information on birth-related and midwifery topics. There are links to other sites and resources throughout the world. Maintained by the Online Birth Center, this is an up-to-date source.

Birth Control Pills   No. 12

🌐 http://www.nau.edu/~fronske/bcp.html

This site discusses birth control pills: how they work, how to take them, and other information related to their use.

Birth Control Trust   No. 13

🌐 http://www.easynet.co.uk/bct/

The BC Trust is a British-based organization that provides online information about contraception, abortion, and reproductive policy in the United Kingdom.

Breast Cancer Home Page   No. 14

🌐 http://www.feminist.org/other/bc/bchome.html

Links to facts you need to know, feminist stories on breast cancer, Internet resources for breast cancer, clinical trials, what you can do, mammography information, and breast cancer events. The Breast Cancer Information Center is maintained by The Feminist Majority and New Media Publishing, Inc.

Breast Center Information Clearinghouse   No. 15

🌐 http://nysernet.org/bcic/

This site is maintained by the New York State Education and Research Network, a partnership of organizations, and the site offers online resources, information, and links for breast cancer patients and healthcare providers.

The Breast Cancer Roundtable   No. 16

🌐 http://www.seas.gwu.edu/student/tlooms/MGT246/
breast_cancer_roundtable.html

Current information about breast cancer from online journals, research studies, and organizations. Includes information on mammography.

C

Canadian Women's Studies Online   No. 17

🌐 http://www.utoronto.ca/womens/hometxt.htm

Site provides information about women's studies programs, resources, and women's organizations in Canada, with links to the Virtual World of Women.

Center for Science in the Public Interest (CSPI)   No. 18

🌐 http://www.cspinet.org/

The Center for Science in the Public Interest is a nonprofit education and advocacy organization that focuses on improving the safety and nutritional quality of our food supply and on reducing the health problems caused by alcohol. Look for the Nutrition Action Healthletter, the CSPI Nutrition Quiz, Just for Kids, What's New, Booze News, and links to other health and nutrition sites.

Circumcision Issues   No. 19

🌐 http://www.eskimo.com/%7egburlin/circ.html

This page has links to sites on female and male circumcision — the alteration or multilation of genitalia. Good link to more pages on female circumcision.

Cyberdiet   No. 20

🌐 http://www.cyberDiet.com/index.html

Offers CyberDiet's interactive nutritional profiler, food facts, menus and meal plans, exercises, and comprehensive links. Maintained by a registered dietician.

D

Depo-Provera   No. 21

🌐 http://users.vnet.net/shae/wissues/depo.html

This site discusses what Depo-Provera is, how it works, and the pros and cons of its use.

Doctor's Guide to Breast Cancer Information and Resources   No. 22

🌐 http://www.pslgroup.com/breastcancer.htm

This site includes information on breast cancer, treatment drugs, and genetic testing. It also has links to other sites and discussion groups.

Doctor's Guide to Osteoporosis   No. 23

🌐 http://www.pslgroup.com/osteoporosis.html

Information as well as links to other sites provided here. Site also offers information on groups and newsgroups. The information is current and written for consumers.

E

Environmental Organization Web Directory!   No. 24

🌐 http://www.webdirectory.com/

Comprehensive site that covers a wide range of topics (health, pollution, agriculture, business, etc.). Has searchable database and extensive links. An excellent general resource. Site is subtitled "Earth's Biggest Environmental Search Engine," and it certainly seems to be that!

F

Food and Drug Administration (FDA)   No. 25

🌐 http://www.fda.gov/

This is the Web site for the Food and Drug Administration. An excellent source of information on food, drug, and cosmetic safety. Updated regularly.

FDA's Center for Food Safety and Applied Nutrition   No. 26

🌐 http://vm.cfsan.fda.gov

This is a page within the Food and Drug Administration's site that specifically focuses on food and nutrition information. It has valuable information and good links to other sites.

Family Health International   NO. 27

🌐 http://www.fhi.org/

This site is sponsored by the Family Health International organization, which is a nonprofit group that works to improve reproductive health around the world, with an emphasis on developing countries. The site includes information on family planning, STDs, and women's studies. It is a good site for international information.

Female Circumcision   No. 28

🌐 http://hamp.hampshire.edu/~mnbF94/clitorectomy.html

An excellent resource for women dealing with this issue. Includes letters from people around the world sharing experiences and information on legal matters pertaining to the subject. Also links to the Marianne Sarkis's (a female genitial multilation researcher) home page, which has extremely timely and extensive links to other sites.

Female Genital Mutilation Research Home Page (FGM)   No. 29

🌐 http://www.hollyfeld.org/~xastur/

This site is dedicated to research pertaining to Female Genital Mutilation (FGM). The practice is presented from a variety of perspectives: psychological, cultural, sexual, human rights, etc. Links to an archive page that is updated daily with new information.

Femina   No. 30

🌐 http:/www.femina.com/femina/health

This is a search engine for health and well-being sites. It includes AIDS, assault prevention, infertility, abortion, and aging. It is a great resource and starting point for searches dealing with women's issues.

Feminist.com   No. 31

🌐 http://feminist.com/health.htm

This is a search engine for women's health. It includes sites on general women's health, breast cancer, and reproductive health. Good starting point and general resource.

Feminist Internet Gateway   No. 32

🌐 http://www.feminist.org/gateway/master2.html

Women's Internet sites by subject. Includes links to global issues, women's health issues and resources, abortion, affirmative action, and women and girls in sports. This is a great site from which to start a general search on women's health.

Fertility Weekly   No. 33

🌐 http://holonet.net/homepage/1f.htm

Maintained by the periodical *Fertility Weekly*, this site includes selected back issues, headlines, and a newsfile on other publications. The information is limited, but the site is a good starting point.

Fibroids (Uterine)   No. 34

🌐 http://www.medicalarts.com/MA_Pages/fibroids.html

Article on fibroids that covers definition, symptoms, treatments, etc. This page is part of a Web site maintained by an Ob/Gyn practice in Utica, New York (http://www.medicalarts.com/MA_Pages/contents.html), and the site has a good section on patient information on Ob/Gyn topics.

Fitness Issues   No. 35

🌐 http://www.inect.co.uk/nsmi/

This site from the United Kingdom provides FAQs on research, publications, and issues related to fitness. Maintained by the National Sports Medicine Institute, it has a fitness glossary and a sports section where you can learn about rowing, tennis, gymnastics, soccer, etc. Not an in-depth site, but it is a good starting point.

FitnessLinks to the Internet   No. 36

🌐 http://www.fitnesslink.com/links.htm

Site developed by an ACE-certified fitness instructor, who has also been a reporter for a financial news organization. FitnessLinks searches the Web for valuable health and fitness resources and rates pages and sites. A well-organized site with comprehensive links provided. Covers general fitness sites as well as medical sites, mind/body/holistic healing and emotional health sites, bodybuilding and weight training sites, sports sites, and more.

Fitness World   No. 37

🌐 http://www.fitnessworld.com/fitnews/news.html

An up-to-date source of news reports on research and events in health and fitness. No links to other research areas, but basic information is provided.

Food Safety and Nutrition Information   No. 38

🌐 http://ificinfo.health.org/fdsninfo.htm

Site consists of an excellent list of links to pages on such topics as adult and child nutrition, dietary fat and cholesterol, sweeteners, additives, pesticides, and FAQs. Links only — there is no descriptive text on nutrition at this site.

A Forum for Women's Health   No. 39

🌐 http://www.healthwire.com/women/

The forum provides a collection of facts, information, advice and suggestions to help women deal with health concerns. It is written by a woman physician. It also provides links to other valuable sites.

Foundation for Women's Health   No. 40

🌐 http://gnomes.org/forward/index.html.

This site has an informational page on female circumcision.

H

Hardin Meta Directory   No. 41

🌐 http://www.arcade.uiowa.edu/hardin-www/md-obgyn.html

Links to sites on obstetrics, gynecology, and women's health. The site originates at the University of Iowa.

Harvard University's Health Publications   No. 42

🌐 http://www.med.harvard.edu/publications/Health_Publications/

This is the site for Harvard University's Health Publications online. It contains information on subscriptions to Harvard's various health-related publications, sample issues, reports on health, as well as articles online.

Harvard Women's Health Watch   No. 43

🌐 http://www.med.harvard.edu/publications/Women/.index.html

The *Harvard Women's Health Watch* seeks to clarify many of the issues surrounding women's health and to provide concise, accurate information to help readers make informed decisions about their own care. The editor's address what is and what is not known, in the absence of scientific research on the female population, about subjects ranging from hormone replacement therapy to weight management to heart disease.

HealthGate   No. 44

🌐 http://www.healthgate.com

A subscriber-based source for information on health, wellness, and biomedical information. It includes *Our Bodies, Ourselves*, access to Medline, and other online databases.

Healthwise — No. 45

🌐 http://www.columbia.edu/cu/healthwise/alice.html

Web site of the Health Services department at Columbia University. Provides comprehensive health-related information for students, good links, and interactive questions and answers on a wide variety of topics, including nutrition, exercise, and weight control.

Highland Park Hospital — No. 46

🌐 http://www.hphosp.org

This site is maintained by Highland Park Hospital in Illinois. It includes information about the hospital, fertility, women's health, menopause, and managed care.

I

Idea Center Health Policy Page — No. 47

🌐 http://epn.org/idea/health.html

Site contains information on current legislation, articles on health care and health reform, as well as links to other sites.

Infertility Resources — No. 48

🌐 http://www.ihr.com/infertility/

Provides information about fertility drugs, treatments, providers, and support organizations. There is also technical information for healthcare providers and the news media. This site is maintained by the Internet Health Resources Company.

Institute of Medical Technology — No. 49

🌐 http://hulda.vta.fi/

This is a general site on cancer genetics from the Institute of Medical technology at the University of Tampere, Finland. It lists recent research and publications on cancer genetics.

The Institute of Medicine of Chicago — No. 50

🌐 http://www.iomc.org

This site has information on and links to the Institute's newsletter and interest areas, including managed care, aging, and ethics, as well as information and summaries of meetings on managed care.

Interactivism — No. 51

🌐 http://www.interactivism.com/

This is an activist-oriented site with political information on abortion rights, censorship, politics, and poverty. Includes discussion groups and links to other sites.

Internet Mental Health Resources — No. 52

🌐 http://www.mentalhealth.com/dis/p20-etol.html

This site contains information and links on anorexia nervosa.

K

Kaiser Permanente — No. 53

🌐 http://www.Kaiserpermanenteca.org/

This site is maintained by Kaiser Permanente of California, a Health Maintenance Organization in California. This site includes general health information, nutrition information, a member's newsletter, and recipes.

M

Male Infertility — No. 54

🌐 http://www.ivf.com/male.html

Maintained by the Atlanta Reproductive Health Center, this page focuses on male factor infertility. It includes information and articles on male infertility as well as information on video tapes. It is a good general site.

Male Infertility Factor — No. 55

🌐 http://www.ihr.com/infertility/male.html

This site is developed and maintained by Internet Health Resources Company. There are articles on how to enhance fertility, male factor infertility, and coping with male infertility. Also discusses the impact of diet, stress, drugs and seasons of the year on male fertility.

Medical Resources — No. 56

🌐 http://www.healthcity.com/

This is a medical resources site for non-medical people. It includes health club information, news articles, alternative medicine, and a library.

Melpomene Institute Home Page — No. 57

🌐 http://www.melpomene.org/

Maintained by a nonprofit research organization dedicated to women's health and physical activity. Links to pages on: osteoporosis, fitness walking, women of color and exercise, and girls and physical activity and self-esteem. Also treats topics on body image, health care decisions, exercise and pregnancy, exercise and menstruation, and much more. Very comprehensive.

Menopause Matters — No. 58

🌐 http://world.atd.com/~susan207/

This site provides information on the treatment of menopausal symptoms. It seeks to empower women through increased knowledge. It is a woman-focused site.

MenoTimes — No. 59

🌐 http://web.gimnet.com/~hyperion/meno/menotimes.index.html

This is a subscriber-based journal that provides information on menopause and osteoporosis.

Mental Health Net — No. 60

🌐 http://www.cmhc.com/mhn.htm

Comprehensive guide to mental health online. It includes numerous resources on depression, substance abuse, journals, and social work. It is a great resource.

Multi-Media Medical Reference Library — No. 61

🌐 http://www.med-library.com

This site is designed to provide access to medical information and resources for professionals, students, and patients. It includes hospitals online, medical schools, Medline abstracts, and various resources on specific health issues. It is put together by an individual, but is sponsored by a variety of private businesses. Excellent resource.

Museum of Menstruation (MUM)   No. 62

◉ http://www.mum.org/

This is the homepage for the Museum, which is in Maryland. The Museum contains a collection of menstrually related products, ads, and articles. The site is informative and entertaining, and somewhat controversial.

N

National Abortion Rights Action League   No. 63

◉ http://www.naral.org/

This site is maintained by the National Abortion Rights Action League (NARAL) and includes information on campus organizing, fact sheets, and publications.

National Agricultural Library, United States Department of Agriculture: Food and Nutrition Information Center   No. 64

◉ http://www.nalusda.gov/fnic

This site offers food and nutrition publications, dietary guidelines for Americans, a healthy eating index, many USDA materials, and links to electronic sources of food and nutrition information.

National Council on Alcohol and Drug Dependence   No. 65

◉ http://www.ncad

This site is maintained by the National Council on Alcohol and Drug Dependence. It offers education, information, and help for people with drug and alcohol problems. It contains information on advocacy, affiliates, publications, and help for parents.

National Council on Alcoholism   No. 66

◉ http://www.health.org/reality/links.htm

Maintained by the National Council on Alcoholism, this site offers links to other sites on alcohol and drugs. It is a good place to start looking for information on this topic.

National Gay and Lesbian Task Force   No. 67

◉ http://www.ngltf.org/

This site is maintained by the National Gay and Lesbian Task Force. It includes general information and publications, press releases, and links to other sites.

National Institute on Mental Health   No. 68

◉ http://www.nimh.nih.gov/

This site is maintained by the National Institute on Mental Health. This is a good general Web site. It includes information about NIMH publications, mental health articles, and educational resources.

The National Institutes on Health (NIH)   No. 69

◉ http://www.nih.gov/

This site offers a listing of various government agencies under NIH, such as the National Cancer Institute. It lists job opportunities and books and resources in the Library of Medicine. It is extremely useful as a search site.

National Women's Health Organization   No. 70

◉ http://gynpages.com/nwho/

Sponsored by the National Women's Health Organization, this site lists abortion clinics that have Web sites and provides facts about abortion.

National Women's Resource Center   No. 71

◉ http://www.nwrc.org/

Resources, articles, and other documents that deal with the prevention and treatment of alcoholism, drug abuse, and mental illnesses.

Natural Medicine   No. 72

◉ http://www.amrta.org/~amrta

This Web site maintains links to alternative or natural health sites on the Internet. It is a great place to start for information on alternative or complementary medicine.

Nutrition HomePage   No. 73

◉ http://www.csbsju.edu/library/internet/nutrition.html

This site is put together by the College of Saint Benedict and Saint John's University in Minnesota. It lists nutrition resources on the Net, general health sites, and electronic journals. It is an excellent resource on nutrition.

Nutrition Sites on the Internet   No. 74

◉ http://wce.uwyo.edu/wctl/high/nutr/default.html

Interesting site because of the wealth of links. A most exciting page that maintains a constantly updated, extensive list of nutrition Web sites, which are rated and fully described. The majority of the sites reviewed are excellent. This site is a good starting point for any research.

O

One Source: Breast Cancer   No. 75

◉ http://www.columbia.net/1source.fall95/breast.html

Maintained by Columbia Healthcare, this site houses *One Source* magazine, a guide to healthy living. Offers current reports on the value of mammograms and advocates women getting to know their bodies, which helps for early detection of malignancy. Also lists trouble spots for most frequent cancers in women. Links to a health manual, physicians, and what's new at Columbia Healthcare.

The Oracle Review   No. 76

◉ http://www.oraclereview.com/

This site presents support for women with breast implants. It includes information on implant risks and current research. It is subscriber-based, but you can get some information without being a subscriber.

Osteoporosis and Related Bone Diseases   No. 77

◉ http://www.osteo.org/

This site provides quality information as well as links to other sites dealing with bone diseases. It is a valuable general site.

Ovarian Cysts   No. 78

◉ http://www.familyinternet.com/peds/scr/001504sc.htm

Site is descriptive and provides links to other sites. Discusses ovarian cysts — the various types and treatment options. Links to other sites that discuss treatment alternatives and prevention.

P

Pap Smears   No. 79
⊕ http://www.neosoft.com/~uthman/

This site is created by Ed Uthman, M.D., a pathologist, and includes articles and resources. It is his homesite and expresses his biases. He does include his curriculum vitae, so you can have an understanding of his background.

Pap Tests   No. 80
⊕ http://erinet.com/fnadoc/pap.htm

This site includes articles about Pap tests and links to other sites.

The Physical Activity and Health Network (PAHNet)   No. 81
⊕ http://www.pitt.edu/~pahnet/

A dynamic list of Internet resources that examine the relationship of physical activity and exercise to health. Maintained by the Department of Epidemiology and the Center for Injury Research and Control at the University of Pittsburgh, this site offers comprehensive links to online journals, cutting edge research topics, and other sites that relate to exercise science and exercise epidemiology. Research oriented.

Planned Parenthood   No. 82
⊕ http://www.ppfa.org/ppfa

This site is maintained by Planned Parenthood. It offers consumer information and education on birth control, sexually transmitted diseases, and a public affairs letter.

Power Surge   No. 83
⊕ http://members.aol.com/dearest/index.html

This site provides information and a means to talk to others about menopause. The site describes hot flashes as power surges. It is a "menopause positive" site.

Psychotherapy, Anxiety, and Suicide   No. 84
⊕ http://www.cyberpsych.org

This site includes information on anxiety, psychotherapy, and suicide. It also includes information on organizations that deal with mental health issues.

R

Rape   No. 85
⊕ http://www.ocs.mg.edu.au/~Korman/feminism/rape.html

A directory of Internet sites that discuss rape. It includes information, resources, and organizations. It was created and is maintained by a woman named Kathy Korman.

S

Sexual Assault   No. 86
⊕ http://www.mes.net/~Kathyw/abuse.html

This site lists essential information on abuse, assault, rape, and domestic violence. It includes links to other sites, information, and resources.

Sexual Assault Information   No. 87
⊕ http://www.cs.utk.edu/-bartley/saInfoPage.html

Information and referrals concerning rape, sexual abuse, and domestic violence can be found at this site. Covers statistics, offers articles, and provides links to other sites.

Sexual Assault Support Services   No. 88
⊕ http://gladstone.uoregon.edu/~service/

This is an Oregon-based service. It provides information on sexual assault, violence, sexual harassment, and help for survivors.

Sexuality Information and Education Council   No. 89
⊕ http://www.siecus.org

This is a nonprofit advocacy agency that affirms that sexuality is a natural and health part of living. Site includes a description of their programs, publications, and activities.

Stress   No. 90
⊕ http://www.uniuc.edu/departments/mckinley/health-info/stress/stress.html

Links to information on coping strategies, goal-setting, relaxation exercises for improved sleep, management strategies for college students, stress skills assessment, taking stock of procrastination, and many other topics. Maintained by the McKinley Health Center at the University of Illinois at Urbana-Champaign.

T

Tobacco BBS   No. 91
⊕ http://www.tobacco.orh/

Excellent resource on tobacco news and information. It includes open debate on tobacco issues, news, and resources.

U

Urinary Tract Infections   No. 92
⊕ http://www.uib.no/isf/people/inkter.htm

This site presents an article on urinary tract infections and treatment options. The information comes from the Universitetet I Bergen in Norway.

W

Web of Addictions   No. 93
⊕ http://www.well.com/user/woa

This site was developed to provide accurate, comprehensive information on alcohol and drug addictions. It is a resource for teachers and students. Includes fact sheets, news, extensive links, and information on support groups.

Wellness Web   No. 94
⊕ http://wellweb.com

This is a great source for health information. It is a collaboration between patients and health care professionals to provide information and support. It includes information on alternative medicine, women's health, smoking, and healthcare products and services.

Women and Health Resources   **No. 95**

🌐 http://www.igc.apc.org/women/activist/health.html

Includes sites from Planned Parenthood, breast cancer, and abortion. Site takes an activist focus.

Women and HIV Infection   **No. 96**

🌐 http://www.cmpharm.ucsf.edu/~troyer/safesex/vanews/vanewswomen.html

A collection of articles on women and AIDS. Articles come form a variety of sources, including the FDA Consumer and various Federal agency reports.

Women and Sport Home Page (Canadian Assoc.)   **No. 97**

🌐 http://infoweb.magi.com/~wmnsport/index.html

The Canadian Association for the Advancement of Women and Sport and Physical Activity (CAAWS) is in business to encourage girls and women to get out of the bleachers, off of the sidelines, and onto the fields, rinks, pools, and locker rooms. This site is working toward a better sport system in Canada so that girls can enjoy all the benefits and sheer fun of sport and physical activity. An informative page with links to CAAWS publications, an action bulletin, a history of women and sport in Canada, physical activity and active living in Canada, and the Canadian Sport and Fitness Administration Centre. Updated regularly.

Women at Wellness Web   **No. 98**

🌐 http://wellweb.com/women/women.htm

This site has information on various issues in women's health as well as links to other sites. Includes information on heart disease, violence, hormone replacement therapy, and ovarian cancer.

Women Leaders Online Website   **No. 99**

🌐 http://www.lm.com/~imann/feminist/abortion.html

Links to information on abortion rights, abuse, sexual orientation, and newsletters.

Women's Health America   **No. 100**

🌐 http://array.womenshealth.com/~wha/

This is a national organization that sells women's health products. Site contains information on PMS, natural hormone replacement therapy, and a company newsletter — *Women's Health Access Newsletter*.

Women's Health Hot Line   **No. 101**

🌐 http://www.softdesign.com/softinfo/womens_health.html

A newsletter providing the media with information on women's health. Published by Beckwith Communications.

Women's Health Interactive   **No. 102**

🌐 http://www.women's-health.com/

This site provides a holistic view of women's health. The site includes information, discussion groups, and links to organizations.

Women's Health Resources Online   **No. 103**

🌐 http://www.web.net/cwhn/resource/resmain.html

Maintained by the Canadian Women's Health Network, this is a listing of Internet resources related to women's health issues. An impressive Table of Contents including: Looking at Our Health, Controlling our Reproductive Health and Fertility, The Medical System and Women, Childbearing, General Women's Health Resources, Medical and Health Conditions, and more. An extensive site with links to other search engines.

Women's Health Resources on the Internet   **No. 104**

🌐 http://www.coil.com/~tsegal/womens_health.html

A site maintained and updated by two women, Tricia Segal and Julie Lea, and affiliated with the University of Michigan School of Information and Library Studies. Links to emotional, physical, and sexual health issues. Also includes a very helpful introduction to their Women's Health Issues guide and how to use the guide.

Women's Health Weekly   **No. 105**

🌐 http://www.newsfile.com/lw.htm

Subscriber-based information. Includes updates on current women's health issues and an international and national calendar of events.

Women's Medical Page   **No. 106**

🌐 http://www.best.com/~sirlou/wmhp.html

This site is managed by a medical student. It includes summaries of scholarly articles from medical journals. It is aimed at health care professionals, but provides interesting information for the layperson as well.

World Health Organization   **No. 107**

🌐 http://www.WHO.ch/

Site is maintained by the World Health Organization, an international health organization. Site includes information on WHO publications and world health issues. General information provided.

WWWomen   **No. 108**

🌐 http://www.wwwomen.com/

This is a search directory for sites related to women. Includes topics on women's health, lesbian issues, diversity, and feminism.

Y

Yahoo: Reproductive Health Links   **No. 109**

🌐 http://www.yahoo.com/health/reproductive_Health/

Links to sites that contain information on birth and pregnancy, infertility, clinics, books on reproductive health, and more.

Yahoo: Urinary Health Links   **No. 110**

🌐 http://www.yahoo.com/health/diseases_and_condition/urinary_incontinence/

This is a Yahoo site with links to information on urinary incontinence and urinary tract infections.

Yahoo: Weight Links   **No. 111**

🌐 http://www.yahoo.com/Health/weight_issues

Links using Yahoo to sites related to weight. Includes sites on weight, eating disorders, and nutrition.

Web Journal

JOURnal Notes

http:// _____ Topic _____

_____

_____

_____

_____

_____

_____

_____

_____

_____

_____

_____

_____

_____

_____

_____

Web Journal

journal Notes

http:// _____ topic _____

_____

_____

_____

_____

_____

_____

_____

_____

_____

_____

_____

_____

Web Journal

JOUrnal Notes

h_{ttp://} _____ topic _____

_____

_____

_____

_____

_____

_____

_____

_____

_____

_____

_____

_____

_____

Web Journal

Journal Notes

http:// _____ Topic _____

_____

_____

_____

_____

_____

_____

_____

_____

_____

_____

_____

_____

_____

_____

Web Journal

Journal Notes

h_{ttp://} _____ Topic _____

_____

_____

_____

_____

_____

_____

_____

_____

_____

_____

_____

_____

_____

Web Journal

Journal Notes

http:// _____ **T**o**p**ic _____

_____

_____

_____

_____

_____

_____

_____

_____

_____

_____

_____

_____

_____

_____

_____

_____

Index